A History of Endometriosis

Ronald E. Batt

A History of Endometriosis

Springer

Author
Ronald E. Batt, M.D., Ph.D.
Professor of Gynecology
State University of New York at Buffalo
Buffalo, New York
USA

ISBN 978-0-85729-584-2 e-ISBN 978-0-85729-585-9
DOI 10.1007/978-0-85729-585-9
Springer London Dordrecht Heidelberg New York

British Library Cataloguing in Publication Data
A catalogue record for this book is available from the British Library

Library of Congress Control Number: 2011928404

Cover design: eStudioCalamar, Figueres/Berlin

Printed on acid-free paper

Springer is part of Springer Science+Business Media (www.springer.com)

To
John Yeh, M.D.
Harold H. Rosenfield Professor of Obstetrics and Gynecology
Harvard Medical School
Chair, Department of Obstetrics and Gynecology
Beth Israel Deaconess Medical Center
Boston, MA

To the Memory of
Kornel Ludwig Terplan, M.D.
Professor and Chairman, Department of Pathology
University of Buffalo School of Medicine (1933–1960)

Foreword by Johannes L.H. Evers

Dr. Ronald Elmer Batt entered the field of endometriosis back in 1968 when he wrote, together with Somers Sturgis, on a still topical issue, adolescents' gynaecologic problems. He went on to contribute many pivotal papers to the literature and was the first to draw our attention to the relationship between endometriosis, peritoneal pockets and the Allen-Masters syndrome. Ron Batt is a meticulous researcher. Instead of taking everything he reads and hears for granted he returns where possible to the original records and primary sources and tries to explain them in the context of the scientific setting of the day. Doing so he stumbles upon little gems of information that would have remained a secret but for his careful literature research. Thanks to him we now know the first occasion that the late great John Albertson Sampson alluded to his legendary transplantation theory: the Transactions of the American Gynecological Society in 1921, where he added the following note-in-print (science publishing was rather unhurried in those days) to his paper on perforating hemorrhagic (chocolate) cysts of the ovary (*Trans Am Gynecol Soc* 1921;46:162–236):

> Two possible sources of the origin of these small tubules or cysts of endometrial type in the ovary present themselves: first, congenital, and second, acquired from the implantation of epithelium escaping from the tube during menstruation and its subsequent invasion of the ovary

John Sampson, clinical professor of gynaecology at Albany medical college, New York, was a great man, although until recently we did not know too much about his professional life. We learn from the present book that he was the only person ever to be elected by unanimous vote to the membership of the prestigious American Gynecological Society, in 1906. Theodore Roosevelt, President of the United States at the time, was his hero. Sampson listed four qualities that he believed were largely responsible for Roosevelt's success in life: his personality, his energy and persistence, the training in learning how to acquire knowledge, and finally, his ability to impress people with his thoughts by his convincing speaking and forceful writing.

Personality, energy, persistence, learning, convincing speaking and forceful writing, all these qualities also pertain not only to Sampson himself, but also to Ron Batt, the author of the seminal work that you are about to read. He illustrates that, as Roosevelt used to put it, "with self-discipline most anything is possible". And this has led to the wonderful historical text now in front of you, allowing us, as armchair travellers, to travel backwards in time and follow the inquisitive author on his expedition into the deep, dark origins of endometriosis. From the Bohemian master macropathologist Carl Freiherr von Rokitansky to his next-generation Westphalian successor Friedrich von Recklinghausen to his student Robert Meyer in Strassburg, and from the – then young and promising – Canadian gynaecological pathologist Thomas Cullen (of ectopic pregnancy fame), via DeWitt Casler's remarkable menstruating ovary to John Sampson himself and his retrograde transplantation theory, a voyage of adventure!

It is both a delight and an honour to have been invited to contribute this foreword to such a significant work, as it is a joy and a privilege to know Ron Batt, if only for the many scientific meetings we attended together. I have an immense admiration for the man and for the effort he put into composing this unique text, and I have great confidence in the quality of this critical work. There was no hesitation in me whatsoever to endorse "A History of Endometriosis". It constitutes a true treasure trove of historical information for endometriosis aficionados, and an extraordinarily diverse source of knowledge for medical historians. The definitive history of endometriosis has finally been written.

Johannes L.H. Evers, M.D., Ph.D., FRCOG

Foreword by Dale C. Smith

This is a monograph a long time in the making, and one I sometimes did not expect to see. Dr. Batt undertook a Ph.D. in history fairly late in life; he already had an international reputation in endometriosis research, and few people that begin such a challenge finish it.

I met Ronald Batt, M.D., at the American Association for the History of Medicine meeting in New York City; he was introduced by a mutual friend as "seriously interested in the history of medicine." We met at meetings for a couple of years and then Dr. Batt told me he was going to enroll in graduate study in history. After a few years he asked if I would serve as a member of his graduate faculty, I consulted the faculty of the University of Buffalo and they confirmed the invitation. It seems Dr. Batt had completed the course work for the Ph.D. while continuing to work as a Professor in Obstetrics and Gynecology at the University. I provided a reading list on the history of diseases and let the issue pass from my mind. I noticed that Dr. Batt had been selected as a History Fellow by the American College of Obstetricians and Gynecologists and when he was in Washington for his fellowship he called to talk about his reading. We met a couple more times and then I was asked to participate in a preliminary examination, then we talked about a thesis, and I cautioned about the magnitude of the project, but Dr. Batt had grown up as a physician with the literature on endometriosis and thought the subject manageable. Chapters followed and I was invited to Buffalo for a defense; Professor Batt had accomplished his goal, he had mastered the discipline of history of medicine at the professional level and completed a study of the history of the disease to which he had devoted his research life. He had retired from practice but been recalled by his University, I was sure the work was finished and while available from electronic thesis publishers – few would care – it made me a little sad that such a nice piece of history would not be read. Again, I had underestimated Ronald Batt, and so, here I sit, writing a forward to a book that does not need an introduction. It is a mature and self-sufficient scholarly monograph on a difficult and important subject; it needs no one to turn up its cuff. Ronald Batt, M.D. and Ph.D., finished the book and did it brilliantly!

In this day of personalized, genome-driven, evidence-based medicine, why read about the wrong ideas of the past? Some (few) readers need only check the index to be satisfied; they made it into the history book; for the rest there must be something more? Why do you take the Hippocratic Oath, it is equally out of date? After all, many readers are gynecologic surgeons, they are (if they take the original oath) swearing "not to cut, not even for the stone" – a promise that would, if followed, reduce the billable procedures in the practice. The oath is tinkered with, it is not the original, but despite the changes it does not reflect the primary concerns of twenty-first century practice. It is a deliberate choice – to select professional ancestors and to honor their contributions to the profession, not so much the science, although that is important, but their shaping of the values that make Medicine in the Western World a thing to be cherished, a calling to be followed, and a commitment to be redeemed. Galen, 400 years after the death of Hippocrates, argued he did something important for medicine and should be remembered. A thousand years later, scholars in the then new medieval university searched the ancients for models and settled on the Hippocratic Corpus and the writings of Galen (often as transmitted through the Islamic world). All three periods understood the same works differently, but all three advocated a deontological ethic: Medicine was about the patient and predicated on a general, rational, and natural understanding of the world, including health and disease. Five hundred years, as but a moment in the history course, and the Scientific Revolution is pushing Galen and the Medieval masters into the obscurity of historic texts – Hippocrates survives, a dynamic textual tradition showing the value of the clinical recorder and epidemiologist.

In Europe of the early modern period the surgeon is most commonly an apprentice trained craftsman, a journeyman or master in an urban guild or a military man in service of the new national armies. They have not been burdened by disease theory, dealing with manipulative procedures, surface pathology and especially wounds. Slowly they are becoming learned, studying anatomy by dissection, asking questions about the procedures and diagnoses they are taught, increasingly walking wards in urban hospitals; by the eighteenth century they were, admittedly in small numbers, becoming engaged in midwifery. Between the Scottish Universities and their American reflections, and the changes in urban extramural teaching programs, especially the hospitals, the surgeons of the eighteenth century became more theory oriented, more physician-like. At the same time, urbanization, public health and democratization of society led physicians to look for patients among the rising middle orders of society who preferred fee for service over retainer relationships. As physicians engaged in anatomical study, especially in southern Europe, they increasingly noticed anatomical variations, some were without obvious clinical correlations but some did seem to be associated with particular syndromes.

The physician, the surgeon, the apothecary and the midwife are drifting toward a single portal of entry profession under different social and scientific pressures in different places. The ancient theories are untenable but a new scientific method, coming from celestial mechanics and optics, is not fully worked out, and it is especially difficult in the diverse biological systems that support medical theories. Under the influence of urban growth and Enlightenment moral philosophy, new social responsibilities are emerging for the physician – in 1793, Thomas Percival of Manchester will argue inmates of hospitals are really patients even though there is no financial relationship with the practitioner, and Benjamin Rush in Philadelphia will urge that practitioners have a larger responsibility to the community in times of epidemic and so should stay in the community to help all comers regardless of risk. The very word "profession" is increasingly taking on a meaning which includes a social responsibility and engagement in addition to traditional learnedness. It is in this environment that Dr. Batt opens his story of endometriosis, an environment much like our own – the meaning of profession is being questioned, the nature of evidence and the understanding of disease causation is under serious debate in preparation for radical change, physicians are managing many diseases but can rapidly and definitively cure very few and so patient satisfaction is frequently low.

The profession of the eighteenth and early nineteenth century look to the past for guidance and values: histories by Daniel LeClerc and John Freind, theses on Hippocrates and the ancients, and then editions of the works from the past, Littre's Hippocrates, the Sydenham Society's reprint of the English master clinician; all served to remind the physicians of the present of a deontological ethic based community of practitioners that they had selected for ancestors. They were reminded that social conditions, theological understandings, and the nature of evidence had all changed before and the profession had not only survived but was currently dynamic and thriving despite the challenges. So as you read the story of the changing nature of explanation and understanding in the disease state we call endometriosis, take comfort – they are "wrong" in our terms but they were doing the best that could be done at the moment. The challenge to do the best you can for the patient in front of you at the moment, while being committed to doing a better job tomorrow, is one of those hallmarks that the history of the profession calls out for affirmation. The histories of the eighteenth and nineteenth centuries affirmed that value for the heroes of Dr. Batt's story, they in turn affirm for our generation.

This is also a story of changes in the nature of evidence, from pathologic anatomy through the rise of histology; it is one of finest English language examples of telling of the power and influence of Rokitansky and the Second Vienna School that I am aware of in the literature. Technology, in this case the microscope, refines the understanding of evidence but so do advances in other sciences, in the case of Cullen and Sampson, physiology, especially endocrinology. Rokitansky, von Recklinghausen, Cullen and Sampson were all committed to practicing "evidence based" medicine, all were committed to doing the best they could for their patients and to advancing knowledge; their struggles caution against hubris while providing inspiration, but most of all they remind us that there is a reality to medicine, it exists in the real time of doctor and patient. Doctor, patient, and health care system are part of a social, cultural and scientific milieu, all are changing and all have a historic trajectory; history helps us understand that the current reality and the trajectory of change are always part of the professional encounter.

Finally, the career researcher and practitioner has, like Osler and Welch a century ago, told the rest of us what he sees as the important points in the history of his discipline. Others will tell other stories but without the insights of one who has devoted his life to the study of the problem, we miss an important dimension. Students of endometriosis will recognize Ronald Batt's name well before they interest themselves in the history of the subject; there is a hint of autobiographical understanding in some of the story telling, but that is okay, it is in fact the way medical history has been initially shaped.

There is something here for everyone: inspiration for tired academics, name recognition for involved researchers, acculturation for innovators, security for practitioners facing demands for improvement, challenge for those advocating reform and understanding for those interested in the progress of the profession. Whatever you wish or hope to find, you will find a good story, well told by an author who is involved and cares; it is hard to image a book paying greater dividends.

Dale C. Smith, Ph.D.
Bethesda, M.D.

Preface

> The production of big pictures is arguably the most significant sign of the intellectual maturity of a field. Ludmilla Jordanova.[1]

The year 2010 marks the sesquicentennial of the discovery and description of adenomyosis and endometriosis by Carl Rokitansky of Vienna. The intervening 150 years have seen intense basic scientific and clinical research and the diagnosis and treatment of millions of women worldwide. Yet there has been no scholarly history, no mention of endometriosis and adenomyosis in historical compendiums of disease. One may ask: Why? I believe the answer lies in the general perception that endometriosis is an enigmatic disease best understood through increasingly sophisticated and reductionistic scientific research. Consequently, historians of science and medicine have felt ill-prepared to engage the subject.

Endometriosis must be understood as the dominant member of five closely related benign müllerian diseases – endometriosis, adenomyosis, endosalpingiosis, endocervicosis, and müllerianosis – and its history is the tale of discovery of each of these diseases and their interrelatedness by a series of pioneering physicians. Further, there is no way to connect the contributions of Carl Rokitansky to Thomas Cullen and John Sampson without reference to those of Hans Chiari and Friedrich von Recklinghausen. And to accomplish this one needs to appreciate the historical relationship of adenomyosis and endosalpingiosis. From a historical perspective, Rokitansky's description of diffuse uterine adenomyosis is more important than his description of ovarian endometriosis. For it is adenomyosis that carries the history of endometriotic diseases for the first thirty-six years from Rokitansky's discovery to Cullen's breakthrough with the caveat that an essential link in the chain of evidence is the description of endosalpingiosis by Chiari. To write the full history, one must know of the existence of the fourth and fifth müllerian diseases, endocervicosis and müllerianosis.

The chief conceptual challenge was to settle on the five benign müllerian diseases as the theoretical trellis for organizing the history. Antecedent to this conceptualization was the research necessary to begin disentangling five distinct but connected sub-histories from within the emerging overarching narrative – a narrative filled with discontinuities and digressions, erroneous theories, and surgical challenges. Further, the historian required deep time, measured in years, to follow the five scent trails like

[1]Jordanova, Ludmilla. Gender and the historiography of science. Brit J History Science 1993;26:469–483.

a bloodhound. These trails ranged and intersected over Central and Western Europe and Eastern North America.

Faced with such a daunting task, the author chose chronological intellectual history with a biographical leitmotif to frame the history of these chronic diseases. A history of ideas enabled me to follow the intellectual development of physician-investigators as they identified and described endometriotic diseases and theories of pathogenesis as well as to trace their influence on one another, all revealed by a patient reading of primary and secondary sources.

Acknowledgments

After a long professional career devoted to treating endometriosis-associated infertility, the author wrote this book to fulfill the requirements for a Ph.D. in history. Over many years in classroom, clinic, laboratory, grand rounds, seminars, national and international meetings, office hours, surgery – innumerable teachers, scientists, professional colleagues, nurses, medical librarians, residents, medical students and patients made contributions that found their way into this work; to all of them I am profoundly grateful.

The author had the extraordinary privilege of a six-member committee, with three professors from the Department of History, State University of New York at Buffalo and three external professors. I wish to thank especially Professor James J. Bono, Chairman of the Department of History, State University of New York at Buffalo for his excellent seminars on the history of science and medicine, his mentoring over a decade, his thoughtful direction of this book, and for his support to completion. He gave his oldest graduate student considerable freedom, such that all academic criticism of this work must fall squarely on the author. I want to acknowledge the invaluable assistance of Professors Andreas Daum and David Herzberg for insights expressed during the early and later stages of this work.

Professor Dale Cary Smith, Senior Vice President and Professor and Chairman of the Department of Medical History in the F. Edward Hebert School of Medicine at the Uniformed Services University of the Health Sciences, Bethesda, Maryland, guided my studies in the history of disease. His sage advice critically informed my thinking as I mapped this work. Professor Philippe R. Koninckx, Department of Obstetrics and Gynecology, University of Leuven, Belgium and Professor John Yeh, former Chairman of the Department of Gynecology-Obstetrics, State University of New York at Buffalo provided invaluable insights toward finalizing the theory of developmental müllerian diseases (müllerianosis).

Dr. Richard A. Smith, Chief of Pathology, Sturdy Memorial Hospital, Attleboro, Massachusetts; Dr. Germaine M. Buck Louis, Chief of Epidemiology Branch, National Institute of Child Health & Human Development, Bethesda, Maryland; Professor Dan Martin, University of Tennessee Health Science Center, Germantown, Tennessee; Professor Charles Chapron, CHU Cochin Saint Vincent de Paul, Pavillon LeLong, Paris, France; and Professors John Yeh and Philippe Koninckx co-authored several articles on the theory of müllerianosis. The five müllerian diseases: endometriosis, adenomyosis, endosalpingiosis, endocervicosis, and müllerianosis provided the conceptual structure for integrating a century and a half of historical evidence.

I am deeply indebted to Dr. Franz Glasauer, Emeritus Professor of Neurosurgery, State University of New York at Buffalo for his meticulous translation from German of the foundational article for the history of endometriosis: Ueber Uterusdrüsen in Uterus- und Ovarial-Sarcomen (*New Growth of Uterine Glands in Sarcomas of the Uterus and Ovaries*) published by Carl von Rokitansky in 1860.

This work was informed by conversations with Professors Myron Gordon and Donald P. Swartz, emeritus Chairmen of the Department of Obstetrics and Gynecology, Albany Medical College, Albany, New York, and with Dr. Arthur Hengerer, the last resident of Dr. John A. Sampson. Karyn J. Connolly, Executive Director of Alumni Relations, Susan Lahey and Jessica Sault Watson, Archival Reference Librarians of Schaffer Library of Health Sciences, Albany Medical College provided valuable archival data on Dr. John A. Sampson.

Prim. Univ. Prof. Dr. Roland Sedivy, Landesklinikum 3100 St. Pölten, Austria, sent the author a generous gift of articles on Rokitansky and Virchow and his short monograph on Carl Rokitansky. I also extend my thanks for valuable information provided by Dr. Hans-Christian Bankl, Institut für Klinische Pathologie, Landesklinikum St. Pölten, Austria; Dr. Douglas Bacon, Department of Anesthesia, The Mayo Clinic; Dr. Ronald Cyr of the University of Michigan Health Center, Brighton, Michigan, and Dr. Salvador M. Udagawa, Department of Colo-rectal Surgery, Sisters of Charity Hospital, Buffalo, New York.

My debt to medical librarians and book sellers extends over a quarter of a century as I amassed scientific articles on endometriosis and an extensive personal library of secondary sources on the history of medicine and disease. For many years, Jacqueline Ciszkowski from my office, searched out and copied journal articles on endometriosis. I wish to give special thanks to librarians at the Health Sciences Library, State University of New York at Buffalo: Lilli Sentz, Curator of the History of Medicine Collection and her successor, Linda Lohr; Dean Hendrix, Coordinator of Educational Services, his predecessor, Steward Brower, now Director of the Schusterman Center, Oklahoma University Health Science Center for locating rare books the author needed and for access to the splendid nineteenth-century history of medicine collection. At the Kaleida Health System, Buffalo, New York: Carolyn Doueck, Linda Freedman, Elaine Mosher, Carolanne Kilichowski, and Gretchen Menifee assiduously responded to numerous request for articles on short notice. Susan M. Sobczak of the Lancaster Book Store, Lancaster, New York and Marta Carney of the Crossroads Book Store in Clarence Center, New York searched and secured needed out-of-print secondary sources.

I am grateful to the Ortho/McNeil Pharmaceutical Company and the American College of Obstetricians and Gynecologists for the generous ACOG-Ortho/McNeil Fellowship in the History of America Obstetrics and Gynecology for 2004 that enabled me to spend many productive and delightfully weeks in the Archives of the American College of Obstetricians and Gynecologists in Washington, DC. Special thanks go to Mary A. Hyde, Director; Debra G. Scarborough, History Librarian and Archivist, and Pamela Van Hine of the American College Obstetricians and Gynecologists Resource Center, Washington, DC.

Raymond Currier Wilson greatly improved this work by his meticulous and sensitive editing of the original manuscript. Paula Batt Wilson provided superb counsel.

The author could wish for no finer editor and editorial assistant than Grant Weston, Senior Editor, Medicine and Cate Rogers, Editorial Assistant at Springer-Verlag. Words cannot express my gratitude for the unwavering support of my wife Kathleen.

Contents

Introduction

This book is an intellectual history, a history of a family of five benign chronic müllerian diseases in women – endometriosis, adenomyosis, endosalpingiosis, endocervicosis, and müllerianosis.[2] A story told from a scientific and clinical perspective within the context of the emerging specialty of morbid pathological anatomy in Austria and Germany and the specialties of gynecology and gynecologic surgical pathology in Germany and the United States of America.[3] Endometriosis, adenomyosis, endosalpingiosis, endocervicosis, and müllerianosis continue to provide intellectual and therapeutic challenges to scientists, clinicians, and patients.[4] To the best of my knowledge, a scholarly history of endometriosis of this scope has not been written. This study fills that void.

For chronic diseases hidden within the interior of the human body during the nineteenth century most nosographic descriptions were founded on morbid pathological anatomy.[5] Only near the turn of the twentieth century was it possible to correlate

---

[2]Joan Wallach Scott, "Gender: A useful category of historical analysis," in *Feminism and History*, ed. Joan Wallach Scott [Oxford: Oxford University Press, 1996], 152–180:156. I use woman as a biological term. The five müllerian diseases occur as biological phenomenon involving the sexual reproductive organs as well as other organs and tissue of biological women. I reject the term gender because as Scott explains: "Its use explicitly rejects biological explanations, such as those that find a common denominator for diverse forms of female subordination in the facts that women have the capacity to give birth and men have greater muscular strength." Scott explains further: "Instead, gender becomes a way of denoting 'cultural constructions' – the entirely social creation of ideas about appropriate roles for women and men."

[3]Karl Sudhoff, "Aims and value of medical history in the self-development and professional life of the physician," in *Essays in the History of Medicine* trans. by various hands and ed. Fielding H. Garrison [New York: Medical Life Press, 1926], 45. "In all branches of science, the need for cultivating the study of their historical development is beyond question. From the literary standpoint, this is equally true of the natural sciences, including medicine. And here, Goethe's dictum is still apposite, - that the history of a science is the science itself."

[4]Endocervicosis refers to the presence of isolated cervical mucosa in the outer wall of the cervix uteri. Adenomyosis refers to the benign invasion of the uterine musculature by the endometrial mucosa. Endosalpingiosis may be defined as the benign invasion of the musculature of the fallopian tube by the endosalpingeal mucosa. Endometriosis refers to presence of ectopic benign invasive endometrial tissue outside the uterus. Müllerianosis may be defined as an organoid structure of embryonic origin; a choristoma composed of müllerian rests – normal endometrium, normal endosalpinx, and normal endocervix – singly or in combination, incorporated within other normal organs during organogenesis.

[5]Knud Faber, *Nosography in Modern Internal Medicine* [New York: Paul B. Hoeber, Inc., 1923], v. Faber defines nosography as "the description of diseases."

clinical observations and surgical pathology. However, at no point was the nosographic description of endometriosis founded on causation.[6] Serendipity, technology, and individual case histories played an inordinate role in the discovery and emergence of the five müllerian diseases.[7] A genealogy of ideas can be traced as investigators in one generation influenced those in succeeding generations.

My central methodological argument insists that only a history of the five müllerian diseases – endometriosis, adenomyosis, endosalpingiosis, endocervicosis, and müllerianosis – can satisfactorily integrate a century and a half of historical evidence.[8]

Judged by their "beginnings" or pathogenesis, endometriosis, adenomyosis, endosalpingiosis, endocervicosis, and müllerianosis are five distinctive diseases.[9] Judged by origins, all five müllerian diseases are related by virtue of their ancestral origin from mesoderm that formed the anlage of the müllerian ducts and urogenital ridge.[10] The central historical question flows from the need for historical synthesis. What were the historical circumstances that permitted endometriosis, adenomyosis, endosalpingiosis, endocervicosis, and müllerianosis to emerge as distinct ontological disease entities?

In sum, this work is based on the vast literature of clinical and scientific articles, monographs, and conference proceedings that accurately reflect cutting edge research and medical care by university-based and university-affiliated physicians, a literature frequently consulted by well-read clinicians with an interest in the disease.

In Chap. 1, the Prelude, I present the philosophical and scientific reorientation that occurred in Europe – particularly in Goethe's Jena Circle – during the late eighteenth and early nineteenth centuries; the reorientation necessary for recognition of the chronic disease endometriosis hidden in the interior of the female body. In Chap. 2, I present the circumstances that permitted the emergence of Rokitansky as the first full-time anatomical pathologist and how he developed his research program that became the foundation for the Second Vienna Medical School. I recount the

---

[6]Knud Faber, 98.

[7]Owsei Temkin, "The Scientific Approach to Disease: Specific Entity and Individual Sickness," in *The Double Face of Janus and Other Essays in the History of Medicine* [Baltimore, MD: Johns Hopkins University Press, 1977], 452-453. "It is not immediately clear why the anatomical interpretation had to follow the road from case histories to disease entities…The role of the case history in a particular phase of medical development elucidates further the notion of the abnormal in medicine…The case history is the form in which the physician links the science, which does not deal with the unique directly, and the patient, who requires attention as an individual."

[8]Brosens JJ, Brosens I. Endometriosis and adenomyosis: a unifying hypothesis. In A Lemay and R Maheux, eds. *Understanding and Managing Endometriosis: Advances in Research and Practice.* New York: The Parthenon Publishing Group, 1999, pp. 11–16. See also: Batt RE, Smith RA, Buck Louis GM, Martin DC, Chapron C, Koninckx PR, Yeh J. Müllerianosis. Histol Histopathology, 2007;22:1161–1166.

[9]O'Brien, Patricia. Michel Foucault's history of culture. In Hunt, Lynn. Editor. *The New Cultural History.* Berkeley, CA: University of California Press,1989;25–46:37. O'Brien notes that Foucault was not interested in evolution. According to O'Brien, Foucault was interested in "beginnings" not origins. "Origins imply causes; beginnings imply differences." The author is interested in both.

[10]While the mesoderm that forms the urogenital ridge and the müllerian ducts is technically not the cause of endometriosis, it is the final common pathway for multifactorial causation. Brosens JJ, Brosens I. Endometriosis and adenomyosis: a unifying hypothesis. In A Lemay and R. Maheux, eds. *Understanding and Managing Endometriosis: Advances in Research and Practice.* New York: The Parthenon Publishing Group, 1999:11–16.

historybehind Rokitansky's magnum opus – his *Handbook of Pathological Anatomy*. In Chap. 3, I relate the long intellectual journey of Rokitansky from macroscopic to microscopic pathological anatomy, a journey that enabled him to discover and describe two new and important diseases – adenomyosis and endometriosis. In Chap. 4, I focus on the amorphous web of investigators from Rokitansky to von Recklinghausen. I relate the story of Rokitansky's important contributions to developmental pathology. How his interest in adenomyosis influenced a generation of European pathologists, including Friedrich von Recklinghausen who formulated a persuasive but controversial Wolffian theory of pathogenesis. From von Recklinghausen the study of adenomyosis jumped the Atlantic Ocean where Thomas Cullen, the young gynecologic pathologist-in-residence at the Johns Hopkins Hospital, challenged his Wolffian theory. I relate the emergence of adenomyosis and endometriosis in North America and the spirited debate between von Recklinghausen and Cullen. Lastly we learn the sad tale of how Robert Meyer, a former student of von Recklinghausen, disproved his old master's Wolffian theory.

In Chap. 5, I present Thomas Cullen's research into cancer, uterine adenomyomas (internal endometriosis) and extrauterine adenomyomas (external endometriosis), and the fruitful collaboration between von Recklinghausen and Cullen. I recount the impact of the Flexner Report on the Department of Gynecology at Johns Hopkins Hospital and on Cullen's research career. In Chap. 6, I relate the history of the discovery, treatment, and complications of treatment of adenomyomas of the rectovaginal septum, vagina, rectum, sigmoid colon, and ovary. In Chap. 7, I present the culmination of Cullen's research over a quarter of a century and his final assessment of the distribution of adenomyomas containing uterine mucosa, including lesions in the ovary. In Chap. 8, I tell the amazing story of DeWitt Casler's menstruating ovary and how his presentation before the American Gynecological Society inspired John Sampson's theory of peritoneal implantation from perforating hemorrhagic (chocolate) cysts of the ovary. And I describe the observations that Sampson made subsequently that inspired his theory of transtubal retrograde menstruation to explain the pathogenesis of ovarian as well as peritoneal endometriosis.

In Chap. 9, I analyze Sampson's research on the life history of ovarian hematomas (endometrial chocolate cysts). In Chap. 10, I present Sampson's explication of his theory of peritoneal endometriosis due to menstrual dissemination and his defense of the theory in the face of increasing influence of the Iwanoff–Meyer theory of coelomic metaplasia. In Chap. 11, I discuss the profound influence of the philosophy of Immanuel Kant on Goethe and his Jena Circle. I summarize the essay: the research of Rokitansky, von Recklinghausen, Cullen, and Sampson, the emergence of surgical pathology in Central Europe and North America, recognition of the clinical symptoms and signs of endometriosis, the different phenotypes of endometriosis, and project trends in clinical and laboratory research into the twenty-first century.

Finally, Chap. 12 places the evolution of endometriotic disease as a clinical entity into historical perspective. The re-emergence of the Hippocratic concept of personal disease places new demands on research and practice in the twenty-first century.

Prelude

1

Goethe, Wilhelm and Alexander von Humboldt, and Johannes Müller

We might venture the statement that the history of science is science itself... One cannot clearly recognize one's own possessions until one knows how to recognize what others possessed before."
Goethe[1]

The Seminal Influence of Johann Wolfgang von Goethe [1749–1832]

The discovery of the diseases endometriosis and adenomyosis in 1860 by Carl Freiherr von Rokitansky (1804–1878) was preceded by a momentous change in scientific perception inspired by the German poet-scientist Johann Wolfgang von Goethe. Goethe perceived science with the holistic eye of the artist.[2] Indeed, many who associate Goethe's greatness with his poetry lament that a lengthy immersion in science diverted him from poetry.[3] He coined the word "morphology" for the study of the structure of plants and animals, and in this scientific pursuit favored the memorialization of careful observation by precise sketching instead of verbal explanation.[4] Goethe saved "the great principle of observation" and rescued natural history and medicine from the influence of followers of the gifted philosopher, Friedrich Wilhelm

[1] Ronold King, "Goethe and the Challenge of Science in Western Civilization," in *Goethe on Human Creativeness and other Goethe Essays,* ed. Rolf King [Athens, GA: University of Georgia Press, 1950], 231. King quoted Goethe from the preface to Goethe's study "On the Theory of Color."

[2] I choose to begin the history of endometriosis with Goethe to capture the initial intellectual heights of the sources of several streams of research that flowed into the twentieth and early twenty-first centuries, a tribute to nineteenth-century German, Austrian, English, and American scholarship in the history of disease. Stephen Jay Gould, "More light on leaves," in *Eight Little Piggies: Reflections in Natural History* [New York: WW Norton & Company, 1993], 157. "In the case of Goethe and science, I advance his second claim of special insight for two reasons. First, I feel that characteristic ways of thinking in the arts – the role of the imagination, holistic vs. reductionistic approaches, for example – might enlighten science (not because scientists never think in this 'artful way' manner, but because the unpopularity of these styles among professionals greatly limits their fruitful use, and an infusion from outside might therefore help). Second, Goethe himself viewed his treatment of biologic problems as different from that of most full time scientists, and he attributed his unconventional approach to his training and practice in the arts. In particular, Goethe argued that his artist's perspective led him to view nature as a unity, to search for integration among disparate parts, to find some law of inherent concord." In this view of the unity of nature Goethe and Alexander von Humboldt were of one mind. See also: Stephen Jay Gould, "A reflective prologue," in *Eight Little Piggies: Reflections in Natural History* [New York: WW Norton & Company, 1993], 19. "Goethe's oracular reduction of all plant form to a leaf archetype needs to be read for its unconventional form of *scientific* excellence."

[3] John George Robertson, *The Life and Work of Goethe: 1749–1832* [New York: Haskell House Publishers, 1973], 312.

R.E. Batt, *A History of Endometriosis*,
DOI 10.1007/978-0-85729-585-9_1, © Springer-Verlag London Limited 2011

Joseph Schelling (1775–1854),[5] "who deduced nature from pure reason."[6] The German medical historian Karl Sudhoff observed that "even the greatest investigators had fallen before the power of this theory and research came to a standstill, as people were chiefly concerned with bringing everything into line with this system."[7] Goethe earnestly disapproved of this system and its underlying teleological reasoning because "in Nature everything exists for its own sake."[8]

While in Italy, Goethe trained himself to observe with the unaided eye, to view objectively and to think systematically. "It was with the eye more than

[4] Stephen Jay Gould, "A tale of three pictures," in *Eight Little Piggies: Reflections in Natural History* [New York: WW Norton & Company, 1993], 427. Goethe: "We should talk less and draw more. I personally would like to renounce speech altogether and, like organic nature, communicate everything I have to say in sketches." For a contrary observation see John George Robertson, *The Life and Work of Goethe: 1749–1832* [New York: Haskell House Publishers, 1973], 307–8. Robertson cited evidence from Goethe's friend Schiller that Goethe proceeded from idea not experience. As Robertson put it: "In all his scientific speculation Goethe went out from the idea; observation and experiment were directed to a degree that would not be countenanced by modern science to supporting and establishing the hypothesis." See also: John George Robertson, *The Life and Work of Goethe: 1749–1832* [New York: Haskell House Publishers, 1973], 306. Robertson, Professor of German Language and Literature at the University of London opined that Goethe's treatise, *Essay in Comparative Osteology, showing that the Intermaxillary Bone of the Upper Jaw is common to Man and the other Animals*, "may well be regarded as a foundation-stone of the new science of comparative anatomy." David L. Hull, *Science as a Process: An Evolutionary Account of the Social and Conceptual Development of Science* [Chicago, IL: University of Chicago Press, 1988], 41. Goethe is ranked among the Continental idealists – along with Lorenz Oken (1779–1851) and Etienne Geoffroy Saint-Hilaire (1772–1844) – who "were partial to explaining natural phenomenon in terms of timeless general patterns or 'archetypes.'" See also Roy Porter, *The Greatest Benefit to Mankind: A Medical History of Humanity* [New York: W. W. Norton & Company, 1998], 249. Lorenz Oken suggested "that nature embodied a transcendental unity of plan, built upon elemental structural archetypes or anatomical building-blocks; this paved the way for philosophical morphology." Stephen Jay Gould, *The Structure of Evolutionary Theory* [Cambridge, MA: Belknap Press of Harvard University Press, 2002], 284. Roy Porter, *The Greatest Benefit to Mankind: A Medical History of Humanity* [New York: W. W. Norton & Company, 1998], 249. Porter noted that Casper Friedrich Wolff (1734–1794) anticipated Goethe. "Comparative studies led by Casper Friedrich Wolff [concluded] that 'all parts of the plant except the stem are modified leaves.'" Goethe's botanical theory of the leaf as an archetypal form probably constitutes his most important contribution to science. Stephen Jay Gould, *The Structure of Evolutionary Theory* [Cambridge, MA: Belknap Press of Harvard University Press, 2002], 284. Scientists like Geoffroy and Oken would apply the same vision to "reduce the great complexity and diversity of [vertebrate] animal … form to the single generating pattern of an archetypal vertebra." See also Gould, page 1101. "Vertebrate homologs in structure and function. So far, the formalist or archetypal content of this discussion has been largely limited to the Goethian theme of common bases for the generation of differentiated serial homologs in a *single* organism - in other words, to internal constraints and channels in the evolutionary history of particular forms and lineages. But the more radical archetypal theories - including both of Geoffroy's derided arguments about vertebral formations and dorso-ventral inversions-postulate the maintenance of such constraints in phyla of distant taxonomic separation and immensely long periods of independent evolution." David L. Hull, *Science as a Process: An Evolutionary Account of the Social and Conceptual Development of Science* [Chicago, IL: University of Chicago Press, 1988], 41. "E. Geoffroy Saint-Hilaire in turn explained all the various parts of the skeleton on vertebrates as modifications of a single structure – the vertebra." Hull also referred to the idealist "Oken."

[5] Karl Sudhoff, "Goethe and Johannes Müller," in *Essays in the History of Medicine* trans. by various hands and ed. Fielding H. Garrison [New York: Medical Life Press, 1926], 371. See also Lorraine Daston and Peter Galison, *Objectivity* [New York: Zone Books, 2007], 69–70. "The typical is rarely, if ever, embodied in a single individual; nonetheless, the astute observer can intuit it from cumulative experience, as Goethe 'saw' the *Urpflanze*. Goethe wrote of his archetype of the animal skeleton: 'Hence, an anatomical archetype [*Typus*] will be suggested here, a general picture containing the forms of all animals as potential, one which will guide us to an orderly description of each animal… The mere idea of an archetype in general implies that no particular animal can be used as our point of comparison; the particular can never serve as a pattern [*Muster*] for the whole.' This is not to say that the archetype wholly transcended experience, for Goethe claimed that it was derived from and tested by observation. However, observations in search of the typical must always be made in series, because single observations made by one individual can be highly misleading: 'For the observer never sees the pure phenomenon [*das reine Phanomen*] with his own eyes; rather, much depends on his mood, the state of his senses, the light, air, weather, the physical object, how it is handled, and a thousand different circumstances.'"

[6] Erna Lesky, *The Vienna Medical School of the 19th Century* [Baltimore, MD: Johns Hopkins University Press, 1976], 80. See also Karl Sudhoff, "Goethe and Johannes Müller," in *Essays in the History of Medicine* trans. by various hands and ed. Fielding H. Garrison [New York: Medical Life Press, 1926], 371. "As if lost in dreams, the medicine and natural history of those days rested quietly in the shadow of the system of Nature Philosophy expounded by the gifted Friedrich Wilhelm Joseph Schelling. This system evolved all natural phenomena from the idea of the absolute and endeavored to spiritualize all natural laws and turn them into laws of perception and cogitation, in consequence of which all natural phenomena seemed to disappear. Even the greatest investigators had fallen before the power of this theory and research came to a standstill, as people were chiefly concerned with bringing everything into line with this

with all other organs that I learned to comprehend the world."[9] Goethe's strength lay in the field of observational science unaided by instrumentation.[10] More the artist and less the mathematician, Goethe, unlike Alexander von Humboldt, "could not recognize the importance of precision measurements in natural science."[11]

Ronold King opined: "If Goethe had possessed a thorough knowledge of mathematics, his keen intellect could have taken him not just to the gateway of natural science, but into its very heart."[12] But then Goethe might have been a specialist and not a universal genius. Goethe's strength in observational science was sufficient to influence a generation of scientists and educators to embrace objective empirical science.[13]

Goethe was the scientific and humanistic genius who inspired Alexander von Humboldt (1769–1859),[14] his brother Wilhelm von Humboldt (1767–1835),[15] and Johannes Peter Müller (1801–1858).[16] This was a time of free intellectual exchange, an age of specialization before separation of the arts from the sciences.[17] Goethe and his three protégés each made seminal contributions to the creative German system of research and scholarship called *Wissenschaft*. "It marked the creative moment when a new type of university came into being, one that promoted research and aimed at the unity of all fields of knowledge."[18] From Goethe's influence on Müller and the brothers von Humboldt three nineteenth-century intellectual streams flowed into the twenty-first century: (1) research on the human Müllerian system, (2) developmental pathology, and (3) environmental and evolutionary biology. These intellectual streams ultimately would shape scientific progress in endometriosis research. This was not

---

system. In this confused era, Goethe, the scientist, had kept himself free from all such philosophic fragments of imagination. Upon him fell the task of saving the great principle of observation." Goethe was never a metaphysician treating from first principles; however, the aging Goethe found the thinking of Schelling harmonious with his deepening pantheism. See: John George Robertson, *The Life and Work of Goethe: 1749–1832* [New York: Haskell House Publishers, 1973], 280, 311.

[7] Karl Sudhoff, "Goethe and Johannes Müller," in *Essays in the History of Medicine* trans. by various hands and ed. Fielding H. Garrison [New York: Medical Life Press, 1926], 371.

[8] Goethe, quoted in Johannes Müller, "Von dem Bedürfnis der Physiologie nach einer philosophischen Naturbetrachtung." Reprinted in Adolf Meyer-Abich, *Biologie der Goethezeit* [Stuttgart: Hippokrates Verlag, 1949], 256–81. Goethe, quoted by Johannes Müller in Owsei Temkin, "Basic Science, Medicine, and the Romantic Era," in *The Double Face of Janus and Other Essays in the History of Medicine* [Baltimore, MD: Johns Hopkins University Press, 1977], 366.

[9] Ronold King, "Goethe and the Challenge of Science in Western Civilization," in *Goethe on Human Creativeness and other Goethe Essays,* ed. Rolf King [Athens, GA: University of Georgia Press, 1950], 223–252:236.

[10] Ronold King, 223–252:240–241. Goethe searched for archetypical phenomena with his unaided eye.

[11] Ronold King, 223–252:243, 247.

[12] Ronold King, 223–252:247.

[13] Ronold King, 223–252:237.

[14] Alexander von Humboldt, "Journey to the equinoctial regions of the new continent," in *The German Mind of the Nineteenth Century: A Literary & Historical Anthology* ed. Hermann Glaser [New York: Continuum, 1981], 273–274.

[15] Wilhelm von Humboldt, "Fragment of an autobiography," in *The German Mind of the Nineteenth Century: A Literary & Historical Anthology* ed. Hermann Glaser [New York: Continuum, 1981], 44–47.

[16] Rothstein, Edward. *Emblems of Mind: The Inner Life of Music and Mathematics* [Chicago, IL: University of Chicago Press, 2006], 150. Rothstein quotes Poincare, a quotation apropos to Goethe: "The Scientist does not study nature because it is useful to do so. He studies it because he takes pleasure in it; and he takes pleasure in it because it is beautiful."

[17] Andreas W. Daum, "*Wissenschaft* and knowledge," in *The Short Oxford History of Germany: Germany 1800–1870* [Oxford: Oxford University Press, 2004], 137–161:140–143.

[18] Andreas W. Daum, "*Wissenschaft* and knowledge," in *The Short Oxford History of Germany: Germany 1800–1870* [Oxford: Oxford University Press, 2004], 137–161:137. Daum equated the German term *Wissenschaft* with scholarship and research which included "the sciences, social sciences, and humanities." For the evolution of the meaning of Wissenschaft in the nineteenth century, see Arleen Marcia Tuchman, *Science, Medicine, and the State of Germany: The Case of Baden, 1815–1871* [New York: Oxford University Press, 1993], 14–15. "*Wissenschaft* [is] a difficult term to define not least because its meaning underwent several changes through the years. Once identified closely with another nebulous term, *Bildung, Wissenschaft* originally signified the search for a holistic understanding of all knowledge aimed at cultivating the individual's personality by developing one's moral and intellectual sensitivities. In this earlier formulation, *Wissenschaft* had an inward focus, but as the century progressed, the focus turned outward and *Wissenschaft* came to refer to the production of new knowledge through in-depth scholarly work in a specialized area of research. Accompanying this transition was an increased appreciation of the importance of acquiring practical experience; by the late nineteenth century, at least in the sciences and medicine, the revered *Wissenschaftler* was one who could manipulate sophisticated instrumental apparatus and gain in this way control over laboratory conditions and, presumably, over nature."

necessarily going to be steady and direct scientific progress but progress, as the eminent German historian Leopold von Ranke explained, more "like a stream that wends its own way."[19]

Goethe's Influence on Alexander and Wilhelm von Humboldt

"Scholars agree that Goethe was the last universal genius."[20] With that statement, Wadepuhl began a short monograph on *Goethe's Interest in the New World*, a monograph dedicated to the American Council of Learned Societies. Goethe's personal influence on Alexander and Wilhelm von Humboldt dates back to 1797 when the three men formed a scientific circle in Jena to investigate the natural sciences important in that era: "anatomy, chemistry, mineralogy, physics, and zoology."[21] The influence was mutual, for it was Alexander von Humboldt who was primarily responsible for redirecting Goethe's interest back to the study of science after a long hiatus. Goethe held an exceedingly high opinion of Alexander and declared: "It is beyond calculation what far reaching contributions Humboldt will one day make to the natural sciences."[22] Humboldt advanced beyond Goethe's empirical naked-eye observations by designing precise instruments with which he measured and recorded observations in the field.[23] Two years later, in 1799, Alexander von Humboldt embarked upon his scientific expedition in South and Central America from which he achieved worldwide fame and, importantly, influenced the young Charles Darwin. At Goethe's request, Wilhelm von Humboldt kept him apprised of the progress of Alexander's scientific expedition.

Goethe's Influence on Johannes Peter Müller

As a child, the introspective Johannes Müller possessed a fertile imagination which he exercised for countless hours "tracing the imaginary figures formed by the crumbling and clinging plaster on the wall opposite the living room"; from them he created new images. As a youth, Müller explored nature in the river valleys near his home in the Rhineland and eagerly read the works of Goethe that had fallen into his possession. Following the teaching of his virtual mentor Goethe, Müller based his scientific studies on exact observation.[24] He was particularly fascinated by Goethe's theory of colors.[25] In an inaugural lecture in 1824, Müller attacked the *Naturphilosophie* of Schelling. Owsei Temkin noted that Müller praised the insights that a biologist gained by carefully observing nature, rather than resorting to teleological reasoning. Karl Sudhoff grasped the crux of Müller's lifelong intellectual fascination with Goethe: "A close sympathy with Goethe and Goethe's many-sided biological activities and a thorough saturation of his mind with Goethe's scientific method of reasoning constituted a real and important step forward for the young biologist."[26] The two met in 1828.

Müller visited Goethe at his home in Weimar. During this memorable visit in a completely darkened

[19] Leopold von Ranke, "How the concept of progress is to be understood in history," in *The German Mind of the Nineteenth Century: A Literary & Historical Anthology* ed. Hermann Glaser [New York: Continuum, 1981], 149–151.

[20] Walter Wadepuhl, *Goethe's Interest in the New World* [New York: Haskell House Publishers, 1973], 7.

[21] Walter Wadepuhl, 77–83. John George Robertson, *The Life and Work of Goethe: 1749–1832* [New York: Haskell House Publishers, 1973], 304. "In his official concern for the development of the University of Jena [Goethe] always showed a greater interest in the professors of science than in those of the humanities." Goethe similarly was concerned with science in his Jena Circle with the von Humboldt brothers.

[22] Walter Wadepuhl, 77–83. Goethe held many of Alexander von Humboldt's books in his private library, now the Goethe National Museum. Two of Humboldt's books are filed under "Botany," four under "Geography," and two under "Geology." Additionally, Goethe had drawn five of Humboldt's books from the "Grand-Ducal Library, now the Landesbibliothek."

[23] Gerard Helferich, *Humboldt's Cosmos: Alexander von Humboldt and the Latin American Journey That Changed the Way We See the World* [New York: Gotham Books, 2004], 232, 332.

[24] Sudhoff, Karl. In Memory of Johannes Müller. *Essays in the History of Medicine.* Translated by various hands and edited, with foreword and biographical sketch, by Fielding H. Garrison. New York: Medical Life Press, 1926: 363–367:364.

[25] Karl Sudhoff, "Goethe and Johannes Müller," in *Essays in the History of Medicine* trans. by various hands and ed. Fielding H. Garrison [New York: Medical Life Press, 1926], 371–3. Laura Otis, *Müller's Lab* [New York: Oxford University Press, 2007], 38.

[26] Karl Sudhoff, "Goethe and Johannes Müller," in *Essays in the History of Medicine* trans. by various hands and ed. Fielding H. Garrison [New York: Medical Life Press, 1926], 372.

room Müller later recalled that Goethe "could see brilliant figures in the 'dark visual field…as a reflex of internal organic conditions in other parts," but that he did not possess Goethe's "gift of being able, with eyes shut, to call up voluntarily into the dark visual field the picture of a flower or some variegated Gothic rose window; the figure thus produced would constantly change its form and color in kaleidoscopic manner from the center outwards." Müller contrasted the difference between their natures: Goethe "possessed the poetic constructive power to the fullest extent." On the other hand, Müller's nature was "directed toward the examination of reality and of that which actually happens in Nature."[27] Both master and pupil possessed extraordinary, though differing, artistic and scientific gifts. Müller recalled the meeting and their similarities and differences in his *Handbook of Human Physiology* published in 1840.[28]

The Influence of Alexander von Humboldt on Johannes Peter Müller

Humboldt returned to Berlin in 1827 from his long residence in Paris where he wrote up his scientific research from South America. Humboldt wanted to strengthen the scientific community in Berlin. In 1828 Johannes Muller was introduced to Humboldt. Humboldt recognized that Johannes Müller's science – his 1826 study *On the Comparative Physiology of Vision in Men and Animals* – was exactly the kind of science that he wanted to promote.[29] The ambitious Müller gladly accepted the patronage of the eminent scientist.[30] Through the direct influence of Alexander von Humboldt, Johannes Müller was called to the chair of anatomy and physiology at the University of Berlin in 1833.[31] That same year Müller began writing his monumental *Handbook of Human Physiology*, which he completed in 1840.[32] His *Handbuch der Physiologie des Menschen* remained the standard text in its field for half a century.[33] Knud Faber believed Müller "ended the domination of Naturphilosophie" with his *Handbook of Physiology*.[34] In the same turn of mind, Karl Sudhoff considered Johannes Müller "the greatest physician who ever taught at the University of Berlin."[35]

Müller served as rector of the University of Berlin in 1847–1848. As rector, he had the authority to close or keep the University open during the Revolution of 1848. Dressed in academic robes, Müller and deans of the faculties walked to the Royal Palace and on behalf of the rebelling students, whereupon he "asked the king to withdraw his troops from the city."[36] Later, Müller marched in the funeral procession for 183 victims of the Revolution that included some students. The funeral march was planned as an exercise in reconciliation between the king and the populace.[37] In this tense situation, the elderly Alexander von Humboldt

[27] Karl Sudhoff, "Goethe and Johannes Müller," in *Essays in the History of Medicine* trans. by various hands and ed. Fielding H. Garrison [New York: Medical Life Press, 1926], 374.

[28] Johannes Müller, *Handbuch der Physiologie des Menschen.* 3rd ed. 2 vols. [Koblenz: J. Holscher, 1838–1840].

[29] Laura Otis, *Müller's Lab* [New York: Oxford University Press, 2007], 9, 11.

[30] Laura Otis, 13–14. While Müller argued for his own candidacy, he did suggest the elder Johann Friedrich Meckel (1781–1833) for the chair.

[31] Laura Otis, 11. Wilhelm von Humboldt (1767–1835) had organized the founding of the University of Berlin in 1810. See also: Arleen Marcia Tuchman, *Science, Medicine, and the State of Germany: The Case of Baden, 1815–1871* [New York: Oxford University Press, 1993], 145. Humboldt was known for intervening on behalf of "talented young scientists." See also Tuchman, page 151. Such an example was his letter on behalf of Hermann Helmholtz in March 1855.

[32] Karl Sudhoff, "In memory of Johannes Müller," in *Essays in the History of Medicine* trans. by various hands and ed. Fielding H. Garrison [New York: Medical Life Press, 1926], 365–366. "In 1833, he was called to Berlin, to become successor of Rudolphi in the chair of anatomy and physiology." "In 1833, at the age of 32, he began his monumental 'Handbook of Physiology,' which he concluded 7 years later."

[33] Peter Gray, *The Encyclopedia of the Biological* Sciences 2nd ed. [New York: Van Nostrand Reinhold Company, 1961], 581–582.

[34] Knud Faber, *Nosography in Modern Internal Medicine* [New York: Paul B. Hoeber, Inc., 1923], 82. *The Great Doctors: A Biographical History of Medicine.* Trans. Eden and Cedar Paul [New York: W. W. Norton & Company, 1933], 309. Müller's *Manual of Human Physiology*, which replaced Albrecht Haller's *Elementa physiologiae*, was "distinguished by its method. As far as Germany was concerned, it denoted a turning away from natural philosophy and towards observation and experiment."

[35] Sudhoff, Karl. Medicine and Art. In *Essays in the History of Medicine* trans. by various hands and edited, with foreword and biographical sketch, by Fielding H. Garrison. New York: Medical Life Press, 1926:305–309:309.

[36] Laura Otis, *Müller's Lab* [New York: Oxford University Press, 2007], 35.

[37] Laura Otis, 36.

marched alongside Müller, undoubtedly to provide moral support for his protégé.[38] Müller was a consummate scientist but he lacked the administrative temperament to handle the frantic negotiations among the military, the aristocracy, the monarch, and the academy; negotiations necessary to defuse the chaos of the 1848 liberal revolution in Berlin. Under threat of drastic measures from the Minister of Culture if he could not control the students, Müller struggled until the end of his term of office as University Rector to reconcile tensions that divided students from the minister and their king.[39] Shortly thereafter he suffered a complete mental breakdown from which he never fully recovered. Ever watchful of his protégé, Alexander Humboldt wrote of his happiness that after several months convalescence with his family in Koblenz and some time spent with Theodor Schwann in Belgium, Müller returned to Berlin in April 1849.[40]

The Influence of Alexander von Humboldt on Charles Robert Darwin [1809–1882]

Alexander von Humboldt shared with Goethe a broad scientific vision which he bequeathed to Darwin in the nineteenth century.[41] Stephen Jay Gould opined that "No one did more to change and enhance science in the first half of the nineteen century than Alexander von Humboldt." It was Humboldt, more than anyone else, who inspired Charles Darwin and Alfred Russel Wallace.[42] Aaron Sachs, professor of history at Cornell University opined: "the closest readers of Darwin realized that large parts of his theories were in fact derived directly from Humboldt, for evolution was essentially ecological."[43] While a student at Cambridge University, Darwin read Humboldt's *Personal Narrative of Travels to the Equinoctial Regions of the New Continent.*[44] In his autobiography, written in his old age, Darwin recalled that J. F. W. Herschel's *Preliminary Discourse on the Study of Natural History* and Humboldt's *Personal Narrative of Travels to the Equinoctial Regions of the New Continent* (1814–29) "stirred up in me a burning zeal to add even the most humble contribution to the noble structure of Natural Science. No one or a dozen other books influenced me nearly so much as these two."[45] Ironically, Darwin seems to have been more influenced by Humboldt's writings than he was by Humboldt in person.[46] Humboldt's writings also influenced Charles Lyell. In turn, Lyell's work in geology influenced Darwin's thinking.[47]

Gould maintained that the travel writings of Alexander von Humboldt were the primary influence that diverted Charles Darwin from the ministry into natural science.[48] Gould also credited Humboldt's view of the importance of travel in the tropics to have directly inspired Darwin to begin negotiations to visit

[38] Laura Otis, 36.

[39] Laura Otis, *Müller's Lab* [New York: Oxford University Press, 2007], 37.

[40] Laura Otis, 36–7.

[41] Gerard Helferich, *Humboldt's Cosmos: Alexander von Humboldt and the Latin American Journey That Changed the Way We See the World* [New York: Gotham Books, 2004], 332.

[42] Stephen Jay Gould, "Art meets science in *The Heart of the Andes:* Church paints, Humboldt dies, Darwin writes, and nature blinks in the fateful year of 1859," in *I Have Landed: The End of a Beginning in Natural History* [New York: Harmony Books, 2002], 93.

[43] Aaron Sachs, *The Humboldt Current: Nineteenth-Century Exploration and the Roots of American Environmentalism* [New York: Viking, 2006], 241.

[44] Janet Browne, *Darwin's Origin of Species* [New York: Atlantic Monthly Press, 2007], 16. Alexander von Humboldt's *Personal Narrative*, the English translation of 1814–1829. Gerard Helferich, *Humboldt's Cosmos: Alexander von Humboldt and the Latin American Journey That Changed the Way We See the World* [New York: Gotham Books, 2004], 306. This work was "packed with scientific data and technical digressions, the books were more a physical description of South America and an account of the social and political conditions that Humboldt had found there." The work ultimately filled four volumes.

[45] Stephen Jay Gould, "Art meets science in *The Heart of the Andes:* Church paints, Humboldt dies, Darwin writes, and nature blinks in the fateful year of 1859," in *I Have Landed: The End of a Beginning in Natural History* [New York: Harmony Books, 2002], 102.

[46] Gerard Helferich, *Humboldt's Cosmos: Alexander von Humboldt and the Latin American Journey That Changed the Way We See the World* [New York: Gotham Books, 2004], 318–9. Darwin recalled in his autobiography "I once met at breakfast at Sir Roderick Murchison's house, the illustrious Humboldt, who honoured me by expressing a wish to see me. I was a little disappointed with the great man, but my anticipations were probably too high. I can remember nothing distinctly about our interview, except that Humboldt was very cheerful and talked much."

[47] Gerard Helferich, 234.

[48] Stephen Jay Gould, "Art meets science in *The Heart of the Andes:* Church paints, Humboldt dies, Darwin writes, and nature blinks in the fateful year of 1859," in *I Have Landed: The End of a Beginning in Natural History* [New York: Harmony Books, 2002], 102.

the Canary Islands, negotiations that, "clearly if indirectly," led to an invitation for Darwin to sail on the *Beagle.*[49] Following his own scientific expedition aboard the HMS Beagle, Darwin published *Journal of the Beagle* in 1839, a book that brought him renown. Alexander von Humboldt wrote to him with praise for his book and correctly predicted "an excellent future" for Darwin, as had Goethe for von Humboldt several decades before.[50]

Gould concluded his argument for the influence of Humboldt on Darwin by stating: "More than mere accident underlies the fact that the twin discoverers of natural selection, Darwin and Alfred Russel Wallace, both cited Humboldt as their inspiration, and both made their most extensive, youthful trips to South America."[51] On the first page of the preface of *Kosmos*, Alexander von Humboldt outlined the grand aim of his entire work that embraced unity in the diversity of natural phenomenon. "The principle impulse by which I was directed was the earnest endeavor to comprehend the phenomena of physical objects in their general connection, and to represent nature as one great whole, moved and animated by internal forces." Gould opined that "this view of life and geology also embodied the guiding principles that…Darwin would tear down with a theory of conflict and balance between internal and external (largely random) forces."[52] Gould went further in his assessment of Darwin's contribution. "Darwin's concept operates as the central organizing principle of all biological science…no one ignorant of evolution can understand science."[53] Gould believed that the scientific theory of evolution posed no threat to religion.[54]

Darwin's book *On the Origin of Species by Means of Natural Selection,* published in 1859, evoked the first truly international debate.[55] Through a century of controversy, a more sophisticated version of Darwin's theory of natural selection emerged in 1959 as the discipline of

[49] Stephen Jay Gould, "Art meets science in *The Heart of the Andes:* Church paints, Humboldt dies, Darwin writes, and nature blinks in the fateful year of 1859," in *I Have Landed: The End of a Beginning in Natural History* [New York: Harmony Books, 2002], 102.

[50] Janet Browne, *Darwin's Origin of Species* [New York: Atlantic Monthly Press, 2007], 38. "The great Alexander von Humboldt wrote to him to call it 'happily inspired', and 'admirable book. … You have an excellent future ahead of you.' Such words from the man whom Darwin had idolized in his Cambridge days, and whose writings were generally regarded as the height of literary style, were praise indeed."

[51] Stephen Jay Gould, "Art meets science in *The Heart of the Andes:* Church paints, Humboldt dies, Darwin writes, and nature blinks in the fateful year of 1859," in *I Have Landed: The End of a Beginning in Natural History* [New York: Harmony Books, 2002], 102.

[52] Stephen Jay Gould, 96. See also: Stephen Jay Gould, *The Structure of Evolutionary Theory* [Cambridge, MA: Belknap Press of Harvard University Press, 2002], 161–2. "All major evolutionary theories before Darwin, and nearly all important versions that followed his enunciation of natural selection as well, retained fealty to an ancient Western tradition, dating to Plato and other classical authors, by presenting a fundamentally 'internalist' account, based upon intrinsic and predictable patterns set by the nature of living systems, for development or 'unfolding' through time." This is why Darwin used the phrase "descent with modification" instead of "evolution." "Darwin's theory, in strong and revolutionary contrast, presents a first 'externalist' account of evolution, in which contingent change (the summation of unpredictable local adaptations rather than a deterministic unfolding of inherent potential under internal, biological principles) proceeds by an interaction between organic raw material (undirected variation) and environmental guidance (natural selection). Darwin overturned all previous traditions by thus granting the external environment a causal and controlling role in the direction of evolutionary change (with 'environment' construed as the ensemble of biotic and abiotic factors of course, but still external to the organism, however intrinsically locked to, and even largely defined by, the presence of the organism itself). Thus, and finally, in considering the validity of extrapolation to complete the roster of essential Darwinian claims, the role of the geological stage becomes an appropriate focus as a surrogate for more overtly biological discussion. If the uniqueness of Darwinism, and its revolutionary character as well, inheres largely to the formulation of natural selection as a theory of interaction between biological insides and environmental outsides – and not as a theory of *evolution*, or intrinsic unfolding – then 'outsides' must receive explicit discussion as well, a need best fulfilled within this treatment of extrapolation." Gould's insight into Darwin's "externalist" view of evolution by natural selection came after the resolution of the antithesis of heredity and environment into the synthesis of heredity and environment achieved by the movement termed EVO–DEVO or evolutionary developmental biology.

[53] Stephen Jay Gould, "Darwin and the munchkins of Kansas," in *I Have Landed: The End of a Beginning in Natural History* [New York: Harmony Books, 2002], 215.

[54] Stephen Jay Gould, 214. "No scientific theory, including evolution, can pose any threat to religion – for these two great tools of human understanding operate in complementary (not contrary) fashion in their totally separate realms: science as an inquiry about the factual state of the natural world, religion as a search for spiritual meaning and ethical values."

evolutionary biology.[56] Initially, elements of the heretofore independent disciplines embryology and evolutionary biology – soon to be followed by developmental pathology, developmental biology, environmental biology, and toxicology – converged to unite heredity and environment in the new discipline of *evolutionary developmental biology*, Evo-Devo.[57] A historical tread of intellectual continuity with Evo-Devo can be traced back through "von Baer and Haeckel … and earlier to … Meckel [the Younger]...." However, the conceptual roots of Evo-Devo grew predominately in the soil of comparative morphology and morphogenesis. Only in the early 1980s did Evo-Devo evolve as a mechanistic science,[58] a new discipline essential to the scientific investigation of the multifactorial etiology of the five benign Müllerian diseases: adenomyosis, endometriosis, endosalpingiosis, endocervicosis, and müllerianosis.[59]

The Influence of Wilhelm von Humboldt on German University Education

Wilhelm von Humboldt's contribution centered on the rehabilitation of scientific and professional training in German universities that had weakened in the latter half of the seventeenth century.[60] As universities became increasingly out of touch with the workaday world, research, open discussion of ideas, experimental science, and the dissemination of new discoveries shifted to the academies, whose members were not distracted with teaching students.[61] By mid-eighteenth century, the emphasis in European universities on humanistic studies had reached down to "secondary schools" or gymnasiums. This humanistic influence reflected – in the German states – a response to the expectations of their growing middle class that the *Gymnasien* would promote *Bildung*,[62] "a lifelong process of self-development inspired through the study of Greco-Roman scholarship and art."[63] By the 1790s, some prominent Prussians held their universities in low regard[64]; and "in France … the very survival of universities was an open question."[65] This nadir in university education was deepened by the demoralizing Prussian defeat at the Battle of Jena in 1806 and the punishing terms Napoleon imposed on Prussia at the Treaty of Tilsit of 1807. Prussia lost all territory east of the Elbe River including its leading University of Halle with its medical school.[66]

Prussian pride demanded reforms and, as part of a broad national program spearheaded by Baron Heinrich Friedrich Karl vom und zum Stein (1757–1821), Karl

55 Janet Browne, *Darwin's Origin of Species* [New York: Atlantic Monthly Press, 2007], 1. Charles Darwin's *Origin of Species* "became the first truly international scientific debate in history." See also: Erna Lesky, *The Vienna Medical School of the 19th Century* [Baltimore, MD: Johns Hopkins University Press, 1976], 471. "When at the beginning of the sixties [1860s], embryology had a stormy period of development under the influence of Darwin and Haeckel, there were young scientists also at Brücke's Institute who made this branch of the sciences their special field of research…In 1873, the Vienna Medical Faculty became the only one in Austria with a separate chair and also a separate institute for embryology." A temporary embryology laboratory was established in the Old Rifle Factory.

56 Janet Browne, 143. "The centenary of publication of the *Origin of Species*, which was coincidently also the 150th anniversary of Darwin's birth [was the occasion when] evolutionary biology was a last a recognizable scientific discipline. Darwin was elevated into its founding father."

57 Sean B. Carroll, *Endless Forms Most Beautiful: The New Science of Evo Devo and the Making of the Animal Kingdom* [New York: W. W. Norton & Company, 2005], 7–9.The first stirring of the synthesis that would become evolutionary developmental biology [Evo–Devo] occurred in the 1970s with the "reunion" of embryology and evolutionary biology. In the 1980s geneticists determined that genes controlled the development of the fly. These studies "revealed a logic and order underlying the generation of animal form… The comparison of developmental genes between species became a new discipline at the interface of embryology and evolutionary biology-evolutionary developmental biology, or 'Evo–Devo' for short." See also: John Maynard Smith, *Genes, Embryos and Evolution* [New Haven, CT: Yale University Press, 1999]. Manfred D. Laubichler and Jane Maienschein eds. *From Embryology to Evo-Devo: A History of Developmental Evolution* [Cambridge, MA: MIT Press, 2007].

58 Gerd B. Müller, "Six Memos for Evo-Devo." In *From Embryology to Evo-Devo: A History of Developmental Evolution*, eds. Manfred D. Laubichler and Jane Maienschein. [Cambridge, MA: MIT Press, 2007], 499–524:501–2.

59 Janet Browne, *Darwin's Origin of Species* [New York: Atlantic Monthly Press, 2007], 153. "The new millennium has consequently begun with Westerners as divided as ever over the implications of a natural origin of species. Despite these challenges, the modern synthesis stands firm at the heart of biological science. No biologist would dream of disregarding the evidence. As Theodore Dobzhansky said in the 1960s, 'nothing in biology makes sense except in the light of evolution.'"

60 John W. O'Malley, *Four Cultures of the West* [Cambridge, MA: Belknap Press of Harvard University Press, 2004], 117.

61 John W. O'Malley, 118–119.

62 John W. O'Malley, 117. Bildung. See Andreas W. Daum, "*Wissenschaft* and knowledge," in *The Short Oxford History of Germany: Germany 1800–1870* [Oxford: Oxford University Press, 2004], 137–161:145. "The 9-year-long *Gymnasium* with

Friedrich Beyme [1765–1832], chief of the Prussian civil cabinet, was appointed to organize the new university at Berlin. He sought advice from scholars, among them Johann Gottlieb Fichte, Friedrich Schleiermacher, and Wilhelm von Humboldt. The first two scholars stressed a new emphasis for *Wissenschaft* that emphasized scholarship and research, the acquisition of new knowledge. However, they felt uneasy with the "careerism" of the professional faculties of medicine, law, and theology and so wished that the university be founded around the discipline of philosophy.[67] In 1809, Humboldt was appointed to the Prussian Interior Ministry with responsibilities for universities. He conceived of a "national university" in Berlin for the middle class that would exert Prussian cultural leadership over central Europe. Humboldt believed that – in time – this "national university" in Berlin would profoundly affect German scholarship by setting the standards of *Wissenschaft* for students and professors at all German universities.[68] Humboldt's emphasis on "*Bildung* and *Wissenschaft*… [was] meant as well to awaken a new spirit in the nation." Reformers such at Wilhelm von Humboldt attributed the "embarrassing defeat of the German states" by Napoleon, which resulted in the formal dissolution of the Holy Roman Empire in 1806, to the indifferent attitude of most Germans toward their absolutist rulers during the eighteenth century. Reformers sought a fundamental revision of the "economic and social structure of the state" as well as the necessity to change "the mentality of the citizens" toward their government.[69]

Wilhelm von Humboldt designed the University of Berlin with the tenets of *Wissenschaft* foremost in mind. He allocated just 25% of the ground floor for ten lecture halls, the remainder for research. As Laura Otis concluded: "In this allocation of space, the institution expressed the aims of its designer, Wilhelm von Humboldt: the inseparability of research and teaching and the acquisition of knowledge for its own sake."[70] By the second half of the nineteenth century, the University of Berlin "had become the unquestioned model for educational reforms in the United States and Japan, and then for other countries as well."[71]

Wilhelm von Humboldt "believed that academic medical education should be exclusively controlled by state controlled university medical faculty; that practical postgraduate medical education should be pursued in a large non-university hospital."[72] Chairs in basic science and clinical specialties would be accorded equal status. Prolonged training combined with independent research in physiology, physiological chemistry, or pathology

an emphasis on training in classical studies and then the university with its philosophical faculty, complemented by faculties for medicine, theology, and jurisprudence, became the places to devote oneself seriously to *Bildung*. Academic scholarship in all fields was expected to serve the higher moral aims laid out by idealism and neo-humanism. Professors therefore had to be more than simply purveyors of knowledge. They were seen as moral models and agents of creativity, restlessly aiming at expanding the limits of knowledge, disregarding any utilitarian purpose or social constraints, and guided only by their free will." See also: Arleen Marcia Tuchman, *Science, Medicine, and the State of Germany: The Case of Baden, 1815–1871* [New York: Oxford University Press, 1993], 41. The *Gymnasia* "were meant to create environments where students would learn, through active participation to think for themselves and develop new ideas. The focus on the individual's creative potential, and more so, on the importance of providing an educational environment aimed at stimulating this potential, is fully consistent with the humanistic conception of *Bildung*."

63 Laura Otis, *Müller's Lab* [Oxford: Oxford University Press, 2007], 6.

64 Thomas H. Broman, *The transformation of German academic medicine 1750–1820* [Cambridge: Cambridge University Press, 1996], 168.

65 John W. O'Malley, 121.

66 Thomas H. Broman, *The transformation of German academic medicine 1750–1820* [Cambridge: Cambridge University Press, 1996], 168. W. Haberling, "German Medicine in the Eighteenth Century: Friedrich Hoffmann, Stahl, Haller, van Swieten," in *German Medicine* translated by Jules Freund Clio Medica [New York: Paul B. Hoeber, 1934], 46. The medical school at Halle was founded in 1694.

67 Thomas H. Broman, 168–70.

68 Thomas H. Broman, 170–173:173. Arleen Marcia Tuchman, Science, Medicine, and the State of Germany: The Case of Baden, 1815–1871 [New York: Oxford University Press, 1993], 4. For Humboldt, "the personal search for knowledge took precedence over the mere acquisition of information. This led ultimately, to a higher estimation of the value of research, and expectations soon arose that a professor should be not only a good teacher but a renowned scholar as well."

69 Arleen Marcia Tuchman, Science, Medicine, and the State of Germany: The Case of Baden, 1815–1871 [New York: Oxford University Press, 1993], 18.

70 Laura Otis, *Müller's Lab* [New York: Oxford University Press, 2007], 16.

71 John W. O'Malley, *Four Cultures of the West* [Cambridge, MA: Belknap Press of Harvard University Press, 2004], 121.

72 Hans H. Simmer, "Principles and Problems of Medical Undergraduate education in Germany during the Nineteenth and Early twentieth Centuries." In *The History of Medical Education*, ed. C. D. O'Malley, No. 12 UCLA Forum in Medical Series [Berkeley, CA: University of California Press, 1970], 180–181.

would become the normal basis for a career in academic clinical medicine.[73] However, Humboldt's plan elicited tension for the discipline of medicine. The requirements of medicine were uniquely different from that of the university at large. Medical education required both academic and clinical teaching as well as research. Medical research comprised the "study of organic nature" in academic laboratories, while clinical teaching required that students examine and treat sick patients in order to acquire a practical knowledge of disease, its diagnosis and medical treatment. In short, clinical teaching required a large nonuniversity teaching hospital to learn the fundamentals of patient care. "Therefore, perhaps more than any other academic discipline, medicine manifested the tensions implicit in the nineteenth-century universities."[74]

One might ask whether or not Wilhelm von Humboldt infused sufficient plasticity into his model for educational reform that it could accommodate mid- and later nineteenth-century scientific laboratories. Tuchman pointed out that the "older historiographic tradition emphasized continuity between the Humboldtian-inspired philological seminars and the research laboratories built during mid-century." More recent revisionist work has challenged this picture of continuity, emphasizing instead the radical differences between the late nineteenth-century laboratories and the early anatomical museums and scientific cabinets.[75] Tuchman's own research supported the revisionist view of German universities.[76] This writer might accept the revisionist argument of discontinuity with respect to laboratory research on the acute infectious diseases, but insists – based on research into the history of endometriosis – on the continuity of laboratory research in pathology for the chronic diseases such as endometriosis.

The Influence of Johannes Peter Müller [1801–1858] on Rokitansky

Along with Johann Lukas Schonlein, Johannes Müller founded scientific medicine in Germany. Henry Sigerist opined that more than any other professor, it was Müller "who trained German doctors to think in terms of natural science."[77] His assistants, all gifted and some brilliant became leaders of German medicine.[78] Johannes Müller, Professor of Physiology and Pathological Anatomy at the University of Berlin, used the microscope to study the "fine structures of tissues as a means of studying physiological function."[79] During most of Müller's academic years which ended with death in 1858, physiology was essentially histology "accompanied by occasional chemical tests and investigations."[80]

In 1830, 3 years before his elevation to professor and chair at the University of Berlin, Müller clearly described the embryology of the Müllerian ducts, the paired embryonic structures that develop into the fallopian tubes, uterus, cervix, and upper vagina. In *Bildungsgeschichte der Genitalien, Embryology of the Genitalia in Vertebrates,* Müller synthesized existing knowledge based on his own observations and those of his contemporaries such as Rathke and Meckel the Younger and his predecessors such as Haller and Wolff.[81] *Bildungsgeschichte*

[73] Hans H. Simmer, "Principles and Problems of Medical Undergraduate education in Germany during the Nineteenth and Early twentieth Centuries." In *The History of Medical Education*, ed. C. D. O'Malley, No. 12 UCLA Forum in Medical Series [Berkeley, CA: University of California Press, 1970], 190.

[74] Thomas H. Broman, *The transformation of German academic medicine 1750–1820* [Cambridge: Cambridge University Press, 1996], 170–173:173.

[75] Arleen Marcia Tuchman, Science, Medicine, and the State of Germany: The Case of Baden, 1815–1871 [New York: Oxford University Press, 1993], 176. This writer believes Tuchman was referring to the era of Johann Peter Frank and his successor, Ludwig Baron von Türkheim of Vienna.

[76] Arleen Marcia Tuchman, 6.

[77] Henry E. Sigerist, *The Great Doctors: A Biographical History of Medicine* trans. Eden and Cedar Paul [New York: W. W. Norton & Company, 1933], 307. See page 311. Müller's assistant, Du Bois-Raymond calculated the literary output of Johannes Müller as "over 15,000 printed pages and about 350 plates drawn by his own hand" during the 37 years of his active life. In contrast, "Johann Lukas Schonlein penned, over and above his dissertations, only two works, one of which extended to three pages and the other to one page."

[78] Laura Otis, *Müller's Lab* [Oxford: Oxford University Press, 2007]. Jakob Henle, Theodor Schwann, Emil du Bois-Reymond, Hermann von Helmholtz, Rudolf Virchow, Robert Remak, and Ernst Haeckel.

[79] Arleen Marcia Tuchman, Science, Medicine, and the State of Germany: The Case of Baden, 1815–1871 [New York: Oxford University Press, 1993], 86–87. Laura Otis, *Müller's Lab* [New York: Oxford University Press, 2007], 8. Müller would succeed to Carl Asmund Rudolphi (1771–1832) to the Chair of Physiology and Pathological Anatomy at the University of Berlin. It was Rudolphi who encouraged Müller to use the microscope in his studies. In 1824, Rudolphi gave Müller his personal Fraunhofer microscope for his research.

[80] Arleen Marcia Tuchman, 86–87.

[81] Harold Speert, 102.

der Genitalien, Müller's treatise on the comparative embryology of genitalia in vertebrates, along with descriptions of some Müllerian malformations that persist into adult life, so impressed the academic community that the anlage of the female reproductive system became known as the Müllerian ducts.[82] Because of the influence of Müller's *Embryology of the Genitalia in Vertebrates* on Rokitansky and the history of endometriosis, a brief digression into the history of embryology will clarify subsequent developments.

A Brief Digression into the History of Embryology

Casper Friedrich Wolff [1733–1794], a German embryologist, was an experimentalist in the age when embryologists had to contend with relatively primitive microscopes. Serial sections of tissue and staining of thin layers of tissue were unknown.[83] Fortunately for Wolff and his contemporaries the technique for hardening soft embryonic tissues had recently been discovered.[84] In 1759, Wolff wrote a defense of epigenesis entitled *Theoria Generationis*, based on a "new experimental foundation of morphogenesis." [85] Wolff demonstrated that the complete chick did not exist preformed in the unincubated egg, but to the contrary the organs formed successively in an epigenetic manner.[86] This work prompted a controversy with Albrecht von Haller of Göttingen, who defended the theory of preformation.[87] Needham opined that Wolff was "undoubtedly an epigenesist-vitalist," which would explain Wolff's concept of *vis essentialis.*[88] Wolff postulated *vis essentialis* as an "immanent formative force" required for epigenesis, "the continual production…of new organs and new relationships between organs already formed." On the other hand, the mechanical preformation theory of Haller – "where embryogeny was little more than a swelling up of parts already there" – required only nutrition for growth and development.[89] Wolff stated his position: "The particles which constitute all animal organs in their earliest inception are little globules, which can always be distinguished under the microscope…How, then, can it be maintained that a body is invisible because it is too small, when the *parts* of which it is composed are easily distinguishable?"[90]

Jacques Roger explained: "Wolff had thought he was seeing animal gluten in the process of organization: in fact, it was already organized since one could make it visible by hardening it with distilled spirits. Wolff had thought he was seeing the formation of the heart: in reality, he had been seeing it appear, for the heart had to exist before acquiring visibility, given that the embryo was already alive….In order to explain what he had seen, and in order not to have recourse to the invisible, Wolff had had to grant living matter a mysterious force, a *vis essentialis*, which was [not acceptable] to Haller."[91] Haller, a physician who debated Wolff, had examined the formation of chicks in eggs minutely for several years, which examinations caused him to renounce epigenesis in 1757 and hold to the idea of preexistent germs "preformation."[92] Haller accepted Wolff's scientific observations; "the facts [Wolff] had observed were beyond debate." But Haller could not accept Wolff's interpretation of the facts observed.[93] In 1768, Wolff published a work based on extensive research: *De formatione Intestinorum* firmly established the epigenetic theory of morphogenesis for the chick intestine and in the process "ruined

[82] Harold Speert, *Obstetric & Gynecologic Milestones: Illustrated* [New York: Parthenon Publishing Group, 1996], 102. Johannes Müller, *Bildungsgeschichte der Genitalien aus anatomischen Untersuchungen an Embryonen des Menschen and der Thiere, nebst einem Anhang über die chirurgische Behandlung der Hypospadia.* [Düsseldorf, 1830]. See also: Zeph J. R. Hollenbeck and John I. Hollenbeck, *Profiles in Surgery, Gynecology and Obstetrics* [Flushing, NY: Medical Examination Publishing Company, 1973], 70.

[83] Joseph Needham, *A History of Embryology.* 2nd ed. [New York: Abelard-Schuman, 1959], 202.

[84] Joseph Needham, 202.

[85] Joseph Needham, *A History of Embryology.* 2nd ed. [New York: Abelard-Schuman, 1959], 220–221.

[86] Francis G. Gilchrist, *A Survey of Embryology* [New York: McGraw-Hill Book Company, 1968], 5.

[87] Joseph Needham, 220.

[88] Joseph Needham, 214.

[89] Joseph Needham, 207. See page 183. In modern terms, preformation corresponds to "growth without differentiation," and epigenesis corresponds to "differentiation plus growth."

[90] Harold Speert, *Obstetric & Gynecologic Milestones: Illustrated* [New York: Parthenon Publishing Group, 1996], 92.

[91] Jacques Roger, *The Life Sciences in Eighteenth-Century French Thought*, ed. Keith R. Benson and trans. Robert Ellrich [Stanford, CA: Stanford University Press, 1997], 498.

[92] Jacques Roger, 493, 495–6.

[93] Jacques Roger, 497. Joseph Needham, *A History of Embryology.* 2nd ed. [New York: Abelard-Schuman, 1959], 116.Wolff relied on empirical observations and experimentation rather than philosophical speculations.

preformation."[94] With respect to *vis essentialis* – the *immanent formative force* – Jacques Roger wrote: "The conclusion of [Wolff's *De formatione Intestinorum*] is particularly specific: 'I am not saying that the parts are produced through a collaboration of particles; through fermentation; through mechanical causes and reasons; through the powers of the soul; but I am saying that they are produced." "By limiting himself to the factual assertions, Wolff avoided the criticisms that Haller directed against *vis essentialis*."[95] Wolff emigrated from Berlin to St. Petersburg in 1769 where he was accepted into the Academy of Catherine the Great at St. Petersburg.[96]

In 1802, in a small pamphlet on the development of the human fetal ovary, Johann Christian Rosenmüller [1771–1820] described the mesonephric remnant in humans which he named the Wolffian body in honor of Casper Friedrich Wolff.[97] Then, in 1812, Johann Friedrich Meckel the Younger translated Wolff's work from Latin into German. This translation proved influential to embryologists such as Christian Heinrich Pander (1794–1865) and von Baer.[98] The great embryologist Karl Ernst von Baer [1792–1876] referred to Wolff's *De Formatione Intestinorum* as "the greatest masterpiece of scientific observation."[99] What particularly impressed Pander and von Baer were Wolff's "observations on derivation of the parts of the early embryo from 'leaf-like' layers" [anticipating the concept of ectoderm, mesoderm, and entoderm].[100] Von Baer discovered the mammalian [dog] ovum in 1827.[101] It was in this expansive period of embryology that in 1830 Johannes Müller wrote his celebrated treatise *Embryology of the Genitalia in Vertebrates*.

As a medical student, Rokitansky was profoundly influenced by Johann Friedrich Meckel's concepts of embryology and comparative anatomy.[102] Given Rokitansky's intense interest in developmental pathology and "Müllerian malformations that persist into adult life," it is inconceivable that he did not read Müller's *Embryology of the Genitalia in Vertebrates*. In the year it was published (1830), Rokitansky became the assistant to Johann Wagner at the University of Vienna autopsy house.[103] Combined with the influence of the great teratologist Johannes Friedrich Meckel, Müller's *Embryology of the Genitalia in Vertebrates* undoubtedly contributed greatly to Rokitansky's "good foundation in embryology [that] helped him to understand aberrant development and to predict what might evolve when development went astray."[104] Müller's embryological treatise – a complete synthesis of vertebrate reproductive embryology with references to the outstanding embryologists including Johann Friedrich Meckel – influenced Rokitansky to investigate anomalies and diseases of the female reproductive tract. Based on his theoretical expertise in embryology and augmented by extensive practical experience in the autopsy house at Vienna, Rokitansky contributed compelling descriptions of Müllerian developmental anomalies.

The most noteworthy of these was his description of partial Müllerian agenesis [Mayer-Rokitansky-Küster-Hauser syndrome],[105] one of the developmental Müllerian diseases characterized by a deficiency of Müllerian tissue. Rokitansky also identified and described uterine and extrauterine endometriosis, which are acquired Müllerian diseases characterized by an excess of Müllerian tissue.[106] In the last decade and a half of his academic life Rokitansky devoted his efforts to the detailed description of developmental anomalies of the cardiovascular system.[107]

[94] Joseph Needham, *A History of Embryology.* 2nd ed. [New York: Abelard-Schuman, 1959], 221.

[95] Jacques Roger, 681–2, n. 153. For a full and sophisticated philosophical discussion of vital forces that is beyond the scope of this work, see Roger, pages 336–353 "IV: The Rebirth of Vital Forces."

[96] Joseph Needham, 220. See also Harold Speert, *Obstetric & Gynecologic Milestones: Illustrated* [New York: Parthenon Publishing Group, 1996], 91.

[97] Harold Speert, *Obstetric & Gynecologic Milestones: Illustrated* [New York: Parthenon Publishing Group, 1996], 92. JC Rosenmüller. *Quaedam de Ovariis Embryonum et Foetuum Humanorum.* [Leipzig: C. Tauchnitz, 1802].

[98] Joseph Needham, *A History of Embryology.* 2nd ed. [New York: Abelard-Schuman, 1959], 223.

[99] Harold Speert, 92.

[100] Joseph Needham, 222.

[101] Harold Speert, 86. See page 96. Von Baer was admitted as a member of the St. Petersburg Academy of Science in 1829.

[102] Venita Jay, "The legacy of Karl Rokitansky," Arch Pathol Lab Med 2000;124:345–346:345.

[103] Harold Speert, 102.

[104] Venita Jay, "The legacy of Karl Rokitansky," Arch Pathol Lab Med 2000;124:345–346:346.

[105] Von Prof. Dr. Rokitansky, Uber die sogenannten Verdoppelungen des Uterus. Medicinische Jahrbucher des kaiserl. konigl osterreichischen Staates 1838;26:S39–77:40.

[106] Carl Rokitansky, Ueber Uterusdrüsen-Neubildung in Uterus- und Ovarial-Sarcomen. Zeitschift Gesellschaft der Aerzte in Wien. 1860;16:577–581.

[107] Venita Jay, 2000;124:345–346:346. Carl Rokitansky, *On Some of the Most Important Diseases of the Arteries* [1852] and *The Defects in the Septum of the Heart* [1875].

Intellectual Development of Carl Von Rokitansky

2

This is indeed an age of specialization. God speed to him who grasps this truth and labors accordingly. Goethe[1]

Emergence of the First Full-Time Anatomical Pathologist

Fortunately, Goethe's scientific philosophy of precise observation spread to Austria as an antidote to Schelling's natural-philosophical system that had retarded medical science in Austria as it had in Germany.[2] Natural scientific pathology emerged out of natural philosophical pathology. In the latter case Sigerist explained, one "tries to work out a system of manifestations abstractly, which is as nearly as possible without gap." On the other hand, in natural scientific pathology "one explains only as much as may be sustained by observation and in experiments." Instead of speculation, one constructs and tests hypotheses to bridge gaps in knowledge, hypotheses which are discarded when new observations make them indefensible.[3]

In 1805, the clinician Philipp Carl Hartmann (1773–1830) criticized the "a-prioristic postulates of the natural philosophers because they lacked empirical foundation."[4] Hartmann was appointed to the Chair of General Pathology, Therapy, and Materia Medica in the Vienna Medical School in 1811.[5] Through Hartmann, Goethe's insistence on precise observation as the basis of science reached his pupil Rokitansky.[6] Rokitansky of Vienna, like Wilhelm and Alexander von Humboldt and Johannes Müller of Goethe's Jena circle, was a man of high endowment.[7]

Rokitansky is the investigator who first identified uterine and ovarian endometriosis. An informed

[1] Johann Wolfgang Goethe, *Wilhelm Meisters Journeyings* I, 4 (1829), 19, 39. Ronold King, "Goethe and the challenge of science in western civilization," in *Goethe on Human Creativeness and other Goethe Essays*, ed. Rolf King [Athens, GA: University of George Press, 1950], 227.

[2] Erna Lesky, *The Vienna Medical School of the 19th Century* [Baltimore, MD: Johns Hopkins University Press, 1976], 78. "True, Brunonianism had collapsed in Vienna as elsewhere in 1804; but as elsewhere, it was succeeded also in Vienna by Schelling's natural-philosophical system which claimed with great confidence that all phenomena in nature could be deduced from reason alone."

[3] Henry E. Sigerist, *Man and Medicine: An Introduction to Medical Knowledge*, trans. Margaret Galt Boise [New York: W. W. Norton & Company, 1932], 116.

[4] Erna Lesky, *The Vienna Medical School of the 19th Century* [Baltimore, MD: Johns Hopkins University Press, 1976], 79.

[5] Erna Lesky, 79.

[6] Erna Lesky, 81. See also Lesky p. 152–4. Ernst von Feuchtersleben (1806–1849), well read in the philosophy of Goethe and who made Goethe's insistence on careful observation based on personal experience his credo, "felt most attracted to Philipp Carl Hartmann," of all his medical teachers. Subsequently, Feuchtersleben was a colleague of Rokitansky, both members of the exclusive circle of the Society of Physicians founded in 1837 by Türkheim.

7 R. J. Rather, Eva R. Rohl. An English Translation of the Hitherto Untranslated Part of Rokitansky's *Einleitung* to volume 1 of the *Handbuch der allgemeinen Pathologie* (1846), with a

R.E. Batt, *A History of Endometriosis*,
DOI 10.1007/978-0-85729-585-9_2, © Springer-Verlag London Limited 2011

appreciation of Rokitansky's remarkable attainments, and their limitations, requires an understanding of the conditions under which he learned and worked: the nature of his medical education, his performance of tens of thousands of autopsies, and his contributions to the field of anatomical pathology. Equally important, by following the tortuous process by which Rokitansky progressed from a – seemingly paradoxical – hematohumoral theory of disease to a cellular theory of disease whilst firmly committed to localistic pathology, one may begin to appreciate the difficulty he faced in discovering a new chronic disease deep in the interior of the female body.[8]

By a state mandate of 1753, all patients dying at the Vienna General Hospital – the Allgemeines Krankenhaus – became subject to autopsy.[9] This was probably the time that the "Leichenhaus," the Vienna autopsy house, was built. The state mandate for autopsy resulted in the accumulation of preserved specimens of disease as well as a continuous stream of fresh corpses.

In 1784, Emperor Joseph II (1780–1790) rebuilt the 2,000-bed Allgemeines Krankenhaus.[10] In 1786, the Emperor initiated academic reforms. The Emperor looked for expert opinion from Pierre-Jean-Georges Cabanis (1757–1808) of France[11] and Johann Peter Frank (1745–1821) of Austria.[12] Both consultants opined that the discipline of anatomy had reached "such a high degree of perfection that only few discoveries of great importance" could be expected.[13] In other words, they believed anatomy was no longer a first-class academic endeavor. Accepting the opinion of these highly regarded physicians, the Emperor reduced anatomy to dissection and elevated the discipline of physiology over anatomy. According to the medical historian, Erna Lesky, "This reform marks the beginning of the unhappy role played by macroscopic anatomy in the Austrian medical curricula far into the nineteenth century."[14] Henceforth, prosectors in the lower discipline of "gross" anatomy performed only macroscopic dissections of cadavers. Demotion to a lower academic status effectively separated gross anatomy from histology and gross anatomical pathology from microscopic pathology.

In 1795, the Emperor Francis II (1792–1835), son and successor of Emperor Leopold II (1790–1792) appointed Johannes Peter Frank (1745–1821), one of the medical consultants to Emperor Joseph II in 1786, as professor of medicine and director of the new Vienna General Hospital.[15] Frank recognized a special opportunity for his medical students to learn by personal experience the entire course of disease in patients from initial diagnosis and subsequent clinical course in Hospital to the terminal disease at autopsy in those who died.[16] Johann Peter Frank, an early specialist in spinal cord diseases and "one of the founders of the pathology of the spinal cord," had a special interest in pathological

Bibliography of Rokitansky's published works. Clio medica 1972;7:215–227:224–227.

[8] Henry E. Sigerist, *Man and Medicine: An Introduction to Medical Knowledge* [New York: WW Norton & Company, 1932], 170. Sigerist, himself a physician, appreciated that chronic diseases are often difficult to define. "Now there are a number of diseases which begin gradually and insidiously, which bring with them no stormy periods of doubtful outcome but which may last a long time, sometimes years, and sometimes decades. These are the *chronic diseases.*"

[9] Sonia Horn, "Vom Leichenoffnen…Beobachtungen zum Umgang mit anatomischen und pathologischen Sektionen in Wien vor 1800," Wiener Klinische Wochenschrift 2004;116/23:792–803:801.

[10] Roy Porter, *Blood and Guts: A Short History of Medicine* [New York: W. W. Norton & Company, 2002], 137–8.

[11] *Webster's New Biographical Dictionary* [Springfield, MA: Merriam-Webster Inc., 1988], 159. Cabanis was a French physician and philosopher, who became Professor of Hygiene in 1794 at the Medical School in Paris.

[12] *Webster's New Biographical Dictionary*, 368. Frank was one of the chief founders of the science of public health.

[13] Erna Lesky, *The Vienna Medical School of the 19th Century* [Baltimore, MD: Johns Hopkins University Press, 1976], 68.

[14] Erna Lesky, 68.

[15] Erna Lesky, *The Vienna Medical School of the 19th Century* [Baltimore, MD: Johns Hopkins University Press, 1976], 4. As professor of medicine, Frank was a clinician. 278.

[16] Erna Lesky, 76. This was the beginning of the comprehensive teaching tradition whereby medical students from the Vienna General Hospital performed autopsies in the morgue followed by physical examinations of patients in the hospital that resulted in a high maternal mortality from puerperal sepsis on the wards attended by medical students. See also pages 181–186. Students would work in the autopsy house and carry infection from corpses back to the Maternity Clinic where they unknowingly infected postpartum patients resulting in many deaths from puerperal sepsis. It was students working in Rokitansky's autopsy rooms that were responsible for epidemics of death from puerperal sepsis when Semmelweis made his discovery of the relationship between contaminated bare hands from autopsy and maternal deaths from puerperal sepsis, a discovery anticipated by Rokitansky.

anatomy.[17] In 1796, when the Pathological-Anatomic Museum was built, Frank appointed the gifted macroscopic pathological anatomist Aloys Rudolph Vetter (1765–1806) to the newly created post of voluntary prosector with instructions to organize the wealth of preserved specimens in the new museum and to coordinate the teaching of pathology with clinical teaching.[18] Given this unusual opportunity, albeit limited to macroscopic pathology, Vetter attempted to organize general pathology into two great classes of disease: acute and chronic.[19] In 1803, Vetter moved to the School of Surgeons in Cracow as Professor of Anatomy and Physiology; from 1796 until 1803 Vetter had been an unpaid prosector in Vienna. Vetter died of pulmonary tuberculosis in 1806.[20] Erna Lesky opined that Aloys Rudolph Vetter, the only thoughtful Vienna prosector "in the years 1796-1832… proved himself a congenial ancestor of Rokitansky."[21] In 1804, Johannes Peter Frank fell into disfavor and was removed from office during a reshuffling of the Vienna Medical School faculty.[22] Lesky records: "Thus the first attempt at establishing pathological-anatomical dissection in Vienna, which had seemed so promising, temporarily came to an end."[23]

Frank was succeeded by his pupil, Ludwig Baron von Türkheim (1777–1846) in 1811.[24] Notwithstanding this favorable appointment, the separation of naked-eye pathological anatomy from microscopy persisted far into the nineteenth century at the University of Vienna. In 1812 after much infighting, Joseph Andreas von Stifft (1760–1836), personal physician to the Emperor and the persecutor who had forced Johannes Peter Frank to leave Vienna, restored pathological-anatomical dissection and appointed Lorenz Biermayer as a salaried prosector. Not unexpectedly, Stifft restored pathological-anatomical dissection but not Frank's pathological-anatomical institute.[25]

Baron von Türkheim, with the support of juridical advisors, restored Frank's institution of pathological-anatomy in 1812 with Biermayer as prosector. From among the "approximately 600 corpses" he dissected annually, Biermayer "recorded, prepared, and conserved at the museum anything that he considered rare or remarkable."[26] In 1816, Biermayer published a catalog of specimens in the museum.[27] As a result of a regulation adopted in 1818 all forensic autopsies in Vienna were assigned to the pathologic-anatomic prosector; consequently all civilian, military, and forensic autopsies in Vienna came under the control of Biermayer.[28] With this increased responsibility performed with "great diligence," Biermayer was rewarded "ad personam" in 1821 when the post of pathologic-anatomic prosector was elevated to a salaried associate

---

[17] Max Neuburger. "Johann Peter Frank as Founder of the Pathology of the Spinal Cord," in *Essays in the History of Medicine*, trans. by various hands and edited with foreword by Fielding H. Garrison [New York: Medical Life Press, 1930], 131–143:142–43. Max Neuburger, Professor of the History of Medicine at the University of Vienna wrote: "May we never forget Frank as one of the founders of the pathology of the spinal cord, even today [1930] when, unexpectedly after the lapse of a hundred years, the seed he sowed has shot up into a flourishing stalk."

[18] Erna Lesky, *The Vienna Medical School of the 19th Century* [Baltimore, MD: Johns Hopkins University Press, 1976], 75. Roland Sedivy, *Carl Freiherr von Rokitansky: Wegbereiter der Pathologischen Anatomie* [Vienna: Verlag Wilhelm Maudrich, 2002], 26.

[19] Erna Lesky, 76. "A scientist of Vetter's caliber was a guarantee that the development of pathological anatomy that was taking place around the medical clinic would not be smothered by pure didactic or by casuistics and museum collections. Vetter, however, also possessed the knowledge required for these fields; as a self-taught man he had acquired the technical skill necessary for making preparations; from Stoll he had learned to apprehend morphological as well as clinical-symptomatic details by keen observation. Thus he, a pathological anatomist, was also firmly rooted in the Hippocratic foundations of Vienna empirical medicine…He attempted to develop a general pathology in which two great classes of diseases would be distinguished on a genetic-morphological basis, "the active or rapidly developing changes" and the "passive, mechanical or chronic ones." This attempt was too early, of course, at a time when pathological anatomy hardly used a microscope." "Vetter proved himself a congenial ancestor of Rokitansky…[he was] the first and only thinker in the series of Vienna prosectors in the years 1796–1832."

[20] Erna Lesky, 77.

[21] Erna Lesky, 76.

[22] Erna Lesky, 20, 58, 87. *Webster's New Biographical Dictionary* [Springfield, MA: Merriam-Webster Inc., 1988], 368. Dismissed by the Austro-Hungarian Emperor, Frank served as physician to Czar Alexander I of Russia from 1805 to 1808.

[23] Erna Lesky, 77.

[24] Erna Lesky, *The Vienna Medical School of the 19th Century* [Baltimore, MD: Johns Hopkins University Press, 1976], 98.

[25] Erna Lesky, 75, 77.

[26] Erna Lesky, 77.

[27] Erna Lesky, 77. It was from one of these museum specimens that Rokitansky was to publish a case of partial müllerian agenesis in 1838.

[28] Erna Lesky, 90–91.

professorship in the University of Vienna.[29] Biermayer, twice rewarded for creativity and due diligence, "grossly neglected" his duties from 1825 to 1829 when he was dismissed. His duties fell to his assistant, Johann Wagner (1800–1832) and to Wagner's "student-apprentice Carl Rokitansky."[30] Wagner was promoted from assistant to associate professor in 1830.[31]

Rokitansky had studied medicine in Prague from 1822 to 1824 and in Vienna from 1824 to 1828.[32] Frustrated by enforced mechanical memorizing of prescribed texts, he began a program of self-instruction, reading the works of Meckel the Younger, Lobstein, and Andral, a program of self-education that he continued his entire professional life.[33] While in medical school he resolved to observe disease first hand at autopsy and draw his own conclusions.[34] On November 1, 1827, during his fifth and last year of medical school,[35] Rokitansky began to work in the "Leichenhaus," the autopsy house or university morgue at the University of Vienna Allgemeines Krankenhaus as an unpaid student-assistant to Johann Wagner.[36] Months earlier, on March 27, 1827, he had assisted Wagner perform the autopsy on Ludwig van Beethoven.[37] Rokitansky performed his first autopsy on October 23, 1827 before he assumed the position of unpaid student-assistant.[38] Shortly after graduation, he was appointed "assistant in the pathologico-anatomical department of the University."[39] Rokitansky became the first physician to eschew clinical practice and devote himself exclusively to general anatomical pathology, a personal decision that may have been influenced by his melancholic personality.[40]

Johannes Wagner, a master at dissection and preparation of autopsy specimens, taught his skills to Rokitansky.[41] The vast number of bodies to be autopsied coupled with lack of refrigeration left no alternative but to develop rapid and disciplined postmortem dissection protocols. An example of his dexterity, Wagner reportedly was able to "open the spinal canal from the lowest end, the sacrum, up to the second vertebra of the neck within 7 minutes."[42] This was undoubtedly a dissecting skill handed down from

[29] Erna Lesky, *The Vienna Medical School of the 19th Century* [Baltimore, MD: Johns Hopkins University Press, 1976], 75, 77.

[30] Erna Lesky, 77.

[31] Erna Lesky, 77.

[32] Ivo Steiner, "Rokitansky in his Bohemian years and his relations with Jan E. Purkyne," *Wiener Klinische Wochenschrift* 2004;116/23: 788–791. This is an excellent source of biographical information on Rokitansky from birth until 1824 when he departed Prague for Vienna.

[33] Erna Lesky, 107. "Mechanical memorizing of prescribed textbooks was all this system could offer him during his years of study in Prague (1822–1824) and in Vienna (1824–1828)." Paul Klemperer. Notes on Carl von Rokitansky's autobiography and inaugural address. *Bulletin of the History of Medicine* 1961;35:374–80:374. "The description which Rokitansky gives of medical education in Prague and Vienna shows the low level of instruction at the time. It was determined by the rule of a bureaucracy which mistrusted talent and aimed at developing a safe mediocrity. The professors were uninspired drill masters of their disciplines." Gilder SSB. Carl von Rokitansky (1804–1878). *Canadian Med J* 1954;71:70–72.

[34] Erna Lesky, 107–108.

[35] Erna Lesky, 77–78. See also pages 18–19: Rokitansky's 5-year medical school curriculum had first been introduced in 1810. The fifth year studies were particularly strong in pathology and included "Special Pathology and Therapy of the Internal Diseases; Practical Medical Instruction at the Bedside; Forensic Medicine, and in the summer session: Medical Police." The curriculum of 1810 was changed in 1833 after Rokitansky graduated.

[36] Erna Lesky, 107.

[37] Hui ACF, Wong SM. Deafness and liver disease in a 57-year-old man: a medical history of Beethoven. *Hong Kong Medical Journal* 2000 Dec;6(4):433–438. The original autopsy report, written in Latin, was found in the Vienna Museum of Anatomical Pathology in 1970.

[38] Gilder SSB. Carl von Rokitansky (1804–1878). *Canadian Med J* 1954;71:70–72.

[39] Carl Rokitansky, *A Manual of Pathological Anatomy*, Volume I. *General Pathological Anatomy*. trans. William Edward Swaine [Philadelphia, PA: Blanchard & Lea, 1855], viii. Editor's Preface to Vol. I.

[40] Carl Rokitansky, *A Manual of Pathological Anatomy*, Volume II. *The Abdominal Viscera*. trans. Edward Sieveking [Philadelphia, PA: Blanchard & Lea, 1855], ix. Editor's Preface. "Rokitansky," as Mr. Wilde correctly remarks, "differs from all other pathologists, in not engaging in the study or treatment of disease during life; he is not a practical physician, and seldom sees one of the many hundreds of cases, whose bodies he dissects." Erna Lesky, *The Vienna Medical School of the 19th Century* [Baltimore, MD: Johns Hopkins University Press, 1976], 107. While in Prague preparatory to the study of medicine, Rokitansky's "basic melancholic disposition became evident, the deep pessimism of his nature, which later made him accept the philosophy of Schopenhauer as the interpretation of the world most appropriate to his nature." See also: Alexander M. Rokitansky, "Ein Leben an der Schwelle," *Wiener Medizinische Wochenschrift* 2004;154/19-20:454–457. Prim. Univ.-Prof. Dr. Alexander M. Rokitansky, Vienna, Austria.

[41] Erna Lesky, *The Vienna Medical School of the 19th Century* [Baltimore, MD: Johns Hopkins University Press, 1976], 77–78.

[42] Erna Lesky, 78.

Johann Peter Frank through Aloys Vetter to Lorenz Biermayer and then to Johann Wagner who would teach it to Rokitansky.[43] While a master prosector, Wagner was not a master pathologist; he failed to understand that the clinician's diagnosis had to be substantiated or disproved based on accurate pathologic diagnosis at autopsy. Like his contemporaries in Paris, Wagner worked in reverse; he tried to explain his findings at autopsy in terms of the clinical findings when the patient was alive.[44] Rokitansky determined to free pathological anatomy from the limitations of museum pathology and Wagner's clinical approach and to "create a new medical science founded on pathological anatomy."[45]

Putting aside Wagner's clinical approach to pathological anatomy, Rokitansky had to teach himself the scientific discipline of anatomical pathology as the foundation for clinical medicine. Daily he encountered a panorama of disease in the morgue. Under such demanding circumstances, Rokitansky developed a sophisticated scanning gaze to detect patterns; patterns different from the usual and mundane.[46] He taught himself macroscopic pathological anatomy, mastering the appearance of disease in the morbid tissues and organs.[47] Rokitansky's career in pathological anatomy commenced at a time when that discipline was in decline at the University of Vienna and when the position of prosector and associate professor of pathologic anatomy was occupied by Johann Wagner.[48] Wagner died in 1832. By that time Rokitansky had long mastered barehand, naked-eye macroscopic pathological anatomy, use of the microscope having been forbidden in 1786 by Emperor Joseph II.[49] Rokitansky resolved to make the most of the situation. Early in his career he had set as his academic goal the complete and systematic classification of general pathology in men and women by synthesis of naked-eye observations at autopsy. He would labor for the next two decades collecting, analyzing, and correlating pathological observations that he would publish as a Handbook of Pathological Anatomy.

Having demonstrated his superior talents and industry, Rokitansky was appointed Wagner's successor in 1834 with the academic rank of associate professor. The task he set for himself was "to arouse German medicine from its natural-philosophical dream and to base it on solid, unchangeable, material facts." As the first full-time pathologist in the Western world, Rokitansky had personal control of an unprecedented flow of thousands of corpses from Europe's largest hospital, the Vienna Allgemeines Krankenhaus. In Rokitansky's hands, this centralization and specialization provided a unique opportunity to study the concept of localization for every disease in the human body, both male and female. This ideal situation in Vienna contrasted sharply with conditions in Paris. For in Paris, not only was medicine decentralized in many hospitals scattered throughout the city, but pathological anatomy was also decentralized; physicians and surgeons performed their own autopsies, which limited the scope of their research.[50]

---

[43] Max Neuburger. "Johann Peter Frank as Founder of the Pathology of the Spinal Cord," in *Essays in the History of Medicine*, trans. by various hands and edited with foreword by Fielding H. Garrison [New York: Medical Life Press, 1930], 131–143: 143. Frank was one of the founders of the pathology of the spinal cord.

[44] Gilder SSB. Carl von Rokitansky (1804–1878). *Canadian Med J* 1954;71:70–72. Erna Lesky, *The Vienna Medical School of the 19th Century* [Baltimore, MD: Johns Hopkins University Press, 1976], 78. "As Rokitansky stated in his autobiography (p. 51), 'notwithstanding the daily contradictions between the results of dissection and the records on disease and diagnosis,' Wagner 'was not able to grasp the lesion beyond casuistics or to form a clear idea of the reforming impact his subject was destined to make…"

[45] Erna Lesky, *The Vienna Medical School of the 19th Century* [Baltimore, MD: Johns Hopkins University Press, 1976], 78.

[46] Gilder SSB. 1954;71:70–72. "[Rokitansky] had a gift for exact observation, and clear exposition."

[47] Paul Strathern, *A Brief History of Medicine from Hippocrates to Gene Therapy* [New York: Carroll & Graf, 2005], 207–211. "Two centuries previously Morgagni had emphasized the organs in which disease is located, and subsequently pathology had very much concentrated on the appearances of diseases" at autopsy. See also: Venita Jay, "The legacy of Karl Rokitansky," *Arch Pathol Lab Med* 2000;124:345–346:345. "At the completion of a postmortem examination, he worked backward to determine what could have led to the observed pathology."

[48] Erna Lesky, *The Vienna Medical School of the 19th Century* [Baltimore, MD: Johns Hopkins University Press, 1976], 77–78.

[49] The marvel of magnification via telescope [Galileo: 1564–1642] and microscope [Leeuwenhoek: 1632–1723] opened for scientific study the vast natural world beyond the visual acuity of humans. Eventually Rokitansky would use the microscope, one of the marvels of technology, but he never mastered the instrument.

[50] Erna Lesky, *The Vienna Medical School of the 19th Century* [Baltimore, MD: Johns Hopkins University Press, 1976], 107.

Once in charge of pathological anatomy, Rokitansky did not proceed blindly. He had been influenced profoundly by the writings of Johann Friedrich Meckel the Younger on embryology and comparative anatomy[51]; the same Meckel had translated Casper Friedrich Wolff's work on embryology from Latin into German in 1812.[52] Meckel the Younger (1781–1833), a third-generation professor from one of the premier medical families in Germany, had studied in Vienna with Johann Peter Frank and in Paris with the comparative anatomist Georges Cuvier.[53] When the University of Halle reopened in 1808, Meckel the Younger assumed the chair and professorship of anatomy, pathological anatomy, surgery, and obstetrics that had been held by his father, Philipp F. T. Meckel (1755–1803).[54] Meckel limited his professional activities to anatomy, pathological anatomy, and physiological research,[55] As a Professor at Halle – and a living force in pathological anatomy when Rokitansky was a student and young prosector – Meckel the Younger became Rokitansky's role model for an academic career in pathological anatomy.[56] Rokitansky emulated Meckel's research program by stressing the *processes* that underlay the anatomical pathology seen at autopsy and by pursuing developmental pathology.[57] Like Meckel, he sought to reconstruct the clinical course of the patient's disease from the terminal state of organs and tissues at autopsy.[58] And like Meckel, Rokitansky studied congenital anomalies and developmental pathology. Meckel had written his doctoral dissertation on developmental abnormalities of the heart.[59] As if in a final tribute to Meckel the Younger, Rokitansky would devote the last 15 years of his academic career to developmental pathology of the heart and cardiovascular system.[60]

---

[51] Venita Jay, "The legacy of Karl Rokitansky," *Arch Pathol Lab Med* 2000;124:345–346:345. Gilder SSB. Carl von Rokitansky (1804–1878). *Canadian Med J* 1954;71:70–72.

[52] Joseph Needham, *A History of Embryology* 2nd ed. [New York: Abelard-Schuman, 1959], 223. Needham wrote: "It was not until 1812 that J. F. Meckel the younger translated Wolff's papers into German." Temkin parses this statement of Needham. Owsei Temkin, "Basic Science, Medicine, and the Romantic Era," in *The Double Face of Janus and Other Essays in the History of Medicine* [Baltimore, MD: Johns Hopkins University Press, 1977], 375. "It is a mistake, though often repeated, that Wolff's *Theoria generationis* was forgotten or failed to make a serious impression and that it took the German translation of Wolff's other work, *On the Formation of the Intestines,* to remind the world of him. It is true that the latter essay remained practically unknown until Meckel's translation in 1812. It is equally true that the emphasis in these two works is placed differently. But I am afraid that Goethe is partly responsible for the misapprehension that in 1790, when he published his *Metamorphosis of Plants,* preformation still prevailed and Wolff was unknown. Goethe learned of the *Theoria generationis* only about 1792, but this was due to his own oversight, not to that of his contemporaries. Moreover, by that time epigenesis, in Germany, had found an even more aggressive and popular protagonist in Blumenbach…At any rate, before the century had passed, epigenesis, though not without qualifications, was accepted by leading German biologists and philosophers, to mention only Herder, Kant, and Schelling among the latter."

[53] Thomas H. Broman, *The transformation of German academic medicine 1750–1820* [Cambridge: Cambridge University Press, 1996], 178. Three generations of Meckel professors: Johann Friedrich Meckel the Elder (1714–1774), his son Philipp F. T. Meckel (1755–1803) and his grandson Johann Friedrich Meckel the Younger (1781–1833).

[54] Arleen Marcia Tuchman, Science, Medicine, and the State of Germany: The Case of Baden, 1815–1871 [New York: Oxford University Press, 1993], 15. "Not until the Napoleonic Wars and the collapse of the Holy Roman Empire were these institutions significantly restructured and redefined." When the University of Halle reopened in 1808, it was in the newly formed Kingdom of Westphalia.

[55] Thomas H. Broman, *The transformation of German academic medicine 1750–1820* [Cambridge: Cambridge University Press, 1996], 178.

[56] Johann Hermann Baas, *Outlines of the History of Medicine and The Medical Profession.* Trans. H. E. Henderson [Huntington, NY: Robert E. Krieger Publishing Co., 1971], 951 n. [Original edition 1889, one volume; Reprint 1971, two volumes]. Erna Lesky, *The Vienna Medical School of the 19th Century* [Baltimore, MD: Johns Hopkins University Press, 1976], 211. Joseph Hyrtl (1810–1894) "like Rokitansky, he was a self-taught man and received his anatomic knowledge from Meckel."

[57] Thomas H. Broman, 186–7. "Pathological anatomy, Meckel observed as early as 1805, had usually been studied in one of two ways. It had consisted either of a catalogue of an organ's possible deviations from its normal form and mixture, without regard for the impaired or defective processes by which the deviation occurred, or it had laid primary weight on the processes, appending a merely supplemental description of the anatomical changes undergone by the organ. In either case, pathological autonomy had studied the degenerative changes of organs that were at one time healthy and normal, an inquiry driven by medical practitioner's desire to know what changes were produced by diseases in the body. Although such goals may be laudable, Meckel argued that the subject need not be restricted to serving clinical needs; it could also serve a "higher interest. This interest, he continued, consisted of 'the developmental history of the organ under normal circumstances,' along with 'the harmonization of various organs and systems with each other."

[58] Erna Lesky, *The Vienna Medical School of the 19th Century* [Baltimore, MD: Johns Hopkins University Press, 1976], 108.

[59] Thomas H. Broman, 178.

[60] Erna Lesky, 112–3.

Rokitansky was also deeply influenced by the Paris School of Pathological Anatomy and Diagnosis.[61] Founded by Corvisart, Dupuytren, and Laennec, who built on the accomplishments of Bichat and Pinel, the Paris School was then at the summit of its influence.[62] Its members were trained as surgeons or like Pinel, Bichat, and Laennec "expressly stated that they handled the data of internal medicine like surgeons," i.e., as localists and anatomists.[63] But it was not until 1836, when Cruveilhier was given the chair of pathological anatomy created in the will of Dupuytren that pathological anatomy became a recognized specialty in Paris.[64] Rokitansky chose to launch his career informed especially by the works of Andral and Lobstein the Nephew.[65]

Johann Georg Lobstein (1777–1835) published a treatise on pathological anatomy in 1829, the year after Rokitansky graduated from medical school. Like Rokitansky's role model Meckel the Younger, Lobstein came from a prominent medical family. He was the nephew of the great J. F. Lobstein who had held the chair of pathological anatomy in Strasbourg since its foundation in 1819. The ideas of Lobstein the Nephew were to exert considerable influence on Rokitansky. As Ackerknecht explained: Lobstein made a "somewhat Germanic attempt to 'lead facts back to ideas and higher views of nature,' in his case a mixture of speculative neuro-and humoral pathology."[66] In other words, in 1829 Lobstein the Nephew sought for an explanation for his pathological findings from autopsies in a combination of neuropathology and humoral pathology. His treatise influenced Rokitansky as he also searched to explain generalized disease without local pathological lesions.

In that same year 1829, Gabriel Andral published a multivolume treatise on pathological anatomy which was the "culminating point of the classic macroscopic pathological anatomy" of the Paris School.[67] Significantly for its influence on Rokitansky, "Andral divided all pathology into lesions of capillary circulation, of nutrition, of secretion, of the blood, and of innervation."[68] Like Lobstein the Nephew, Andral's work contributed to the hematohumoral theory of the origin of generalized disease as an explanation for death when the autopsy showed no significant pathology. Rokitansky would embrace this theory in his Handbook of Pathological Anatomy of 1845.

Rokitansky's Research Program – Second Vienna Medical School

Appointed associate professor of pathological anatomy in 1834 by Baron von Türkheim, Rokitansky found himself in a position to formally establish his research program. In the 8 years since assisting at the autopsy of Beethoven, Rokitansky had acquired a wealth of experience and a clear and comprehensive grasp of the potential for research at the Vienna autopsy house. First, he justified the separate existence of the discipline of anatomical pathology by "sorting [clinical] facts scientifically" – based on the morbid pathological anatomy found at autopsy.[69] In his quiet and determined way, Rokitansky "proved himself" a master "pathological anatomist" both by his systematic classification of pathological lesions visible to the naked eye and by his identification of new

[61] Venita Jay, "The legacy of Karl Rokitansky," *Arch Pathol Lab Med* 2000;124:345–346:345.

[62] Roswell Park, *An Epitome of the History of Medicine* 2nd ed. [Philadelphia: F. A. Davis Company, 1908], 244–245. Venita Jay, "The legacy of Karl Rokitansky," *Arch Pathol Lab Med* 2000;124:345–346:345. Erwin H. Ackerknecht, *Medicine at the Paris Hospital 1794–1848* [Baltimore, MD: Johns Hopkins Press, 1967], 83–4, 166–7.

[63] Erwin H. Ackerknecht, *Medicine at the Paris Hospital 1794–1884* [Baltimore, MD: Johns Hopkins Press, 1967], 25. See also: 89. Laennec "and his teacher Bichat both emphasized the fact that *pathological anatomy was imported into medicine by surgeons.*"

[64] Erwin H. Ackerknecht, 164, 167. Cruveilhier (1891–1873) was the most celebrated member of the Paris School. Roswell Park, *An Epitome of the History of Medicine* 2nd ed. [Philadelphia: F. A. Davis Company, 1908], 244. The American surgeon and medical historian Roswell Park (1852–1914) wrote of the Paris School of Pathological Anatomy and Diagnosis: "It made it the duty of the physician to search for changes in the human body, to investigate the local products of disease, and assigned to medicine the duty of removing these products. The tendency of its teaching was to treat the patient rather as a living cadaver than as a sentient being endowed with vital forces." Park went on to quote an author named Kratzmann. "Kratzmann wrote some years ago: 'In France every one experiments on the sick, less to attain the best method of cure than to enrich science with an interesting discovery and to advance the accuracy of diagnosis by some new physical sign."

[65] Gilder SSB. Carl von Rokitansky (1804–1878). Canadian Med J 1954;71:70–72

[66] Erwin H. Ackerknecht, *Medicine at the Paris Hospital 1794–1884* [Baltimore, MD: Johns Hopkins Press, 1967], 167.

[67] Erwin H. Ackerknecht, 168.

[68] Erwin H. Ackerknecht, 167–8.

[69] Erna Lesky, *The Vienna Medical School of the 19th Century* [Baltimore, MD: Johns Hopkins University Press, 1976], 107.

diseases.[70] He introduced new descriptive metaphors to describe his findings at autopsy, such as: "'a raspberry jelly,' 'a puree of peas,' or 'coffee grounds.'"[71] By observing quantitative and qualitative changes and recurrent patterns of disease in many thousands of autopsies, Rokitansky constructed objective pictures of common diseases and recognized new diseases.[72] By comparing various stages of pathological change over time for each disease, he established a scientific basis for the concept of "disease process."[73] Rokitansky demonstrated the applicability of this scientific clinical-pathological experience to accurate diagnosis in living patients.[74] He fulfilled this second goal of benefiting living patients by teaching pathological anatomy to clinicians such as the German internist Kussmaul,[75] and by collaborating with his clinical colleagues on the faculty of the Second Vienna Medical School: the internist Skoda,[76] the dermatologist Hebra, and the surgeon Schuh.[77]

Simultaneously with the inauguration of the Medical Yearbooks of the Imperial Royal Austrian State in 1836, the Second Vienna Medical School was founded by Baron von Türkheim. By centering the medical school on "Carl von Rokitansky's autopsy table," Ludwig Freiherr Baron von Türkheim initiated "one of the most fruitful and brilliant epochs of Viennese medicine."[78] Then in 1837, Türkheim organized the Vienna Society of Physicians which facilitated lively scientific discussion and resulted in publications by the younger members of the faculty.[79] Perhaps stimulated by such discussions, Rokitansky scanned the wealth of pathological material preserved in specimen jars in Vetter's pathological anatomy museum or perhaps he first scanned Lorenz Biermayer's catalog of specimens in the museum.[80] Among the specimen jars he found a developmental anomaly of the female reproductive organs, an anomaly that one day would bear the name Mayer-Rokitansky-Küster-Hauser syndrome.

Deficiency of Müllerian Tissue (1838)

In the course of human history, diseases and disorders affecting the body exterior or obvious abnormalities of organs in the body interior were identified long before diseases with more subtle pathological manifestations. Such was the case with partial müllerian agenesis, a müllerian *deficiency* disorder characterized by absence of the vagina and malformation of the uterus, the former readily detected on external physical examination in the living and the latter readily detected at autopsy.[81]

[70] Erna Lesky, 108.

[71] Erna Lesky, 108.

[72] Erna Lesky, 108. Henry E. Sigerist, *The Great Doctors: A Biographical History of Medicine.* Trans. Eden and Cedar Paul [New York: W. W. Norton & Company, 1933], 292, 294.

[73] Erna Lesky, 108. See also: R. J. Rather, Eva R. Rohl. An English Translation of the Hitherto Untranslated Part of Rokitansky's *Einleitung* to volume 1 of the *Handbuch der allgemeinen Pathologie* (1846), with a Bibliography of Rokitansky's Published Works. *Clio medica* 1972;7:215–227:215. "Rokitansky, too, believed that the task facing the general pathologist centered on the explanation of the disease process."

[74] Erna Lesky, 107.

[75] Owen H. Wangensteen and Sarah D. Wangensteen, *The Rise of Surgery: From Empiric Craft to Scientific Discipline* [Minneapolis, MN: University of Minnesota Press, 1978], 440. Kussmaul worked at Rokitansky's side for 4 months while they performed autopsies. Kussmaul returned to Germany. He taught Robert Meyer at the German University of Strassburg. At Strassburg, Friedrich von Recklinghausen performed autopsies for Kussmaul.

[76] Erna Lesky, *The Vienna Medical School of the 19th Century* [Baltimore, MD: Johns Hopkins University Press, 1976], 109. Skoda remained at the University of Vienna where he and Rokitansky became dominant figures in the specialties of medicine and pathological anatomy in the Second Vienna Medical School.

[77] Gilder SSB. Carl von Rokitansky (1804–1878). *Canadian Med J* 1954;71:70–72.

[78] Erna Lesky, 106. This would not be the only time that a yearbook or journal was to be intimately associated with the rise of a University Medical School; the same occurred 10 years later, in 1845–1846 in Buffalo, New York, USA with the publication of the Buffalo Medical Journal and the incorporation of the University of Buffalo Medical School and in 1889 with the opening of Johns Hopkins Hospital and the inauguration of The Bulletin of Johns Hopkins Hospital.

[79] Erna Lesky, 99. The Vienna Society of Physicians which met in Türkheim's apartment published its own "house organs," *Verhandlungen* (Transactions) commencing in 1842 and the *Zeitschrift der k.k.Gesellschaft der Arzte zu Wien* (Journal of the Imperial Royal Society of Physicians in Vienna) commencing in 1844.

[80] Roland Sedivy, *Carl Freiherr von Rokitansky: Wegbereiter der Pathologischen Anatomie* [Wien: Verlag Wilhelm Maudrich, 2002,] 26. The pathological anatomy museum, where Rokitansky found his specimens, was constructed in 1796 on the personal order of Kaiser Joseph II. An illustration of this pathological anatomy museum is rendered on page 27 of Sedivy's monograph.

[81] Ghirardini G, Popp LW. The Mayer-von Rokitansky-Küster-Hauser syndrome (uterus bipartitus solidus rudimentarius cum vagina solida): the development of gynecology through the history of a name. *Clin Exp Obstet Gynecol* 1995;22:86–91. These authors state that partial müllerian agenesis with solid vagina was known to Avicenna and Albucassis in the middle ages.

Diseases characterized by *excessive* müllerian tissue were much more subtle and identifiable only at autopsy before the advent of safe abdominal and pelvic surgery.

In 1829 Professor Mayer of Bonn, Germany observed a developmental anomaly at autopsy in a 53-year-old woman. This anomaly would become known as partial müllerian agenesis or Mayer-Rokitansky-Küster-Hauser syndrome.[82] He published this case as illustrative of one of four different duplications of the uterus.[83] Mayer found an absent vaginal canal and two rudimentary uterine buds widely separated except where connected inferiorly. Both tubes and ovaries were normal.[84] The very next year (1830), Johannes Müller published his treatise on the embryology of vertebrate genitalia, entitled *Bildungsgeschichte der Genitalien aus anatomischen Untersuchungen an Embryonen des Menschen und der Thiere*.[85] In this celebrated work, Müller skillfully integrated his own observations with those of distinguished embryologists, describing normal embryonic formation as well as common developmental malformations, especially those "involving the distal ends of the genital tube, the urinary duct, and the intestinal canal."[86] Müller's work placed developmental anatomy and pathology of the müllerian organs on a new and higher scientific plane.

Following Müller's scientific tour de force, Rokitansky reported 20 cases of uterine duplication. He retained the classification proposed by Mayer in 1829, referring to Mayer by name in the text and citing his paper in a footnote.[87] Only the first of the 20 cases represented uterus bipartitus with solid vagina and normal tubes and ovaries.[88] The patient was a 60-year-old woman named Magdalena Fischer[89] who had died of cancer in the "allgemeinen Krankenhaus" on July 30, 1828. Possibly Rokitansky was present at her autopsy on that summer day and remembered the case. The specimen was then preserved for a decade in Vetter's pathologic-anatomic museum where Rokitansky retrieved it for description in his 1838 paper.[90]

[82] The various lenses through which scientists, clinicians, and patients have viewed endometriosis will be described and evaluated from a chronologic perspective beginning in the early nineteenth century with Mayer's description of vaginal agenesis, the first contribution in a nearly two-century long evolution of the Mayer-Rokitansky-Küster-Hauser [M-R-K-H] syndrome further clarified by Fedele et al. in 2007. The M-R-K-H syndrome may serve as a *Rosetta stone* for understanding the classic theories of pathogenesis of endometriosis.

[83] Mayer, Ueber Verdoppelungen des Uterus und ihre Arten, nebst Bemerkungen uber Hasenscharte und Wolfsrachen. *Journal der Chirurgie und Augen Heilkunde* 1829;13:525–564. Mayer's cases were not true duplications of the uterus as described by Joe Leigh Simpson. See: Simpson JL. Genetics of the female reproductive ducts. *Am J Med Genet* (Semin Med Genet) 1999;89:224–39:235. True duplication of the uterus "is very rare and almost always misclassified. Affected women must have two separate uteri, each of which can have *two* fallopian tubes….Embryogenesis presumably involves division of one or both müllerian ducts early in embryogenesis…True duplication should be distinguished from incomplete müllerian fusion, the much more common condition in which each of two hemiuteri is associated with only a single fallopian tube."

[84] Mayer, Ueber Verdoppelungen des Uterus und ihre Arten, nebst Bemerkungen uber Hasenscharte und Wolfsrachen. *Journal der Chirurgie und Augen Heilkunde* 1829;13:525–564. See also: Ghirardini G, Popp LW. The Mayer-von Rokitansky-Küster-Hauser syndrome (uterus bipartitus solidus rudimentarius cum vagina solida): the development of gynecology through the history of a name. *Clin Exp Obstet Gynecol* 1995;22:86–91.

[85] Johannes Müller, *Bildungsgeschichte der Genitalien aus anatomischen Untersuchungen an Embryonen des Menschen und der Thiere* [Düsseldorf: Arnz, 1830].

[86] Harold Speert, "Johannes Müller and the Müllerian Ducts," in *Obstetric & Gynecologic Milestones Illustrated*, 2nd ed. rev. [Parthenon Publishing Group, 1996], 102.

[87] Von Prof. Dr. Rokitansky, Uber die sogenannten Verdoppelungen des Uterus. Medicinische Jahrbucher des kaiserl. konigl osterreichischen Staates 1838;26:S39–77:40. Later their names became associated with the syndrome of partial müllerian agenesis, the Mayer-Rokitansky-Küster-Hauser syndrome.

[88] Von Prof. Dr. Rokitansky, 1838;26:S39–77.

[89] Parenthetically, it is interesting to see that patient anonymity was not preserved, nor were the identities of other patients Rokitansky presented. He identified some by their full name, others by their first name and the first letter of their family name. Presumably this was standard practice in Vienna in 1828 because Rokitansky would not have had the authority to initiate such a practice during his first year in the autopsy house in 1827–1828. In 1829 in Bonn, (Germany) Mayer identified his cases by the noun "subject" or "person" instead of the patient's proper name.

[90] Partial müllerian agenesis is relatively uncommon, 1 in 5,000 births or autopsies. See: Aittomaki K, Eroila H, Kajanoja P. A population-based study of the incidence of müllerian aplasia in Finland. *Fertil Steril* 2001;76:624–5. There are two forms of müllerian aplasia: partial müllerian agenesis, Mayer-Rokitansky-Küster-Hauser syndrome and complete müllerian aplasia characterized by absence of the vagina, uterus, and fallopian tubes. Complete or total müllerian aplasia may occur in XX females and in XY phenotypic females when it is called androgen insufficient syndrome. "Most women with müllerian aplasia are otherwise healthy and have normal female chromosome constitution, hormonally active functioning ovaries, and normal female secondary sexual characteristics. However müllerian aplasia also occurs in specific syndromes such as androgen insensitivity." In Finland, the incidence of vaginal aplasia over a period of 10 years [including Mayer-Rokitansky-Küster-Hauser syndrome and complete müllerian agenesis] was 1:5,000 newborn girls. In Finland, most patients had Mayer-Rokitansky-Küster-Hauser syndrome.

Partial müllerian agenesis is characterized by *deficiency* of müllerian tissue – absent vaginal canal and deformed uterus. An absent vagina is easily recognized on physical examination of the body exterior; a deformed uterus is readily recognized by cursory examination of the body interior. At first the syndrome of partial müllerian agenesis was named the Rokitansky syndrome,[91] but in time Mayer's contribution would be recognized with successive renaming as the Mayer-Rokitansky-Küster syndrome[92] and finally as Mayer-Rokitansky-Küster-Hauser syndrome.[93] Only years later in 1860, would Rokitansky identify and describe the more subtle müllerian diseases – uterine and ovarian endometriosis – characterized by an *excess* of müllerian tissue associated with a normally developed uterus and ovary situated in the interior of a female corpse.

In 1846, Rokitansky made further observations on partial müllerian agenesis and summarized his leading-edge knowledge of developmental anomalies of the human female reproductive tract: "The vagina may be totally absent, or partially deficient; in the latter case there is a cul-de-sac opening externally, or the vagina terminates blindly at a greater or less distance from the labia, or opens posteriorly into the urethra – in this instance the development takes place from both points, but an intervening portion is deficient, thus forming a transition to congenital atresia." "The presence of blood assumes particular importance when it is retained by a redundant hymen or by congenital or acquired obturation…"[94]

"Complete absence of the uterus must be considered as extremely rare; in most cases in which the uterus was found deficient in the dead or living subject, rudiments of a uterine organ of different forms were discovered." "The most common case of arrest, which is generally considered as absence of the uterus, is that in which the fold of the peritoneum, which is destined for the reception of the internal sexual organs, contains, on one or both sides, posteriorly to the bladder, one or two small, flattened solid masses, or larger hollow bodies, with a cavity of the size of a pea or a lentil, which is lined with mucous membrane. They are to be viewed as rudiments of the uterine horns, and the Fallopian tubes bear an exact relation to their development. These may either be totally deficient, or terminate in the vicinity of the uterus in the peritoneum as blind ducts, or they may communicate with the uterus with or without an open passage."

"This formation of the uterus, and especially the existence of two lateral, hollow, elongated and rounded uterine remnants, each of which is connected with a corresponding Fallopian tube and ovary, constitutes what Mayer terms the uterus bipartitus. From each of the uterine rudiments a flattened, round cord of uterine tissue ascends within the fold of the peritoneum, and the two from each side coalesce. The place of the uterus is occupied by cellular tissue, in which a few uterine fibres, derived from the just-mentioned cord, may be traced; it presents the general outline of a uterus, and reaching downwards, rests upon the arch of a short vaginal cul-de-sac. The external sexual organs and the mammary glands, as well as the general sexual character of the individual, attain a normal development."[95] Rokitansky distinguished between congenital and acquired anomalies[96] but acknowledged that a good classification of malformations was lacking "owing to the difficulty of establishing a principle of division generally applicable."[97]

[91] Ramirez JC, Puerta AJ, Rebollo A, Benitez R, Pena A, de la Macorra JC. Rokitansky's syndrome in association with renoureteral abnormalities. Teratogenic period. *Eur Urol* 1987;13:346–50.

[92] Acien P. Lloret M, Chehab H. Endometriosis in a patient with Rokitansky-Küster-Hauser syndrome. *Gynecol Obstet Invest* 1988;25:70–72.

[93] Griggs JA, Rudoff J, Coddington CC. Mayer-Rokitansky-Küster-Hauser syndrome with splenosis. A case report. *J Reprod Med* 1990;35:821–3.

[94] Carl Rokitansky, A Manual of Pathological Anatomy, Volume II. The Abdominal Viscera. trans. Edward Sieveking [Philadelphia, PA: Blanchard & Lea, 1855] Chapter III. Abnormalities of the Female Sexual Organs, 201–202. Note how Rokitansky intuits the importance of retained blood that ordinarily would have been expelled. Only in 1921 would John Sampson recognize the significance of retrograde menstruation as one mode of pathogenesis of endometriosis.

[95] Carl Rokitansky, *A Manual of Pathological Anatomy*, Volume II. The Abdominal Viscera. trans. Edward Sieveking [Philadelphia, PA: Blanchard & Lea, 1855]. Chapter III. Abnormalities of the Female Sexual Organs, 206–207.

[96] Carl Rokitansky, A Manual of Pathological Anatomy, Volume I. General Pathological Anatomy. trans. William Edward Swaine [Philadelphia, PA: Blanchard & Lea, 1855], 23. [Author's] Introduction. "XVI. With reference to the period during which anomalies originate, we have to distinguish congenital, or such as have become established during intra-uterine life, and acquired, or such as have arisen during extra-uterine life. The former comprehend primitive anomalies." "XVII. Primitive anomalies comprise malformations. These are deviations of the organism, or of an organ, so intimately blended with its primary development, as to occur only at the earliest periods of embryonic life, or at any rate before that of mature fœtal existence."

[97] Carl Rokitansky, *A Manual of Pathological Anatomy*, Volume I. General Pathological Anatomy. trans. William Edward Swaine

Rokitansky's Autopsy Experience (1828–1844)

Rokitansky continued the tradition of barehand and naked-eye examination of the bodies and viscera of corpses at autopsy set by the founder of modern pathological anatomy, Morgagni. Giovanni Battista Morgagni (1682–1771) became Professor of Anatomy at the University of Padua in 1715; a successor to Versalius, Fallopius, Fabricius, and Spigelius. Morgagni, a clinician as well as an anatomist, developed the anatomical concept of disease. Symptoms were "the cry of the suffering organs."[98] At autopsy Morgagni traced the patient's symptoms to a deranged organ which he identified as the seat of disease. As Nuland, surgeon and medical historian, observed: "his book's title is a summary of its message: *The Seats and Causes of Disease Investigated by Anatomy* (*De Sedibus et Causis Morborum per Anatomen Indagatis*)."[99] Morgagni's investigations "shifted the emphasis from *symptoms* to the *site* of disease...from a physiological theory [of] disease [as] an abnormal condition of the whole organism to an ontological theory of disease" as an entity with a locus in a particular part of the body.[100] Morgagni established anatomical pathology when he localized disease to organs.

The other barehand, naked-eye pathological anatomist of note was Matthew Baillie (1761–1823). Like the Italian Morgagni, the Englishman Baillie was both clinician and pathologist. Baillie described the gross pathologies of human emphysema, cirrhosis of the liver, and gastric ulcers in *Morbid Anatomy of Some of the Most Important Parts of the Human Body* (1793), the first English book on pathology.[101] Baillie arranged disease in his *Morbid Anatomy* by organs.[102] As had Morgagni and Baillie before him, Rokitansky observed the appearances of morbid disease at varying stages and correlated them with clinical symptoms.[103] Rokitansky was not satisfied to trace Morgagni's "cry of a suffering organ" to identify disease in the deranged organ as the terminal event. He proceeded to reconstruct the process of disease in each patient – from its beginning to its end – in order to permit earlier diagnosis, treatment, and possible recovery.[104]

The physical conditions under which Rokitansky and members of his department worked tax the imagination of twenty-first-century readers. Not many years after Rokitansky died, Roswell Park, the American surgeon, medical historian, and founder of Roswell Park Cancer Hospital, described working conditions within the Leichenhaus, the Vienna autopsy house. He wrote: "von Rokitansky worked for a long time in miserable quarters in Vienna...[where]...he performed more than thirty thousand autopsies."[105] Apparently, poor working conditions for pathological anatomy were not uncommon during that era. During his tenure

[Philadelphia, PA: Blanchard & Lea, 1855], 25. [Author's] Introduction. See also page 30 where Rokitansky discussed the classification of malformations according to Bischoff. "First Class. – Malformations deficient in some essential attribute of their kind." "At this day, however, so much in this assumption is still hypothetical that we are compelled to deal with it cautiously, addressing ourselves, where it is possible, to other causes, more especially to interrupted evolution of an organ out of its germ, or to its development being impeded through external influences, such as impression wrought upon the mother; destruction of the organ, in the progress of its development, through disease, particularly through dropsical accumulation; finally, destruction of an organ through mechanical influence-for example, the amputation of a limb by means of the umbilical cord or a pseudomembranous formation with the ovum, etc."

[98] Sherwin B. Nuland, "The New Medicine: The Anatomical Concept of Giovanni Morgagni." In *Doctors* [New York: Alfred A. Knopf, 1988], 145–170: 147.

[99] Sherwin B. Nuland, 147–149.

[100] Roy Porter, *Blood and Guts: A Short History of Medicine* [New York: W. W. Norton & Company, 2002], 73.

[101] Roy Porter, ed. *The Cambridge Illustrated History of Medicine* [Cambridge: Cambridge University Press, 1996], 652, 707, 1112.

[102] Roy Porter, *Blood and Guts: A Short History of Medicine* [New York: W. W. Norton & Company, 2002], 73.

[103] Steven I. Hajdu, Pathologists who attained fame without using microscopy. *Annals of Clinical & Laboratory Science* 2003;33:119–122. Both Morgagni and Baillie had clinical practices; Rokitansky did not. Henry E. Sigerist, *The Great Doctors: A Biographical History of Medicine.* Trans. Eden and Cedar Paul [New York: W. W. Norton & Company, 1933], 236. Morgagni's "ideas of general pathology were entirely conventional. His chosen field was that of special pathological anatomy, and, as a matter of course, naked-eye pathological anatomy." Sherwin B. Nuland, "The New Medicine: The Anatomical Concept of Giovanni Morgagni." in *Doctors* [New York: Alfred A. Knopf, 1988], 145–170: 152. Morgagni, the clinician practiced anatomy without the benefit of microscopy. Nuland, page 161: Historians consider Morgagni as the founder of modern medical diagnosis.

[104] Sherwin B. Nuland, "The New Medicine: The Anatomical Concept of Giovanni Morgagni." In *Doctors* [New York: Alfred A. Knopf, 1988], 145–170:241–2.

[105] Roswell Park, *An Epitome of the History of Medicine*, 2nd ed. [Philadelphia: FA Davis Company, 1908], 250-1. See also: Rickman John Godlee, *Lord Lister* [Oxford: Clarendon Press, 1924], 346. The Allgemeines Krankenhaus in Vienna as well as

at the University of Berlin from 1833 to 1858, Johannes Müller's and his assistants performed their most crucial microscopic research in "small, dark, foul-smelling rooms."[106] In a memorial address for Müller, one of his former assistants described the Berlin Anatomical Institute as "a foul-smelling hole."[107]

Erna Lesky reproduced an illustration of Rokitansky's postmortem rooms in her book, *The Vienna Medical School of the 19th Century.*[108] In 1997, the Austrian pathologist, Bankl, published an original photograph of the old autopsy house.[109] The drawing and photograph show a long rectangular single-story building with a dormered roof that doubled the height of the building. Facing the building, one observes on the left, a large pair of arched wooden "barn doors" that provided entry for wagons bearing corpses from the Allgemeines Krankenhaus. To the right of the arched wooden door, four narrow windows with six panes of glass alternated with four doors surmounted by ventilation windows. One narrow dormer with windows rose immediately above the second doorway and a large dormer with eight windows occupied a position midway between the crest line of the roof and the third doorway. These windows provided the principle source of natural light which, judging from a contemporary photograph of the dissection room in the Old Rifle Factory, was augmented by diffuse artificial light from gas lamps suspended from the ceiling.[110] Judging from the deep shadows, most of the light came through windows.[111] Based on the position of the large dormer near the right end of the autopsy house where most of the natural light was concentrated, it is probable that this larger dormer provided light directly above the autopsy table where Rokitansky worked. Two chimneys, one in the center of the building and one to the right of the large dormer near the end of the building, perhaps not far from Rokitansky's work site, indicate that the Leichenhaus was heated by stoves during the winter.

Lacking refrigeration to preserve corpses and air conditioning to ameliorate summer's heat, optimum working conditions in the Leichenhaus for that era were confined to moderate weather of spring and autumn; heat in summer hastened deterioration of corpses and the coldest winters of the Little Ice Age stiffened the fingers of Rokitansky, his assistants, and the medical students.[112] Evisceration of the corpses, dissection, interpretation of findings, and dictation were necessarily confined to hours of daylight. One cannot help but be impressed with the volume of first-rate research and teaching that Rokitansky accomplished under these trying conditions until 1862 when new quarters were provided.

Rokitansky is generally credited with having performed 30,000 autopsies during his career.[113] Autopsy

Rokitansky's autopsy house were "hopelessly out of date" in the 1860s. "About 1865 the most celebrated hospitals on the continent, the Allgemeines Krankenhaus at Vienna, the Hotel-Dieu at Paris, the Charite at Berlin, The Julius Hospital at Würzburg, and others…were hopelessly out of date."

[106] Laura Otis, *Müller's Lab* [Oxford: Oxford University Press, 2007], 19.

[107] Laura Otis, 19.

[108] Erna Lesky, *The Vienna Medical School of the 19th Century* [Baltimore, MD: Johns Hopkins University Press, 1976], illustration number 20.

[109] Bankl H. Die Prosektur Rokitanskys: Historische Erinnerungen zu den Jubilaumsjahren der Wiener Pathologie 1996 und 1997. (The Rokitansky morgue. Historical retrospect on the occasion of the anniversary years of Vienna pathology 1996 and 1997) Wien Kin Wochenschr 1997;109:858–60.

[110] Laura Otis, *Müller's Lab* [New York: Oxford University Press, 2007], 15. Berlin had gas lighting in 1829. Considering that Berlin was still a provincial city compared to Vienna, it is reasonable to assume that the Leichenhaus, the Vienna autopsy house, had gas lighting in 1829 or within a reasonable time thereafter.

[111] Erna Lesky, *The Vienna Medical School of the 19th Century* [Baltimore, MD: Johns Hopkins University Press, 1976], illustration number 41. "Dissection room in the "Alte Gewehrfabrik" ("Old Rifle Factory")

[112] Doug Macdougall, *Frozen Earth: The Once and Future Story of Ice Age* [Berkeley, CA: University of California Press, 2004], 217. "The Little Ice Age lasted from approximately 1300 to 1850, and its coldest period was near its end." Macdougall is Emeritus Professor of Earth Sciences at the Scripps Institution of Oceanography, University of California, San Diego. See also: Brian Fagan, *The Little Ice Age: How Climate Made History 1300–1850* [New York: Basic Books, 2002].

[113] Carl Rokitansky, *A Manual of Pathological Anatomy*, Volume II. The Abdominal Viscera. trans. Edward Sieveking [Philadelphia, PA: Blanchard & Lea, 1855], vii–ix. Editor's Preface. "The immense fund of material thus placed at his disposal [the number of corpses dissected by him is summed up at 30,000] was almost entirely reserved for the elaboration of that grand work on pathological anatomy, which, in the consciousness of having thoroughly mastered the subject, he gave to the world between the years 1842 and 1846; which has passed, unaltered, through three reimpressions; and which, under the auspices of the Sydenham Society, has been translated into the English language." See also: Roswell Park, *An Epitome of the History of Medicine*, 2nd ed. [Philadelphia: FA Davis Company, 1908], 250-1. The Sydenham Society translation of Rokitansky's 1846 Handbook of Pathological Anatomy that I reviewed at the Health Sciences Library, State University of New York at Buffalo was owned and signed by Roswell Park with his surname *Park*. It is a reasonable assumption that Park derived his estimate of over 30,000 autopsies from that source.

lay at the heart of the practice of anatomical pathology until the end of the nineteenth century. But what were the circumstances that permitted such a Herculean performance? How could these bodies be studied before refrigeration became available to preserve them? The answer lay in rapid dissection before the bodies decomposed. The need for speed coupled with an inexhaustible supply of human anatomical specimens permitted Rokitansky to develop a most remarkable pathological gaze – the ability to scan a vast anatomical panorama and find patterns, differentiate between normal and abnormal, and detect the abnormal. This required mature judgment.

Lester King asserted that pathology at its origins "could be considered an attitude of mind, a search for inner connections within the realm of disease." The physician dissector simply took a look for himself at a body's exterior and interior and tried to correlate what he saw with the patient's signs and symptoms. King continues: "The good pathologist, seeking the hidden causes of disease, must have this critical attitude. He must be able to select, and select wisely; he must judge, and judge fairly; he must evaluate, and evaluate logically. All these processes we can sum up as constituting *judgment*." In sum, differentiating normal from abnormal (pathological) organs and tissues came from experience, seeing, touching, smelling, in some cases tasting (urine); the accumulation of empirical knowledge and testing that knowledge against the judgment and conclusions of others.[114] By the beginning of the seventeenth century, the ontological conception of diseases was well established. In the ontological view, disease enters the body from without to damage bodily organs. Thus Morgagni in the eighteenth century, and Rokitansky in the nineteenth century, practiced pathological anatomy within the framework of the ontological conception of disease.[115]

Canguilhem developed a sophisticated argument regarding the concept of the normal and the pathological. In some respects the argument for such a differentiation remains problematical. For as Canguilhem explains, "every conception of pathology must be based on prior knowledge of the corresponding normal state, but conversely, the scientific study of pathological cases becomes an indispensable phase in the overall search for the laws of the normal state."[116]

---

[114] Lester S. King, *The Medical World of the Eighteenth Century* [Huntington, NY: Robert E. Krieger Publishing Co., 1958, Reprint 1971], 276-277. Henry E. Sigerist, *Man and Medicine: An Introduction to Medical Knowledge.* Trans. Margaret Galt Boise [New York: W. W. Norton & Company, 1932], 127. Anatomical pathology may be divided into "two great lines of research; the study of deformities called *teratology*, and the study of disease, [called] *nosology*." Henry E. Sigerist, *Man and Medicine: An Introduction to Medical Knowledge.* Trans. Margaret Galt Boise [New York: W. W. Norton & Company, 1932], 120. "In order to relate causally an anatomical change to a disease symptom one must first know the normal function of the organ. Only then is it possible to judge in how far a symptom is an expression of disturbed function. An anatomical pathology not only presupposes anatomy but also physiology. Before the eighteenth century's new physiology [when Morgagni practiced] had gained a certain point in progress pathological anatomy could be of no great importance." Henry E. Sigerist, *Man and Medicine: An Introduction to Medical Knowledge.* Trans. Margaret Galt Boise [New York: W. W. Norton & Company, 1932], 123. Marie-Francois-Xavier Bichat [1771–1802], working in late eighteenth century and within the ontological conception of disease, took anatomical pathology to a new and finer level; he explained that "each separate tissue may be attached by disease." Carl Rokitansky [1804–1878] working in the nineteenth century, performed pathological anatomy within the ontological conception of disease, except when he tried to explain disease with minimal or no localized pathology, then he reverted to the ancient physiological conception of disease and formulated his hematohumoral theory. Henry E. Sigerist, *Man and Medicine: An Introduction to Medical Knowledge.* Trans. Margaret Galt Boise [New York: W. W. Norton & Company, 1932], 124. Rudolf Virchow [1821–1902], working also in the nineteenth century and within the ontological conception of disease, championed the cell as the seat of disease in his famous *Cellular Pathology* published in 1858.

[115] Henry E. Sigerist, *Man and Medicine: An Introduction to Medical Knowledge.* Trans. Margaret Galt Boise [New York: W. W. Norton & Company, 1932], 119.

[116] Georges Canguilhem, *The Normal and the Pathological.* Trans. Carolyn R. Fawcett in collaboration with Robert S. Cohen [New York: Zone Books, 1991], 51. Canguilhem continues, "The observation of pathological cases offers numerous, genuine advantages for actual experimental investigation. The transition from the normal to the abnormal is slower and more natural in the case of illness, and the return to normal, when it takes place, spontaneously furnishes a verifying counterproof." Canguilhem wrote while in prison during World War II and this last sentence was not operative when Rokitansky wrote his *Handbook of Pathological Anatomy*; in 1846, the year when the final volume was published, anesthesia had just been discovered. Without anesthesia there was not surgical pathology, that is, examination of tissues removed from a patient who survived surgery and hence the ability to visualize and examine microscopically to ascertain whether or not the diseased organ or tissues had indeed "returned to normal."

If 30,000 autopsies during one career strains the imagination; 60,000 seems incredible. Nevertheless, 60,000 autopsies is the estimate given by John Talbott[117] and Roy Porter.[118] Arriving at a reasonably accurate estimate of the number of autopsies for which Rokitansky was responsible would serve to approximate his actual experience.[119]

The editor's preface to the Sydenham Society translation of Rokitansky's Handbook provides solid contemporary evidence. "The principal hospital of the Austrian capital, the largest in the world, offers very extensive opportunities and unusual facilities for the cultivation of Pathological Anatomy. Exclusive of the Lying-in Hospital and the Lunatic Asylum, which occupy the same range of buildings, the Kaiserlich-Koniglich-Allgemeine-Krankenhaus (Imperial Royal General Hospital) contains 104 wards, capable of receiving 2,214 patients; 1,247 beds being destined for males, and 967 for females. We find that, in 1838, the number of patients treated amounted to 20,545; of these, 2,678 died, giving a mortality of 12.03%, or one death in 7.6 cases. As I am not proved with tables of mortality for other years, I am unable to state the annual average mortality in the hospital; but it does not appear, by a comparison with the mortuary tables of the Viennese Foundling Hospital, that the year 1838 was marked by peculiar endemic or epidemic influences. By the laws of the hospital, postmortem examinations may be made of all who die within its walls. 'To examine all, or one-half would be impossible'; but as 'generally from four to six bodies are opened daily', the extent of the field presented for cadaveric research may easily be estimated. For a series of years, the Professorship of Pathological Anatomy has been held by Dr. Carl Rokitansky, and the numbers of medical men of all nations who are attracted to Vienna by him, are the best evidence in which he has availed himself of the opportunities at his disposal...Records of every case, taken down at the dictation of the Professor, are kept, and all interesting specimens are preserved for the Pathological Museum. Rokitansky has embodied the facts observed, and the conclusions deduced from them, in his 'Handbuch der Pathologischen Anatomie', published in Vienna during the years 1841–1846."[120]

Taking the median of 5 autopsies/day multiplied by 6 work days/week equals 30 autopsies/week. Multiplied by 50 weeks/year equals 1,500 autopsies/year; multiplied by 18 years (1828–1846) equals 27,000 autopsies, close to the editor's approximation of 30,000 autopsies performed by 1846. Talbott's estimate of a lifetime experience of 60,000 autopsies was probably obtained by multiplying by a factor of two to account for autopsies performed between from 1846 to 1874, a period of 28 years when Rokitansky was busy with numerous administrative duties.[121] So considering the contemporaneous testimony of the editor for the Sydenham Society edition of Rokitansky's Handbook, Talbott's estimate of 60,000 autopsies is not unreasonable – if put into perspective. Jay's comment is pertinent: "By the time Rokitansky retired, after having spent an active career in Vienna, he had performed more than 30,000 postmortem examinations and had several thousands more available for his review."[122] All patients who died in the Vienna General Hospital were subject to autopsy but not all bodies were necessarily autopsied. Thus, Rokitansky's experience was based on examination of specimens obtained from 4 to 6 autopsies per day on patients who had died at the

[117] John A. Talbott, *A Biographical History of Medicine: Excerpts and Essays on the Men and Their Work* [New York: Grune & Stratton, 1970], 586. John Talbott was the author's professor of medicine at the State University of New York at Buffalo and later editor of the Journal of the American Medical Association.

[118] Roy Porter, *The Greatest Benefit to Mankind: A Medical History of Humanity* [New York: W. W. Norton & Company, 1998], 315. "Rokitansky was the age's champion dissector-his institute did over 1,500 necropsies a year and he supposedly performed 60,000 autopsies in the course of his career."

[119] Prim. Univ.-Prof. Dr. Roland Sedivy, e-mail message to author, September 2, 2007. "Rokitansky had no refrigeration and there was no ice-box. I checked most of all autopsy books where he signed all reports of autopsy. This fact does not certify that he performed the autopsies...I am convinced that he discussed each case and signed the report."

[120] Carl Rokitansky, *A Manual of Pathological Anatomy*, Volume II. The Abdominal Viscera. trans. Edward Sieveking [Philadelphia, PA: Blanchard & Lea, 1855], vii – ix. Editor's Preface.

[121] Erna Lesky, *The Vienna Medical School of the 19th Century* [Baltimore, MD: Johns Hopkins University Press, 1976],113. "He held the highest academic office and executed the most responsible corporative and administrative functions in the spirit of progress: as the first freely elected dean of the medical collegium of professors (1849–1850, 1856–1857, 1859–1860), as the first freely elected chancellor of the Vienna University (1852–1853), as president of the Society of Physicians (1850–1878) and as president of the Academy of Sciences (1869–1878)."

[122] Venita Jay, "The legacy of Karl Rokitansky," *Arch Pathol Lab Med* 2000;124:345–346:345.

Wiener Allgemeines Krankenhaus. He performed some autopsies personally and some autopsies were performed by his assistants or medical students under his supervision.[123]

To summarize: if we take the estimate of the editors of the Sydenham Society in 1855, that by 1846 Rokitansky had performed 30,000 autopsies and the estimate of John Talbott[124] that he had performed 60,000 autopsies in his lifetime, we perhaps have a more reliable estimate than that of Erna Lesky's 2,000 autopsies annually for 43 years plus 25,000 forensic autopsies. Still, the sum of 60,000 autopsies requires an explanation. First, Rokitansky's training as a medical-student prosector enabled him to work rapidly. Second, Rokitansky concentrated on macroscopic pathology and dictated his findings; time-consuming histology was not routinely done. Third, Rokitansky did not personally perform all the autopsies; many were done by his assistants and medical students that he and his assistants trained. Fourth, he was devoted to the lifetime goal of cataloguing human morphologic pathology that he had set early in his career. Fifth, he concentrated all his daylight efforts on his work. He was not talkative and did not waste time in idle conversation. Erna Lesky described his temperament as "gloomy fundamental pessimism"[125] and the eminent German Professor of Medicine Kussmaul, who worked side by side with Rokitansky for 4 months, described it as taciturn.[126] His introspective personality aside, Rokitansky was a happy man. It is reasonable to assume that he was happy at work as he was at home. He was blessed with good health until his final years. He was blessed with a happy marriage, four successful sons – two musicians like his wife and two physicians and sufficient money that he had no financial worries before he retired.[127] Rokitansky's academic life and research were richly fulfilling. He could take satisfaction from having led efforts that made lasting reforms in the structure of the university. On his 70th birthday he was showered with honors as the entire University of Vienna and the City of Vienna celebrated his accomplishments.[128]

Rokitansky's Handbook of Pathological Anatomy

> An age that specializes exclusively in analysis and is as it were, afraid of synthesis is not on the right path, for only both together, like breathing in and out, make up the life of science in its broadest sense. Goethe[129]

Rokitansky's Historic Trip to Paris in 1842

Türkheim continued to advance Rokitansky's career. Based on his cumulative experience Rokitansky was preparing his magnum opus, the Handbook of Pathological Anatomy. Knowing that this great scientific work represented the culmination of French

[123] Arleen Marcia Tuchman, Science, Medicine, and the State of Germany: The Case of Baden, 1815–1871 [New York: Oxford University Press, 1993], 160. Medical students were supervised in their autopsies under Rokitansky who was interested in morbid macroscopic pathological anatomy. However, that was apparently not the case with medical students in Berlin under the direction of Johannes Müller who was interested in microscopic anatomy and physiology rather than autopsies. "In Müller's dissection courses … the students [were] left to their own devices, hacking away at corpses without any guidance."

[124] Dr. John A. Talbott was the author's professor of medicine at the State University of New York at Buffalo in the 1950s. He later became Editor-in-Chief of the Journal of the American Medical Association. For many years Dr. Talbott had had an interest in the history of medicine. The estimate of 60,000 autopsies attributed to Rokitansky is contained in his *Biographical History of Medicine* published in 1970.

[125] Erna Lesky, *The Vienna Medical School of the 19th Century* [Baltimore, MD: Johns Hopkins University Press, 1976], 115.

[126] Owen H. Wangensteen and Sarah D. Wangensteen, *The Rise of Surgery: From Empiric Craft to Scientific Discipline* [Minneapolis, MN: University of Minnesota Press, 1978], 440. Kussmaul worked at Rokitansky's side for 4 months while they performed autopsies. The Wangensteen's recorded that "Kussmaul wrote that he spent four months working daily beside Rokitansky, assisting with autopsies. During all that time the only words Rokitansky spoke to him occurred during an interruption of work while the two stood together for a few minutes in the doorway on a fine autumn morning. Said Rokitansky, "Today we have beautiful weather." The astounded Kussmaul pulled himself together and replied, "Yes, it is truly a beautiful day."

[127] Gilder SSB. Carl von Rokitansky (1804–1878). *Canadian Med J* 1954;71:70–72.

[128] Harvey Cushing, *The Life of Sir William Osler* [Oxford, UK: Clarendon Press, 1926], 113.

[129] Ronold King, "Goethe and the Challenge of Science in Western Civilization," in *Goethe on Human Creativeness and other Goethe Essays,* ed. Rolf King [Athens, GA: University of Georgia Press, 1950], 223–252:229.

pathological anatomy, Türkheim sent Rokitansky and his medical colleague Skoda to Paris in 1842 to study the "achievements of French medicine."[130] However, the Paris School that Rokitansky saw was in decline.[131] An 1875 history of French surgery described the frantic state of Paris Medicine between 1835 and 1847. "This was the moment when…the scientific level began to decline in France, and all the writings of the time carry the imprint of this sort of discouragement which follows epochs of agitation and struggle. Medicine, fatigued by the storms raised by the doctrines of Broussais, disgusted with theories and systems, turned toward experimental research and abandoned itself to the cult of individual facts. Each one ploughed his furrow alone, followed his own ideas, his formulas, moved straight ahead without looking to the right or the left, without concerning himself with the work of others; each dreamed of finding his place in the sun, to achieve his own fame, and there resulted a general free-for-all of research without direction."[132]

Türkheim, founder of the Second Vienna Medical School, undoubtedly knew that when Johann Peter Frank, the organizer of pathological anatomical dissection in Vienna, was dismissed in 1804, pathological anatomy had migrated from the First Vienna Medical School to Paris where it flourished under Bichat, Laennec, Cruveilhier, and others.[133] According to Ackerknecht, the era of Paris "hospital medicine" of Bichat, Laennec, and Cruveilhier extended from 1794 to 1848 when it had come "to a dead end" and was replaced by the new "laboratory medicine" of Louis Pasteur, Claude Bernard, and members of the Societe de Biologie.[134] Thus, the Paris trip held great symbolic significance for Rokitansky, for Türkheim and for the Second Vienna Medical School. However, behind the symbolism of Rokitansky's journey to Paris lies a more complicated story than his simple retrieval of the pathological anatomical legacy of Vienna's first medical school. Parisian anatomical pathology was derivative; Paris borrowed sequentially from Leyden, Edinburgh, Vienna, and Pavia.[135] Even Bichat's massively influential *Traite d'anatomie generale* that revolutionized pathological anatomy by focusing on diseased tissues may have been derivative. In an essay that examines the debate surrounding the genesis of tissue pathology, Othmar Keel may have found an explanation for the phenomenally short period of two and a half years in which Bichat revolutionized pathological anatomy (1799–1802)[136]; the groundwork had been laid elsewhere. "But, as for the beginnings of tissue pathology in France, it is still inadequate to speak of a 'derivation' from foreign development; what we are really speaking about is a veritable appropriation by French clinicians of an entire body of knowledge produced by the English and others."[137] Notwithstanding the genesis of his ideas, Bichat's monumental contributions were appreciated throughout Europe.[138]

Importantly, Rokitansky purchased a microscope, but more significantly he retrieved the pathological anatomic heritage of the First Vienna Medical School – so enriched by the French – and brought it back home to the Second Vienna Medical School. There Rokitansky would complete the macromorphological classification of human pathological anatomy. Rokitansky was fully

[130] Erna Lesky, *The Vienna Medical School of the 19th Century* [Baltimore, MD: Johns Hopkins University Press, 1976], 99.

[131] Ann La Berge and Caroline Hannaway, "Paris Medicine: Perspectives Past and Present," in *Constructing Paris Medicine*, ed. Caroline Hannaway and Ann La Berge [Amsterdam, NL: Editions Rodopi B. V., 1998], 1–69:19.

[132] Ann La Berge and Caroline Hannaway, 1–69:18.

[133] Erna Lesky, 16–20. As the result of the aggressive and repressive "restoration program" that Joseph Andreas von Stifft began in 1803, Johann Peter Frank – the physician who had reorganized pathological anatomy at the University of Vienna – was dismissed in 1804 as part of Stifft's unrelenting spirit of persecution. See Erna Lesky, p 77. Frank left Vienna in 1804. "Thus the first attempt at establishing pathological-anatomical dissection in Vienna, which had seemed so promising, temporarily came to an end." Klemperer reference is more explicit. See: Paul Klemperer, Notes on Carl von Rokitansky's Autobiography and Inaugural Address. Bulletin History of Medicine 1961;35:364–80:377. "It was deplorable for the glory of Vienna that this exceptional man [Johann Peter Frank] was forced to abandon his office in 1803, but pathological anatomy found another home in Paris where it could grow beyond the scope of descriptive correlation of Morgagni into the rational science of medicine."

[134] Erwin H. Ackerknecht, *A Short History of Medicine* [New York: Ronald Press, 1968], xiii.

[135] Ann La Berge and Caroline Hannaway, "Paris Medicine: Perspectives Past and Present," in *Constructing Paris Medicine,* ed. Caroline Hannaway and Ann La Berge [Amsterdam, NL: Editions Rodopi B. V., 1998], 1–69:7.

[136] Erwin H. Ackerknecht, 51.

[137] Othmar Keel, "Was Anatomical and Tissue Pathology a Product of the Paris Clinical School or Not?" in *Constructing Paris Medicine,* ed. Caroline Hannaway and Ann La Berge [Amsterdam, NL: Editions Rodopi B. V., 1998], 117–183: 133–4.

[138] Ann La Berge and Caroline Hannaway, 1–69:25.

aware of the symbolic nature of his trip from Vienna to Paris and his return to Vienna. In his great Handbook of Pathological Anatomy, he acknowledged the noble heritage transmitted by those who had contributed to the field of pathological anatomy.[139]

Two years before his death in 1844, Türkheim, aware of Rokitansky's academic prowess, promoted him to full professor and Chair of Pathological Anatomy.[140] In the process he elevated the status of pathological anatomy from a 4-year-term associate professorship to a permanent full professorship.[141]

Full Professor at the Height of His Fame

The year 1844 proved momentous for Rokitansky. He had completed two volumes of his monumental three-volume *Handbuch der Pathologischen Anatomie,* and pathological anatomy became a compulsory subject at the University of Vienna. Rokitansky – a newly appointed full professor – "stood at the height of his fame, attracting physicians from numerous foreign countries."[142] Volumes two and three of the *Handbuch* focused on anatomical lesions of specific organs and completed the nosological classification of macroscopic pathological anatomy of humans, this building on the foundations of anatomical pathology "which had originated in the French school at the beginning of the century."[143] Such was his international reputation that the Sydenham Society would translate and publish Rokitansky's *Handbuch* into English between 1849 and 1854.

Rokitansky's Handbook of Pathological Anatomy

In 1846 Rokitansky published the final volume of his Manual of Pathologic Anatomy [*Handbuch der Pathologischen Anatomie*].[144] He modeled his magnum opus after the 1829 *Traite d'anatomie pathologique* of Lobstein the Younger of Strasbourg, following an anatomical classification of the pathological material.[145] Rokitansky explained the significance of this work. He opined that pathological anatomy "assumed the dignity of an independent science...only of late years."[146] He described his reliance on close observation of his autopsy material. "The appearance of this first volume brings the publication of my 'Pathological Anatomy' to a close...The same self-reliance that characterized the commencement of my pathologico-anatomical studies has stood by me whilst engaged in observing and interpreting the facts of which the said materials are composed: for, each individual discovery encouraged me more and more to pin my faith upon Nature alone. Still I have never failed to watch and to appreciate the achievements of other men."[147]

Rokitansky then explained his interest in pathological chemistry as an integral part of his hematohumoral

[139] Carl Rokitansky, *A Manual of Pathological Anatomy*, Volume I. *General Pathological Anatomy.* trans. William Edward Swaine [Philadelphia, PA: Blanchard & Lea, 1855], 17–19. [Author's] Introduction.

Rokitansky presented a brief historical review of an "occasional, fragmentary, indeterminate study of pathological anatomy" that commenced in the sixteenth century. However, he believed pathological anatomy to be "modern science." "It is indeed only of late years that it has assumed the dignity of an independent science at all."

[140] Erna Lesky, *The Vienna Medical School of the 19th Century* [Baltimore, MD: Johns Hopkins University Press, 1976], 99. "With Türkheim's assistance, the laboratory of pathological-chemical examinations was established in [1842] at the General Hospital, under the direction of Johann Florian Heller, and thus became the nucleus of the subsequent medical-chemical institute.

[141] Erna Lesky, 77, 99. Vienna was the second university to establish a Chair of Pathological Anatomy. The first Chair of Pathological Anatomy was established at the University of Strasbourg, France in 1791, 2 years after the onset of the French Revolution.

[142] Erna Lesky, *The Vienna Medical School of the 19th Century* [Baltimore, MD: Johns Hopkins University Press, 1976], 109. Lesky noted also that Virchow, at the end of the nineteenth century, wrote that Rokitansky's *Handbuch der Pathologischen Anatomie* "of all existing textbooks in this discipline ... immediately proved to be the best and the actual basis of practical medicine."

[143] Erna Lesky, 109.

[144] Rokitansky acknowledged the pathological anatomical contributions of Johannes Müller. Carl Rokitansky, *A Manual of Pathological Anatomy*, Volume I. *General Pathological Anatomy.* trans. William Edward Swaine [Philadelphia, PA: Blanchard & Lea, 1855], 168, 193, 206, 219.

[145] Henry E. Sigerist, *The Great Doctors: A Biographical History of Medicine.* Trans. Eden and Cedar Paul [New York: W. W. Norton & Company, 1933], 295–296.

[146] Carl Rokitansky, *A Manual of Pathological Anatomy*, Volume I. *General Pathological Anatomy.* trans. William Edward Swaine [Philadelphia, PA: Blanchard & Lea, 1855], 17–19. [Author's] Introduction.

[147] Carl Rokitansky, *A Manual of Pathological Anatomy*, Volume I. *General Pathological Anatomy.* trans. William Edward Swaine [Philadelphia, PA: Blanchard & Lea, 1855], ix, x. Author's Preface.

theory of disease. "The present work will at any rate tend to show, how thorough is my conviction that Pathological Anatomy must constitute the groundwork, not alone of all medical knowledge, but also of all medical treatment; nay, that it embraces all that medicine has to offer of positive knowledge, or at least of what is fundamental to it. Its domain will here, however, be found more extended, and more nearly approximated to the confines of Pathological Chemistry than has generally been the case in pathologico-anatomical writings."[148] In other words, Rokitansky the macropathologist, on his own initiative had explored the world of microscopic pathology while holding to his hematohumoral theory of disease.

The German medical historian, Henry Sigerist, wrote one of the best explanations of Rokitansky's search for the explanation of generalized diseases without local pathologic lesions. "Rokitansky, however, did not limit himself to the description of what he actually saw, for he transcended the limits of anatomy. In a great many diseases the anatomical conditions found on postmortem examination were so trivial that they failed to explain the severity of the illness. Obviously, then, in addition to localized maladies of the organs, there must be generalized diseases. Rokitansky was too much the anatomist not to seek a local habitat for these diseases. Their habitat must be the blood, the only tissue which is universally present in the body – a tissue just as much as muscular tissue or nervous tissue, although the intercellular substance of the blood is fluid. Thus, Rokitansky was brought back into the domain of the old humoral pathology, and he tried, by means of his doctrine of 'crasis,' to combine the teachings of humoral pathology with anatomical views. He called in chemistry to his aid. The blood contains fibrin and albumen. Morbid changes in these, caused especially by oxidation, gave rise to a crasis, a pathological condition. But a general disease had a tendency to localize itself. Thus diseases of the organs resulted from a dyscrasia. Nevertheless, the converse was possible. An organ might be primarily diseased, and, as a sequel, a generalized malady might arise. The doctrine of crasis was erroneous and could not be maintained because its chemical presuppositions were unsound. Here Rokitansky had left the field of observation and had wandered off into speculation. Virchow, who greatly admired those parts of the *Handbuch* which dealt with Rokitansky's direct observations, subjected the doctrine of crasis to ruthless criticism."[149]

Rokitansky's hematohumoral theory, an attempt to explain the seat of otherwise inexplicable disease by chemical means, was not an outlandish theory. Unfortunately, he was ahead of his time theoretically, chemistry had not developed to the level that it could be helpful and immunology was yet to be discovered as a new science. As Lester King noted, "Had chemistry made tremendous strides in the eighteenth century, then the pathologist, or student of disease, would have been primarily a chemist. But as it was, the data to explain disease came principally from autopsy dissection," and sometimes that data were insufficient.[150]

Rokitansky's Handbook of Pathology was translated into English and Italian with considerable difficulty because of Rokitansky's linguistic style and his controversial hematohumoral theory of disease, "the so-called Krasenlehre, which rested upon humoral doctrines."[151] Between 1827 and 1846 Rokitansky had developed his hematohumoral theory of disease

[148] Carl Rokitansky, ix. Author's Preface. Vienna, July, 1846.

[149] Henry E. Sigerist, *The Great Doctors: A Biographical History of Medicine.* Trans. Eden and Cedar Paul [New York: W. W. Norton & Company, 1933], 296–297.

[150] Lester S. King, *The Medical World of the Eighteenth Century* [Huntington, NY: Robert E. Krieger Publishing Co., 1958, Reprint 1971], 264.

[151] Castagnoli L, Jonjic N, Rizzardi C, Melato M. Carl von Rokitansky and the Italian translation of the Handbuch der Pathologischen Anatomie: a linguistic and doctrinal enigma. *Pathologica* 2001;93:654–61. Carl Rokitansky, *A Manual of Pathological Anatomy*, Volume I. *General Pathological Anatomy.* trans. William Edward Swaine [Philadelphia, PA: Blanchard & Lea, 1855], 20. [Author's] Introduction.

Rokitansky explained some general points before embarking on his discussion of the anomalies of organization. "IV. This demonstration of general disease is indeed a step in advance for pathological anatomy. It threatens, however, to mislead us into the error of exclusive, transcendental, all-pervading humoralism-into the error of denying all local disease, by deducing the latter in every instance from a corresponding general affection,-not but that many diseases really are but the localization of a pre-existent general disease." Next, note how in the editor's preface, the English editors respectfully chose to use Rokitansky's own word "transcendental" to skillfully avoid the subject of "all-pervading humoralism" which was not acceptable in England in 1846. Carl Rokitansky, *A Manual of Pathological Anatomy*, Volume I. *General Pathological Anatomy.* trans. William Edward Swaine [Philadelphia, PA: Blanchard & Lea, 1855], viii. Editor's Preface to Vol. I. "The editor has felt the necessity of abridging somewhat the author's general introduction, partly because, totally unlike the general tendency of the work, it is too "transcendental" a character either to suit the English language or to harmonize with English ideas; but more particularly because it is interwoven with a train of speculative reasoning upon the relation between power and matter, which might, in this country, very possibly give rise to misinterpretation and rebuke."

because organ-based anatomical pathology failed to explain diseases of a general nature; those diseases where "the anatomical lesion was too insignificant to explain the fatal outcome."[152] He needed a unified theory of pathogenesis, to complement his unified classification of human pathological anatomy.

"Rokitansky...believed that the task facing the general pathologist centered on the explanation of the disease *process* [for] clinical medicine."[153] In a number of patients, Rokitansky could find no local pathology at autopsy to explain the patients' deaths. He postulated a hematohumoral theory on the assumption that the otherwise unexplained cause of death in these patients without local pathologic lesions "must lie in some chemical change in the universal tissue, the blood."[154] Hampered by a weak foundation in theory and basic sciences,[155] it appears that Rokitansky cobbled together his hematohumoral theory of dyscrasis from ideas formulated by several contemporaries. Rokitansky's professor, Philipp Carl Hartmann (1772–1830), was appointed to the Chair of General Pathology, Therapy and Materia Medica in Vienna in 1811. Hartmann differentiated dynamic "endogenous diseases" such as "disturbances in blood formation," from "organizational diseases" diagnosed by morphological pathology.[156] Erna Lesky contends that it was from Hartmann's concept of dynamic, endogenous diseases that Rokitansky, his pupil, "was to develop his system of crasis."[157] Rokitansky was also influenced by his reading of Francois Magendie (1783–1855), Gabriel Andral (1797–1876), and Lobstein the Younger (1777–1835) of France.[158] Francois Magendie and Andral, while studying tissues as the seat of disease, went beyond descriptive pathological anatomy and tried to explain disease by studying structural and functional changes in tissues.[159] Magendie and Andral believed they were working on the cutting edge of medical knowledge.[160]

Magendie held to a dual classification of disease: disease caused by alterations in the blood "subject to the laws of hydraulics and physics," and disease in solid tissues "explicable in terms of the vitality and the nervous system."[161] Magendie decided that the nervous system "could be understood only through vivisection [and proceeded to undertake] the most comprehensive program of vivisection yet known to medicine."[162] Coulter noted that Magendie's research exerted substantial influence on medical thought.[163] In his *Essai*

[152] Erna Lesky, *The Vienna Medical School of the 19th Century* [Baltimore, MD: Johns Hopkins University Press, 1976], 110.

[153] R.J. Rather, Eva R. Rohl. An English Translation of the Hitherto Untranslated Part of Rokitansky's *Einleitung* to volume 1 of the *Handbuch der allgemeinen Pathologie* (1846), with a Bibliography of Rokitansky's Published Works. *Clio medica* 1972;7:215–227:215, 218.

[154] Gilder SSB. Carl von Rokitansky (1804–1878). *Canadian Med J* 1954;71:70–72.

[155] Erna Lesky, 18. "Stifft [the reformer] decreed to his students a ready made, precisely regulated textbook knowledge based on Boerhaave's old aphorisms and Stoll's humoral pathology. The student who memorized these best was classified as eminent. This procedure was likely to reduce a generation of physicians to the level of mechanical medical artisans, and to "encourage general regimentation instead of developing individuality, which is so very desirable in medicine."

[156] Erna Lesky, 81.

[157] Erna Lesky, *The Vienna Medical School of the 19th Century* [Baltimore, MD: Johns Hopkins University Press, 1976], 81.

[158] Robert J Miciotto, Carl Rokitansky: a reassessment of the hematohumoral theory of disease. *Bulletin History Medicine* 1978;52(2):183–99:185. Gilder SSB. Carl von Rokitansky (1804–1878). *Canadian Med J* 1954;71:70–72. Henry E. Sigerist, *The Great Doctors: A Biographical History of Medicine.* Trans. Eden and Cedar Paul [New York: W. W. Norton & Company, 1933], 295. Lobstein the Younger was the first professor of Pathological Anatomy in France. The Chair of Pathological Anatomy at Strasbourg, France founded in 1819 was the first chair of pathological anatomy in Europe; Lobstein the Younger was the first professor of pathological anatomy in Europe.

[159] Arleen Marcia Tuchman, Science, Medicine, and the State of Germany: The Case of Baden, 1815–1871 [New York: Oxford University Press, 1993], 64.

[160] Harris L. Coulter, Divided Legacy: A History of the Schism in Medical Thought. Volume II: The Origins of Modern Western Medicine: J. B. Van Helmont to Claude Bernard [Berkeley, CA: North Atlantic Books, 1977, 2000], 706. Magendie and Andral "came to feel that medicine was in its infancy and destined to make a precipitate advance." Ann La Berge and Caroline Hannaway, "Paris Medicine: Perspectives Past and Present," in *Constructing Paris Medicine*, ed. Caroline Hannaway and Ann La Berge [Amsterdam, NL: Editions Rodopi B. V., 1998], 1–69:22. When Rokitansky visited Paris in 1842, Andral was a powerful force, one of the young "triumvirate of the Paris School: Andral, Chomel, and Louis."

[161] Harris L. Coulter, 628.

[162] Harris L. Coulter, 618. Coulter, page 620. Magendie's experimented on the nervous system of animals and discovered the "distinction between motor and sensory nerves."

[163] Harris L. Coulter, *Divided Legacy: A History of the Schism in Medical Thought. Volume II: The Origins of Modern Western Medicine: J. B. Van Helmont to Claude Bernard* [Berkeley, CA: North Atlantic Books, 2000], 620. Erwin H. Ackerknecht, *A Short History of Medicine* [New York: Ronald Press, 1968], 165. Claude Bernard (1813–1878) was a pupil of Magendie.

d'Hematologie Pathologique, Andral acknowledged his indebtedness to Magendie. Prophetically Andral wrote: "Thus where anatomy no longer finds changes, chemistry shows them to us, and I don't doubt that it will become more and more one of the foundations of pathogenesis."[164] Andral, Magendie, and many others participated in the debate of the 1820s and 1830s between humoralism and solidism. Humoralism was first exposited by Hippocrates, and Morgagni originated solidism.[165] Andral influenced Rokitansky, by "resolv[ing] the humoralism/solidism conflict in favor of the humors – as improved by chemistry."[166]

Andral's *Precis d'Anatomie Pathologique* (1829) helped to "shift medicine from a solidist to a neo-humoralist basis.[167] Coulter explains that in this work Andral "aimed to fuse the two strands of thought in the molecular exchange between the blood and the solids which take place in the capillaries; he elaborated a complex disease classification on the basis of this primordial physiological function…In his 1843 *Essai d'Hematologie Pathologique* [Andral] located pathological causes in the fluids alone, initiating the neo-humoralism which was thereafter official doctrine of the Paris School."[168]

Rokitansky drew from the "chemical" theories of disease of both his Parisian contemporaries, Magendie and Andral.[169] Lobstein the Younger, professor of pathological anatomy at Strasbourg, wrote a treatise on pathological anatomy in 1829. Not only did this work serve Rokitansky for a model of his own *Handbook of Pathological Anatomy*, Lobstein also contributed to Rokitansky, as had Magendie and Andral, his "mixture of speculative neuro- and humoral pathology.[170] But it was the 1840 memoir by Andral and Gavarret, *Recherches sur les modifications de proportion de quelques principes de sang,* that proved decisive in favor of hemopathology to explain the pathogenesis of disease and was "seized upon" by Rokitansky for his hematohumoral theory.[171] Erwin Ackerknecht summarized the situation in the 1840s. "It was only logical that Andral, after his demonstrations of symptoms without lesions in the solid organs, should develop in the direction" of hemopathology. Rokitansky "eagerly seized upon and copied" Andral's contribution to hemopathology which led to the misadventure with his theory of crasis.[172] Magendie and Andral were alive in 1842 when Rokitansky visited Paris, though Lobstein the Younger had died in 1835.

Meanwhile in Germany, Theodor Schwann, an assistant of Johannes Müller, had postulated that cells were formed from precipitation of "an amorphous basic substance, the blastema"; in other words, Schwann conceptualized cell formation as a process of crystallization from its solution.[173] Schleiden and Schwann judged that cells "were the fundamental units of zoological and botanical action."[174] Schleiden and Schwann made the crucial discovery that "cells… were the ultimate units of structure, and probably function."[175] They pondered the origin and growth of cells. Porter noted that Schleiden and Schwann's conceived

[164] Erwin H. Ackerknecht, *Medicine at the Paris Hospital 1794–1848* [Baltimore, MD: Johns Hopkins Press, 1967], 107.

[165] Erwin H. Ackerknecht, 106. "After an eclipse of almost forty years, humoralism had a comeback in the 1830s in, of course, a new and scientific vein and mostly in the form of hemopathology." Ackerknecht gave some of the names prominent in this movement: Lobstein, Prevost (1820s), Dumas (1820s), Magendie (1820s), Gaspard (1820s), Denis (1830s), Lecanu (1830s), Rochoux (1823), Velpeau (1824), Piorry (1840), and Bouillaud (1853), all in support of hemopathology.

[166] Harris L. Coulter, *Divided Legacy: A History of the Schism in Medical Thought. Volume II: The Origins of Modern Western Medicine: J. B. Van Helmont to Claude Bernard* [Berkeley, CA: North Atlantic Books, 2000], 538.

[167] Harris L. Coulter, 534.

[168] Harris L. Coulter, 537.

[169] Robert J Miciotto, Carl Rokitansky: a reassessment of the hematohumoral theory of disease. *Bulletin History Medicine* 1978;52(2):183–99:185. Erwin H. Ackerknecht, *Medicine at the Paris Hospital 1794–1848* [Baltimore, MD: Johns Hopkins Press, 1967], 106. "It was only logical that Andral, after his demonstrations of symptoms without lesions in the solid organs, should develop in [the] direction of … humoralism … mostly in the form of hematopathology."

[170] Erwin H. Ackerknecht, *Medicine at the Paris Hospital 1794–1848* [Baltimore, MD: Johns Hopkins Press, 1967], 167.

[171] Erwin H. Ackerknecht, 106.

[172] Erwin H. Ackerknecht, *Medicine at the Paris Hospital 1794–1848* [Baltimore, MD: Johns Hopkins Press, 1967], 106.

[173] Erna Lesky, *The Vienna Medical School of the 19th Century* [Baltimore, MD: Johns Hopkins University Press, 1976], 110, 220.

[174] Roy Porter, *The Greatest Benefit to Mankind: A Medical History of Humanity* [New York: W. W. Norton & Company, 1998], 330.

[175] Arleen Marcia Tuchman, Science, Medicine, and the State of Germany: The Case of Baden, 1815–1871 [New York: Oxford University Press, 1993], 59.

of cell reproduction as a "kind of spontaneous generation"; new cells arose from a nurturing fluid – a blastema – as crystals grow in solution.[176] Following Schwann's line of reasoning, Rokitansky "speculated that conditions affecting the blood sometimes caused the blastema to spawn abnormal cells, leading to disease." According to his hypothesis, "diseases originated in an imbalance of protein substances such as fibrin and albumin in the blood." Rokitansky was attempting to explain the cause of death at autopsies where he found no gross pathological lesions.[177] Rokitansky "made blastema theory the cornerstone for a comprehensive haemato-humoral pathogenesis."[178]

However, Schwann was unaware that cells developed only from cells, which would thwart the application of his *blastema* theory to pathological anatomy.[179] While Schwann's biological cell theory was correct, his hypothesis regarding the formation of cells was not. Unaware that Schwann's *cytoblastema* theory was erroneous,[180] Rokitansky chose to follow his "blastema doctrine of cellular genesis."[181] In conclusion, Rokitansky seems to have had every reason to believe that he had built on a solid foundation when he constructed his hematohumoral theory to explain the pathogenesis of disease. He had drawn directly on the work of a prominent German investigator – Theodor Schwann – and the work of prominent French investigators – Lobstein the Younger, Magendie, and Andral.

Nonetheless, the young pathologist Rudolph Virchow immediately attacked Rokitansky's theory, calling it a "monstrous anachronism."[182] The medical historian Erna Lesky recounted the basis of Virchow's

---

176 Roy Porter, *The Greatest Benefit to Mankind*, 330.

177 Roy Porter, *The Greatest Benefit to Mankind: A Medical History of Humanity* [New York: W. W. Norton & Company, 1998], 330–1.

178 Roy Porter, 331. Porter's explanation of the blastema theory and Rokitansky's employment of same is the clearest exposition the author has found.

179 Erwin H. Ackerknecht, *A Short History of Medicine* [New York: Ronald Press, 1968], 160.

180 Robert E. Fechner, "The Birth and Evolution of American Surgical Pathology," in *Guiding the Surgeon's Hand: The History of American Surgical Pathology*, ed. Juan Rosai [Washington, DC: Armed Forces Institute of Pathology, 1997], 9. "However Schwann erroneously viewed cells as continuously being generated out of a primitive body fluid (a lingering hold-over of the humoral theory of disease)."

181 Carl Rokitansky, *A Manual of Pathological Anatomy*, Volume I. *General Pathological Anatomy.* trans. William Edward Swaine [Philadelphia, PA: Blanchard & Lea, 1855], x. Author's Preface. Vienna, July 1846. Rokitansky drew singular attention to his "doctrine of a primitive diversity in blastemata, as the only tenable basis for a humoral pathology." See also Robert J Miciotto, Carl Rokitansky: a reassessment of the hematohumoral theory of disease. *Bulletin History Medicine* 1978;52(2):183–99:185. Erna Lesky, *The Vienna Medical School of the 19th Century* [Baltimore, MD: Johns Hopkins University Press, 1976], 222. In effect Rokitansky's theory was a direct "application of Schwann's theory of blastema to pathology."

182 Carl Rokitansky, *Handbuch der allgemeinen Pathologischen Anatomie* [Wien: Braumüller & Seidel, 1846]. Quotation from Robert J Miciotto, Carl Rokitansky: a reassessment of the hematohumoral theory of disease. *Bulletin History Medicine* 1978;52(2):183–99: 184. Miciotto quoted Rudolph Virchow: "Rudolph Virchow, who later became the doyen of nineteenth-century medicine, characterized Rokitansky's hematohumoralism as an *ungeheurer Anachronismus* – monstrous anachronism – in his famous review of December 1846 in the *Preussische Medizinal-Zeitung.*" Rudolph Virchow, "Rokitansky, Handbuch der pathologischen Anatomie," Medizinische Zeitung des Vereins fur Heilkunde in Preussen, Literarische Beilage zur medicinischen Zeitung, December 1846, no. 49, pp. 237f.; no. 50. pp. 243f. See also R.J. Rather, Eva R. Rohl. An English Translation of the Hitherto Untranslated Part of Rokitansky's *Einleitung* to volume 1 of the *Handbuch der allgemeinen Pathologie* (1846), with a Bibliography of Rokitansky's Published Works. *Clio medica* 1972;7:215–227:219–221. Rather quoted Rokitansky regarding why he developed a theory known as the crasis or hematohumoral theory of disease: "The goal of the anatomical treatment of nosology: to furnish definite material foundations for the investigation of the nature of a disease process and thereby reliable premises throughout, to widen the scope of the investigation of disease and to offer therein objects worthy of and accessible to the human understanding – in short, to furnish pathology a broader and more secure basis, to elevate it to physiological pathology. Just as pathology can no longer dispense with an anatomical basis (an anatomical component) so also can pathological anatomy be treated with a steady regard for clinical observation, as follows from much of what has already been said; indeed she [pathology] must take this practical course if she is to achieve an anatomical description of the disease-process as broad as possible, in addition to the expansion of her field already noted. The following points contain the most essential foundations of such a workup: 3. She must be determined by general phenomena in such a way as to base disease not on changes in the solids but instead, and primarily, on anomalies of the blood mass, the more so the harder it becomes for her to discover strict localization in general, or alternatively disturbances therein that are sufficient in degree and kind. Here she joins up with an allied pathological chemistry, which cannot be pursued without her in a manner at all fruitful…Since pathological anatomy studies are the disease-process in the most varied stages of its advance and retreat from the very beginning, where the organic changes characterizing it just become noticeable, the supposed objection therefore really involves the following one in addition, namely it is thought: *That the earliest beginnings of disease, the dynamic factor, has not successfully been demonstrated in the material substrate by pathological anatomy,* that there are still very many diseases which run their course and become lethal without a palpable disturbance of organization."

criticism. According to Virchow, Rokitansky "had attempted to explain matters of anatomy by matters of chemistry."[183] But what could explain the supreme self-confidence and temerity of the 25-year-old Virchow to launch such a scathing criticism? The medical historian Lester King offered an opinion: Virchow, "arrogant and authoritative…became thoroughly expert in a way that older pathologists like Rokitansky (1804–1878), raised in an earlier tradition, could never achieve."[184] For a fuller explanation we look to Virchow's professional education.[185]

Rudolf Virchow (1821–1902) entered the Friedrich-Wilhelm Institute of the University of Berlin in 1839, where he studied under Johannes Müller.[186] In that year Müller's assistant, Theodor Schwann, published his foundational research into cell biology in *Microscopical Researches into the Accordance in the Structure and Growth of Animals and Plants*.[187] With Schwann assisting, Müller had been applying Schwann's cell theory to the microscopic anatomy of tumors since 1838.[188] Müller established pathologic histology as a scientific discipline when he recognized the "cell as the principal element of…neoplasms." He differentiated types of tumors based on cytologic differences as the diagnostic criterion.[189] Virchow took every advantage of his association with Müller.[190] As Müller's new assistant, Virchow became aware of the research of Müller and Schwann on cells. Otis opined that this was likely the time that Virchow developed an interest in cell theory.[191] 1839 was also the year that Virchow became aware of Schwann's *cytoblastema* theory of the origin of cells.

Otis wrote: "Schwann came to his cell studies in late 1837…His proposal that all living organism consist of cells (the cell theory) was part of his greater scientific aim."[192] Schwann wanted to show that living phenomena had physical, material causes and were not the manifestations of some mysterious life force.[193] This idea

[183] Erna Lesky, *The Vienna Medical School of the 19th Century* [Baltimore, MD: Johns Hopkins University Press, 1976], 111.

[184] Lester S. King, *Medical Thinking: A Historical Preface* [Princeton, NJ: Princeton University Press, 1982], 48.

[185] Laura Otis, *Müller's Lab* [New York: Oxford University Press, 2007], 162. "Ultimately, the best indication of Virchow's regard for Müller, is not what the student said but what he did… Through his rigorous microscopic and chemical studies of the blood, Virchow disproved Karl Rokitansky's dominant pathological theory that blood disorders underlay all diseases, which had been based on the assumption that blood produced the raw material that gave rise to sick cells."

[186] Laura Otis, 132.

[187] Alexander Hellemans and Bryan Bunch, *The Timetables of Science: A Chronology of the Most Important People and Events in the History of Science*, Touchtone Edition [New York: Simon & Schuster, 1988], 304. Harold Speert, "Johannes Müller and the Müllerian Ducts," in *Obstetric & Gynecologic Milestones Illustrated,* 2nd ed. rev. [Parthenon Publishing Group, 1996], 104. "In Müller's youth there had been no knowledge of cells, no microtome, no histologic staining methods, no binocular microscope. Schwann became known as the founder of the cell theory, and Rudolph Virchow, another of [Müller's] disciples, as the father of cellular pathology." See also Henry E Sigerist, *The Great Doctors* [New York: WW Norton, 1931], 307-11. Quoting Virchow: Müller "did not make original discoveries of primary importance in any of these fields, but whatever subject he touched was given by him an added depth."

[188] Laura Otis, 138.

[189] Harold Speert, "Johannes Müller and the Müllerian Ducts," in *Obstetric & Gynecologic Milestones Illustrated,* 2nd ed. rev. [Parthenon Publishing Group, 1996], 104. Karl Sudhoff, "In Memory of Johannes Müller." *Essays in the History of Medicine.* Translated by various hands and edited, with foreword and biographical sketch, by Fielding H. Garrison. New York: Medical Life Press, 1926:363–367:365. Sudhoff notes in his discussion of the extensive research of Müller that "of greatest importance were his investigations of the blood."

[190] Paul Strathern, *A Brief History of Medicine from Hippocrates to Gene Therapy* [New York: Carroll & Graf, 2005], 207–211. In 1840, Virchow's master, Johannes Müller, published the last volume of his magnum opus, *The Handbook of Human Physiology* based on microscopic studies. Virchow took meticulous notes in Müller's physiology course in the summer of 1840, as he did in Müller's embryology lectures. In 1841 he attended Müller's comparative anatomy course and in the summer of 1842, he attended Müller's pathological anatomy course where Müller discussed his research on tumors. Laura Otis, *Müller's Lab* [Oxford: Oxford University Press, 2007], 135–137.

[191] Laura Otis, *Müller's Lab* [Oxford: Oxford University Press, 2007], 42. "For thirty years, Müller attracted some of Europe's brightest young scientists." Virchow's biological theory of disease was based on microscopic observations, research that easily flowed from the emphasis on microscopy and exact observation that Johannes Müller fostered among his assistants.

[192] Laura Otis, 62.

[193] Robert P. Hudson, *Disease and Its Control: The Shaping of Modern Thought* [Westport, CT: Greenwood Press, 1983], 130–2. Claude Bernard (1813–1878) demonstrated the material cause of fluctuations in the level of blood sugar. In 1861 he demonstrated by experiments that the liver metabolized sugar into glycogen which was released as the body required it. He also demonstrated that the blood normally contained sugar, that it was not present only as a sign of pathology. Of even broader physiological (material) significance, Bernard established the concept of the internal fluid environment which he termed *milieu interieur.* In his classic book *An Introduction to the Study of Experimental Medicine* (1865) he explained his

contradicted Müller's most fundamental scientific views."[194]

Müller believed that "living organisms possess a life force for which physical laws cannot account."[195] After he moved to Berlin in 1833, he became increasingly focused on comparative anatomy.[196] Intent on building and controlling a world-class comparative anatomical collection in Berlin, Müller spent large sums of his annual salary for 25 years to acquire rare specimens.[197] Using his collection Müller studied the "organizing principles of life."[198] A Roman Catholic Rhinelander in Protestant Berlin,[199] he believed in a *life force*. Müller wrote that "everything that feels and moves itself voluntarily according to its own desires has a soul."[200] By collecting as many animals in his Anatomical Museum as he could afford and arranging them to "show patterns and relationships", Müller "hoped to learn what life was."[201]

Laura Otis summarized the fundamental conflict between Schwann and Müller as Schwann explained it in 1858 to du Bois-Reymond, another assistant of Müller. According to Schwann, "Müller believed organisms contained a life force that made them fundamentally different from inorganic matter." He conducted "important physiological experiments, but for the wrong reason: to understand this non-existent life force." Nonetheless, the experimental methods that Müller established were appropriate for German physiology.[202] Otis explained that Schwann believed Müller's simultaneous acceptance of his cell theory and life force made no sense.[203] "In a lecture of 1878, Schwann stated that he never believed in vital force, seeking final causes 'not in the creature, but in the creator.'"[204] Ackerknecht explained that the concept of life force or vitalism developed in the eighteenth century as a "necessary corollary to the tremendous development of physics, which accentuated the vast gulf between living and nonliving things."[205]

In view of this fundamental dispute, one might not believe that Schwann, after Jakob Henle, was Müller's favorite assistant.[206] What excited Schwann, as a young assistant of Müller, was the latter's expertise with the microscope and his expertise in experimental physiology.[207] Like Müller, Schwann did not practice medicine, devoting all his energy to scientific work.[208] In a memorial address for Schwann, Henle recalled Schwann's circumstances when they lived and worked in the same building: He lived in a "narrow, rather dark rear room on the third floor of a less than second-rate

---

experimental method. Bernard demonstrated repeatedly that bodily functions, physiological and pathological could be investigated by chemical and physical experimentation. Erwin H. Ackerknecht, *A Short History of Medicine* [New York: Ronald Press, 1968], 165. With Claude Bernard's "discovery of the glycogen-forming function of the liver [he demonstrated] for the first time that the body plays a synthesizing role in the metabolic process as well as a decomposing one." Timothy Lenoir, *The Strategy of Life: Teleology ad Mechanics in Nineteenth-Century German Biology* [Chicago, IL: University of Chicago Press, 1989], 124, 126. Lenoir gives a more nuanced interpretation: "Schwann argued that there are two frameworks within which to conceive organic phenomena: 'The first view is that a special 'force' lays at the basis of each class of organ which forms them in accordance with an immaterial idea, and arranges the molecules in the manner necessary for achieving the purpose intended by this idea. … The other view is that the elementary forces of the organism are in fundamental agreement with the forces of inorganic nature to the extent that they operate blindly according to the laws of necessity independently of any particular purpose; in short that they are forces which are presupposed with the existence of matter, just like physical forces."

[194] Laura Otis, *Müller's Lab*, 62.

[195] Laura Otis, 21.

[196] Laura Otis, 20.

[197] Laura Otis, 13–14, 26.

[198] Laura Otis, 20, 27. Otis, p. 23. Classification of marine life bordered on an obsession and consumed much of his vacation time.

[199] Karl Sudhoff, "In Memory of Johannes Müller." *Essays in the History of Medicine.* Translated by various hands and edited, with foreword and biographical sketch, by Fielding H. Garrison. New York: Medical Life Press, 1926:363–367:363.

[200] Laura Otis, 21. For an erudite discussion of vital forces, see Jacques Roger, *The Life Sciences in Eighteenth-Century French Thought*, ed. Keith R. Benson and trans. Robert Ellrich [Stanford, CA: Stanford University Press, 1997], 336–53.

[201] Laura Otis, 27.

[202] Laura Otis, *Müller's Lab* [Oxford: Oxford University Press, 2007], 73.

[203] Laura Otis, 22. In 1838, [Müller] applied Schwann's cell theory to the pathology of tumors in his book *On the Fine Structure of Pathological Tumors,* "demonstrating…that tumors consist of cells."

[204] Laura Otis, 73.

[205] Erwin H. Ackerknecht, *Medicine at the Paris Hospital 1794–1848* [Baltimore, MD: Johns Hopkins Press, 1967], 54.

[206] Laura Otis, 34. Loved in the sense they shared the ability to work closely together, scientific intimacy, combined with Müller's paternalistic affection for Henle and Schwann.

[207] Laura Otis, 50.

[208] Laura Otis, 60.

restored building… which he often failed to leave for days at a time. [He was] surrounded by only a few books but by innumerable glass bottles, flasks, test tubes, and homemade primitive apparatus."[209] Schwann became an expert microscopist.[210] Henle recalled that "Schwann had an 'inborn drive' to experiment and a special gift for handling technical apparatus." Schwann received advice on construction of his physiological and electrical apparatus from his brother, a goldsmith. "According to Henle, no one who ever saw Schwann at work and watched 'his sober gaze' could doubt the reliability of his findings."[211] Schwann conducted controlled experiments and recorded his experiments in a laboratory notebook.[212] In his publications, he wrote his methodology and experimental design in detail "so that readers [could] repeat his experiments."[213]

Fortuitously, Matthias Jacob Schleiden (1804–1881) discovered cells in plants in 1837 while collaborating with Johannes Müller on a study of plant development. Schwann had earlier seen similar cells in the chorda dorsalis (notochord).[214] Otis quotes Schwann's dramatic awakening which illustrates the role of analogy in the formulation of his biological cell theory: "One day when I was having dinner with Schleiden (in October 1837) that illustrious botanist indicated to me the important role that the nucleus plays in the development of plant cells. Suddenly, I remembered having seen a similar structure [*un organe pareil*] in cells of the chorda dorsalis, and at that very instant I grasped the extreme importance the discovery would have if I succeeded in showing that, in the cells of the chorda dorsalis, the nucleus plays the same role that it plays in the development of plant cells…This fact, if solidly established through observation, would imply the negation of a vital force common to animals and would make it necessary to admit the individual life of the elementary parts of other tissues and a common means of formation through cells. This recognition of a principle, later verified by observation, constitutes the discovery I had the good fortune to make…I invited Schleiden to accompany me to the Anatomical Theater, where I showed him the nuclei in the chorda dorsalis cells. He saw [reconnut] a perfect resemblance to the nuclei of plants."[215]

In 1837 Schwann, a very religious man, wrote to his brother of the tension that existed between Müller and himself over "the question of the soul's location."[216] When Schwann wrote *Microscopical Researches into the Accordance in the Structure and Growth of Animals and Plants* (1839), he argued "that like crystals – which are inorganic and cannot be driven by any life force – all plant and animal cells follow 'one common principle of development.'"[217] "According to Schwann, all cells grew out of a formless, extracellular substance that he called the *cytoblastema.* The analogy to crystal growth served as a leitmotif throughout his work, although he warned readers about its limitations. He employed it to convey his most essential point: the common cellular, crystal-like structure of all living things suggested that physical and chemical laws, not some indefinable life force, controlled life functions."[218] Schwann's scientific views diverged fundamentally from those of Müller.[219] Nevertheless, and to his credit, Müller wrote in the second volume of his Handbook of Human Physiology in 1840 that "Schwann's discovery of animal cells constituted 'some of the most important progress ever made in physiology.'"[220]

In time Virchow would become famous for his revolutionary cell theory that transformed pathology by recognizing the cell as the seat of disease.[221] Notwithstanding

[209] Laura Otis, 53.

[210] Laura Otis, 59. "Quiet, serious Theodor Schwann used the microscopes of the mid-1830s better than just about anyone."

[211] Laura Otis, *Müller's Lab* [Oxford: Oxford University Press, 2007], 60.

[212] Laura Otis, 60.

[213] Laura Otis, 61, 64.

[214] Laura Otis, 63. *Illustrated Stedman's Medical Dictionary* 24th ed. [Baltimore, MD: Williams & Wilkins, 1982], 962. "Notochord 1. In primitive vertebrates, the primary axial supporting structure of the body, derived from the notchordal or head process of the early embryo; an important organizer for determining the final form of the nervous system and related structures. 2. Chorda dorsalis or vertebralis; in embryos, the axial fibrocellular chord about which the vertebral primordial develop; vestiges of it persist in the adult as the nuclei pulposi of the intervertebral disks."

[215] Laura Otis, *Müller's Lab* [Oxford: Oxford University Press, 2007], 63.

[216] Laura Otis, 65.

[217] Laura Otis, 63.

[218] Laura Otis, 64.

[219] Laura Otis, 62–64.

[220] Laura Otis, *Müller's Lab* [Oxford: Oxford University Press, 2007], 67. Erwin H. Ackerknecht, *A Short History of Medicine* [New York: Ronald Press, 1968], 160. Medical historians often refer to the Schleiden–Schwann cell theory.

[221] Paul Strathern, *A Brief History of Medicine from Hippocrates to Gene Therapy* [New York: Carroll & Graf, 2005], 207-211. Robert Meyer, *Autobiography of Dr. Robert Meyer (1864–1947):*

his later fame, Virchow was relatively unknown in 1846 when he criticized Rokitansky.[222] As Owsei Temkin noticed that Virchow did not publish his famous formula *omnis cellula a cellula* [all cells from other cells] until 1855. However, the principle upon which Virchow based *omnis cellula a cellula* had been developed by Robert Remak 3 years earlier in 1852.[223] Virchow's fully developed cell theory was not to be published until 1858,[224] 2 years after he succeeded his mentor, Johannes Müller, as professor of pathological anatomy in Berlin.[225] So on what basis did Virchow criticize the blastema theory of Rokitansky?

Virchow's criticism was based on solid research unrelated to his famous cell theory. In 1844, 1 year after he had defended his dissertation for a PhD degree under the guidance of Johannes Müller and received his medical degree from the University of Berlin,[226] Virchow left Müller's laboratory. Virchow became the assistant to Robert Froriep, associate professor at the University of Berlin and prosector of pathological anatomy at the Charite Hospital.[227] Under Froriep's guidance Virchow began his *Habilitation*, "a kind of second dissertation that allowed [him] to teach at a university."[228] Virchow studied the cause of blood poisoning. This led him to systematic microscopic study between 1844 and 1847 of the blood, blood clotting, and phlebitis – inflammation of vein walls.[229] In the process, he discredited the blastema theory of disease causation. Virchow was jubilant when this study, his *Habilitation*, was accepted for publication in 1845 in *Scientific and Medical Notes*, a journal edited by his new mentor, Robert Froriep.[230]

In 1846, Virchow succeeded Froriep as prosector at the Charite.[231] It was from this platform as prosector at the Charite Hospital in Berlin and his newly acquired academic credentials that Virchow launched the attack

---

A Short Abstract of a Long Life [New York: Henry Schuman, 1949], 38-9. In his autobiography, Meyer stated that Virchow is known, or should be known, "the world over as the founder of cellular pathology. ... It was a logical continuation from Schleiden, who recognized the cell as the element of the development and morphology of plants (1838), to Schwann, who recognized the cell as the element of the normal tissue in animals (1839), and to Virchow (about 1852) who was the first to describe the pathological proceedings as change of the cells. In 1858, he published his *Cellular Pathology*, in which he called the cell the ultimate formative element of all life and, at the same time, designated illness as due to physical and chemical changes of the cells. This ingenious doctrine was revolutionary. It brought medicine out of the humoral way of thinking to the realization that we must look for physico-chemical changes in the cells themselves. This was a concrete theory on which everyone could build. It was the localization of disease in special cells which first gave medicine a firm basis."

[222] Erwin H. Ackerknecht, *A Short History of Medicine* [New York: Ronald Press, 1968], 171. Virchow became better known in 1847 when he and Reinhardt established a new journal, the *Archives for Pathological Anatomy, Physiology, and Clinical Medicine,* which later became known as Virchow's Archives. Virchow and the German School of Pathologic Physiology believed that the disease *process* could not be ascertained at the autopsy table, but only "by a study of disturbed function."

[223] Owsei Temkin, "Basic Science, Medicine, and the Romantic Era," in *The Double Face of Janus and Other Essays in the History of Medicine* [Baltimore, MD: Johns Hopkins University Press, 1977:396. See also Laura Otis, *Müller's Lab* [Oxford: Oxford University Press, 2007], 170 and note #32 on page 281. Otis: 171. Robert Remak, an assistant of Johannes Müller, was internationally known for his embryologic studies. Remak identified the three embryonic germ cell layers and the organs that developed from each layer. According to Otis, some authors believe that Remak deserves credit for the principle of *omnis cellula a cellula,* not Virchow. Otis: 165. Despite support from Johannes Müller and Alexander von Humboldt, Remak never received an appointment as professor in any Prussian university, but continued his research and practiced from his home. Erwin H. Ackerknecht, *A Short History of Medicine* [New York: Ronald Press, 1968], 159-60. "Since the beginning of the [nineteenth] century medical scientists such as Oken and Meckel, and later Raspail, Dutrochet, and other, had claimed that living bodies consisted basically of 'vesicles,' 'cells,' or 'globules.'... The formulation of the cell theory was crystallized through the efforts of Theodor Schwann (1809-1885)...That cells developed from cells, and only from cells, was demonstrated by Hugo von Mohl, John Goodsir, Robert Remak, and preeminently by Rudolf Virchow in 1854."

[224] Rudolf Virchow, Die Cellularpathologie in ihrer Begründung auf physiologische und pathologische Gewebelehre [Berlin: Hirschwald, 1858].

[225] Harris L. Coulter, *Divided Legacy: A History of the Schism in Medical Thought. Volume II: The Origins of Modern Western Medicine: J. B. Van Helmont to Claude Bernard* [Berkeley, CA: North Atlantic Books, 1977, 2000], 607.

[226] Robert E. Fechner, "The Birth and Evolution of American Surgical Pathology," in *Guiding the Surgeon's Hand: The History of American Surgical Pathology*, ed. Juan Rosai [Washington, DC: Armed Forces Institute of Pathology, 1997], 10. Laura Otis, *Müller's Lab* [Oxford: Oxford University Press, 2007], 140. Johannes Müller acted as official advisor for his thesis.

[227] Laura Otis, *Müller's Lab* [Oxford: Oxford University Press, 2007], 141.

[228] Andreas W. Daum, "*Wissenschaft* and knowledge," in *The Short Oxford History of Germany: Germany 1800–1870* [Oxford: Oxford University Press, 2004], 137–161: 143.

[229] Laura Otis, 143.

[230] Laura Otis, *Müller's Lab* [Oxford: Oxford University Press, 2007], 141–3.

[231] Laura Otis, 141.

that destroyed the blastema theory, the theory of crasis, and exudates upon which Rokitansky had based his explanation for the cause of disease.[232] Rokitansky was well aware of the scientific advantages of German medical education and of *Wissenschaft*, advantages that he and his fellow faculty members at the University of Vienna never enjoyed.[233] Until the Revolution of 1848, the professors at the Vienna Medical School were subordinate to medical practitioners. In the Revolution of 1848, Rokitansky and the other professors of the Vienna Medical Faculty were among the "avant-garde in the battle for a new university constitution in Austria."[234] These circumstances help to explain Rokitansky's acceptance of Virchow's criticism. When Rokitansky rewrote the first volume of his textbook, *Lehrbuch der pathologischen Anatomie,* published in 1855,[235] he eliminated his theory of blastema. In its place the scholarly Rokitansky wrote "in natural scientific terms, and in doing so, encouraged Virchow to further develop the natural scientific conception of disease."[236] This would not be the last time that Virchow influenced Rokitansky along the tortuous path to the discovery of endometriosis.

Like Andral and Schwann's theory of cell origin, Rokitansky's general theory of disease was published prematurely. Later in the nineteenth century a debate ensued, arraying Elie Metchnikoff's antigens, antibodies, and resistance against the immunological theories of Emil von Behring and Paul Ehrlich, who argued that "immunological warfare was waged less by the white blood cells than by the blood serum."[237] Miciotto, a scholar of Rokitansky's hematohumoral theory, opined in 1978 that: "There are few indications that Rokitansky's theory met with instant rejection, or that Virchow's review was immediately accepted as the final word on Rokitansky's ideas."[238]

232 Erna Lesky, *The Vienna Medical School of the 19th Century* [Baltimore, MD: Johns Hopkins University Press, 1976], 111.

233 Andreas W. Daum, "*Wissenschaft* and knowledge," in *The Short Oxford History of Germany: Germany 1800–1870* [Oxford: Oxford University Press, 2004], 137–161: 159. "In fact, the revolution of 1848 marked the beginning of a fundamental transformation of the Austrian universities, which were now restructured according to the model of the Prussian reforms a generation earlier and experienced massive increases in the number of students up to 1871."

234 Erna Lesky, 96. See also Laura Otis, *Müller's Lab* [Oxford: Oxford University Press, 2007], 148. The impetuous genius Virchow actually manned the barricades in Berlin during the 1848 revolution. Rokitansky and Virchow were cut from the same liberal cloth, only they enacted reform differently.

235 Carl Rokitansky, *Lehrbuch der pathologischen Anatomie*, Vol. I [Wien: Braumüller, 1855]

236 V. Becker, [Rokitansky and Virchow: throes about the scientific term of disease] Wien Med Wochenschr 2005;155:463–7. See also Byers JM 3rd. Rudolph Virchow – father of cellular pathology. *Am J Clin Pathol* 1989 Oct;92 (4 Suppl 1):S2–8.

237 Roy Porter, *Blood and Guts: A Short History of Medicine* [New York: W. W. Norton & Company, 2002], 93.

238 Robert J Miciotto, Carl Rokitansky: A reassessment of the hematohumoral theory of disease. *Bulletin History Medicine* 1978;52(2):183–99:185.

3 Microscopy and the Discovery of Endometriosis and Adenomyosis

Reconstructing the history of the discovery of the condition we today call adenomyosis is neither simple nor easy because for almost 90 years adenomyosis and endometriosis were considered – with the exception of ovarian endometriosis – as one disease: 'adenomyoma.' As such, the early history of adenomyosis is interwoven with the early history of endometriosis, and it was not until the mid-1920 that the two conditions were finally separated.

Benagiano and Brosens[1]

Emergence of Microscopy in Rokitansky's Department

Study of histologic sections of uterine tissue was essential to discover the new disease uterine endometriosis (adenomyosis) and to differentiate it from a degenerating uterine leiomyoma (fibroid) and from uterine cancer. Unfortunately, the Imperial reform of 1786 had demoted the mission and status of pathological anatomy by transferring microscopy to the department of physiology and thus deprived all subsequent pathological anatomic prosectors – including Rokitansky – use of the microscope.[2] Then two publications appeared in the 1830s that demonstrated the importance of microscopy in pathological anatomy. Between 1835 and 1840 Johannes Müller of Berlin published his highly acclaimed *Handbook of Human Physiology*. Between 1837 and 1844, Joseph Berres of Vienna published the first atlas of the histology of the human body entitled *Anatomy of the Microscopic Formations of the Human Body*.[3] Both works appeared at a crucial point in Rokitansky's career and they undoubtedly aroused his interest in microscopy.

In 1834, Rokitansky had been appointed associate professor of pathological anatomy by Baron von Türkheim, an appointment that put Rokitansky in a position to formally establish his research program. In rapid succession, von Türkheim founded the Second Vienna Medical School, inaugurated the Medical Yearbooks of the Imperial Royal Austrian State in 1836, and in 1837 organized the Vienna Society of Physicians to stimulate scientific research, discussion, and publication.[4] The fact that von Türkheim built the

[1] Benagiano G, Brosens I. History of adenomyosis. *Best Pract Res Clin Obstet Gynecol* 2006;20:449–63:450.

[2] Erna Lesky, *The Vienna Medical School of the 19th Century* [Baltimore, MD: Johns Hopkins University Press, 1976], 68. Arleen Marcia Tuchman, *Science, Medicine, and the State of Germany: The Case of Baden, 1815–1871* [New York: Oxford University Press, 1993], 86–7. Physiology amounted to "little more than microscopical anatomy accompanied by occasional chemical tests and investigations" until mid-nineteenth century when slowly the development of sophisticated instrumental techniques led to "a methodical approach to the study of function."

[3] Erna Lesky, 73–4. Berres (1796–1844), a Moravian surgeon-macroscopic-anatomist, stimulated by the work of a Viennese optician, had learned microscopy after he was appointed to Vienna.

[4] Erna Lesky, *The Vienna Medical School of the 19th Century* [Baltimore, MD: Johns Hopkins University Press, 1976], 99, 106.

R.E. Batt, *A History of Endometriosis*,
DOI 10.1007/978-0-85729-585-9_3,

Second Vienna Medical School around Rokitansky's autopsy table gave Rokitansky space for innovation; incrementally he reintroduced microscopy into pathological anatomy at the University of Vienna.

As Rokitansky began gathering material for his *Handbook of Pathological Anatomy*, the need for histologic illustrations became pressing, given the illustrated treatises of Müller and Berres. While on an academic pilgrimage to Paris in 1842, arranged by Baron von Türkheim, Rokitansky not only bought a Brunner microscope, he availed himself of an opportunity to visit England.[5] There he was entertained in the home of Joseph Jackson Lister, famous for improving the achromatic microscopic lens system.[6] Between the years 1826 and 1830, Joseph Jackson Lister, the father of Joseph Lord Lister, had discovered the "law of aplanatic foci"[7] which enabled him to construct an achromatic microscope lens system that was virtually freed from spherical and chromatic aberrations.[8] Lister joined two achromatic lenses together with Canadian balsam by which process effective light was increased by nearly 100%.[9]

It is reasonable to infer from references in the 1846 edition of his *Handbook of Pathological Anatomy* that upon his return to Vienna Rokitansky made principal use of his microscope when he suspected cancer.[10] The microscope did not live up to his expectations. "Microscopic analysis, therefore, from which important disclosures in relation to the diagnosis of benignant and of malignant growths, and tenable grounds for the establishment of a system were expected, has in reality thrown but an uncertain light upon the subject."[11] However, when studying the development of cancer, he found the microscope more satisfying. *"Cancer-cyst* varies in respect to size from the microscopic, to the circumference of the colossal cysts, in the compound cystoid...Within the encysted parenchyma, again, is sometimes lodged a smaller, filial cyst...Upon this point and upon the development of the cancer-cyst

[5] Prim. Univ.-Prof. Dr. Roland Sedivy, e-mail message to author, September 2, 2007. "In his autobiography Rokitansky mentioned that he bought 1842 Brunner microscope (fig. attached!). More details are currently not known. But I found in one archive the free-hand graphics of some histological figures he used in his second edition of his textbook. The size of cells in these figures allow [one] to get some idea of what magnification he might have used. I presume that he referred to a magnification in total (ocular × objective) between 50–100x." See Erna Lesky, *The Vienna Medical School of the 19th Century* [Baltimore, MD: Johns Hopkins University Press, 1976], 99.

[6] Rickman John Godlee, *Lord Lister* [Oxford: Clarendon Press, 1924], 55: "the Rokitanskys...had dined at Upton [with Joseph Jackson Lister and his family] fourteen years earlier (1842)."

[7] Sherwin B. Nuland, *Doctors: The Biography of Medicine.* New York: Alfred A. Knopf, 1989:351.

[8] Michael J. O'Dowd and Elliott E. Philipp, *The History of Obstetrics and Gynaecology* [New York: Parthenon Publishing Group, 1994], 220. Nuland, Sherwin B. *Doctors: The Biography of Medicine.* New York: Alfred A. Knopf, 1989:352. Nuland quoted from Joseph Lister's 1900 Huxley Lecture. In 1900, when surgical pathology was a reality, Lister recalled that his father's investigations "had raised the compound microscope from little better than a scientific toy to the powerful engine for investigation." See also: Rickman John Godlee, *Lord Lister* [Oxford: Clarendon Press, 1924], 11–12. "Between 1824 and 1843, whilst actively engaged in business, he found time to make his mathematical calculations, actually to grind the glasses himself, and to supply the necessary data to Tulley, Ross, and Smith, who were the manufactures. This work gained for him the Fellowship of the Royal Society in 1832, and brought him into contact with a large scientific circle." He wrote a paper in 1842–3 entitled "On the Limit to Defining Power, in Vision with the Unassisted Eye, the Telescope and the Microscope" that remained unpublished until it appeared in Journal of the Royal Microscopical Society, 1913, Part I: 34–55.

[9] RM Allen, *The Microscope* [New York: D. Van Nostrand Company, 1940], 8. Arleen Marcia Tuchman, Science, Medicine, and the State of Germany: The Case of Baden, 1815–1871 [New York: Oxford University Press, 1993], 57. The Frenchman, Charles Chevalier is credited with having improved resolution at high magnifications by "inserting a biconcave lens between several achromatic lenses." E. M. Tansey, "From the Germ Theory to 1945," in *Western Medicine,* ed. Irvine Loudon [Oxford: Oxford University Press, 1997], 108. Subsequent improvements in microscopes "were matched by advances in the techniques of preserving, cutting, and selectively staining sections for histological examination....Improvements in microscopes for static observations and measurements were also made, especially after the invention of the achromatic lens by Joseph Lister (1786–1869), father of the surgeon Joseph (Lord) Lister. These were matched by advances in the techniques of preserving, cutting, and selectively staining sections for histological examination." Erna Lesky, *The Vienna Medical School of the 19th Century* [Baltimore, MD: Johns Hopkins University Press, 1976], 171–2. However, "staining and hardening techniques were still undeveloped in the late 1850s." Alexander Hellemans and Bryan Bunch, *The Timetables of Science: A Chronology of the Most Important People and Events in the History of Science*, Touchtone Edition [New York: Simon & Schuster, 1988], 362–4. However, some advances such as the microtome to slice thin tissue sections were not invented until 1885. The microtome was invented by Charles Darwin, son of Charles Darwin, author of *The Origin of Species.*

[10] The 1855 translation of the 1846 edition by the Sydenham Society

[11] Carl Rokitansky, *A Manual of Pathological Anatomy*, Volume I. *General Pathological Anatomy.* trans. William Edward Swaine [Philadelphia, PA: Blanchard & Lea, 1855], 76.

microscopic inspection throws much light."[12] He discussed microscopic examination of "excrescences occurring upon the inner surface of the cyst."[13] In 1846 Rokitansky was aware of cell-nuclei and had a rudimentary idea of the role of the cell in development, most likely from reading the microscopic research of Schwann on the notochord and of Müller and Virchow on cancer. He mentioned Virchow by name. "This history of cyst-development is essentially corroborated by the expansion of the cell-nuclei, of so frequent, although by no means exclusive, occurrence in *cancer-cells;* an expansion first pointed out with precision by Virchow, but which, owing to the identity of development of the normal gland vesicle, and of the cyst, cannot be regarded as heteroplastic. It consists in the development of the cell-nucleus into a comprehensive cyst, identical with that evolved out of the naked nucleus."[14]

Rokitansky had long recognized malignancies by their macroscopic characteristics. "They reveal their cancerous nature by their external medullary characters, as well as by their vigorous growth. In the capillaries the coagulation assumes the form of the cancerous depot-so called metastasis (capillary phlebitis)."[15] In the next passage, Rokitansky seems to be comparing his 19-year total immersion in macropathology with his emergent 4-year experience with histopathology. "We have the following forms, some more or less recognizable with the naked eye. (a) A medullary carcinoma etc."[16] Nonetheless, even in 1846, there can be little doubt that Rokitansky appreciated the benefit of microscopy for diagnosis and study of cancer. "The differences, however, discoverable with the naked eye in carcinoma, are slight compared with those revealed in the elementary texture of medullary carcinoma, with the aid of a magnifying power."[17] Furthermore, even at this early stage of his experimentation with microscopy, Rokitansky can be seen studying not only development of mononuclear and multinucleated cells but also cellular "dissilience" or cell fragmentation. "Under a magnifying power of 90 diameters, the substance of fungus haematodes exhibits a stroma, consisting of two distinct webs, which appear to interlace each other in all directions...Further examination shows this wreath-like tissue, which at first seemed opaque and granular, to be studded with crowds of minute nucleated cells, which, under a magnifying power of 400, are distinctly set forth as round or oval cells, many, although not all, containing one or several nuclei, others engaged in the act of elongation, others again in process of dissilience."[18]

Though Rokitansky never mastered the microscope personally, he used his considerable administrative and scientific influence to ensure that microscopy flourished in his department and the other departments of the University of Vienna. His assistant Joseph Engel was the first person in Vienna to give lectures on pathological histology.[19] The question may be raised why Rokitansky did not send more of his tissues for histological examination by his assistants or colleagues. The answer may lie in a clash of personalities. Joseph Engel, an accomplished microscopist in the early 1840s, and "undoubtedly the most gifted and versatile" of Rokitansky's assistants, quarreled with Rokitansky as he did later with colleagues in pathology in Prague and the St. Joseph's Academy in Vienna. Unfortunately "this highly gifted man died in resigned isolation."[20] Had their relationship been more cordial, Rokitansky might have been persuaded to send more of his interesting autopsy specimens for histologic examination and by so doing have discovered endometriosis earlier in his career. On the other hand, "staining and hardening techniques were still undeveloped" in the 1850s; this may be another reason why Rokitansky was not fully appreciative of the potential benefits from applying histology more widely in his personal research.[21]

Rokitansky and certain able assistants had some noteworthy accomplishments at the University of Vienna in the middle years of the century. Rokitansky appointed Carl Wedl (1815–1891) in 1846 and Carl Stellwag von Carion (1823–1904) in 1847 to perform histological work in his department. Then in 1853 he was responsible for

[12] Carl Rokitansky, 174.

[13] Carl Rokitansky, 176.

[14] Carl Rokitansky, 184.

[15] Carl Rokitansky, 197.

[16] Carl Rokitansky, *A Manual of Pathological Anatomy*, Volume I. *General Pathological Anatomy.* trans. William Edward Swaine [Philadelphia, PA: Blanchard & Lea, 1855], 209.

[17] Carl Rokitansky, 208.

[18] Carl Rokitansky, 220.

[19] Erna Lesky, *The Vienna Medical School of the 19th Century* [Baltimore, MD: Johns Hopkins University Press, 1976], 112.

[20] Erna Lesky, *The Vienna Medical School of the 19th Century* [Baltimore, MD: Johns Hopkins University Press, 1976], 115–6.

[21] Erna Lesky, 171–2.

the appointment of Carl Wedl as associate professor to an endowed Chair of Histology at the University of Vienna, the first in "German-speaking territories."[22] By 1854, Wedl had his own two-room Institute of Histology on the second floor of the Old Rifle Factory, another first of its kind in German-speaking lands. Wedl soon became "a very popular and prominent histopathologist of the Second Vienna Medical School."[23] In 1855, Wedl published a comprehensive 825 page work entitled *Rudiments of Pathological Histology*.[24]

Leo Graf v. Hohenstein Thun, successor to von Türkheim, carried on the latter's reforms. He appointed the physiologist Ernst von Brücke, an assistant of Johannes Müller of Berlin, to the University of Vienna faculty to develop experimental methods "in order to bring the predominantly morphologically oriented Vienna Medial School completely up-to-date."[25] Even with these innovations, the University of Vienna was far behind developments in pathological anatomy in German universities.[26] In 1855, Virchow first enunciated his cell theory in the famous formula "*omnis cellula a cellula*"[27]; 1855 was also the year that Rokitansky published the revised second and final edition of his *Handbook of Pathological Anatomy*. With the second edition of his *Handbook*, Rokitansky completed his primary research objective – the classification of human pathological anatomy begun decades before by the French. At this stage in his career, Rokitansky was also occupied by many high-level administrative duties in the University of Vienna.

Several unrelated events in these years combined to make Rokitansky see the inevitability of microscopic histopathology. Joseph Lister married April 23, 1856 and after spending a month in England, started a tour of Europe during which the couple visited many celebrated medical schools including Vienna. Since the Listers and Rokitansky's were family friends,[28] Rokitansky invited young Lister and his new wife to supper that evening in his home.[29] In so doing, Rokitansky returned the courtesy of Joseph Jackson Lister in 1842 when Joseph Lister was yet an unknown.[30] Considering that happy memory and the fact that young Lister had just published two papers on microscopy in 1853,[31] it is not improbable that they discussed the topic of microscopy. Also in 1853 came unexpected praise from Rudolph Virchow for Rokitansky's own work and that of the Second Vienna Medical School.[32] In 1858, Rudolph Virchow again influenced Rokitansky when he expanded his cell

[22] Erna Lesky, 112, 219. Lesky, p. 465. "However, the true home and source of microscopists in Vienna, despite the existence of an official Chair of Histology was the Institute of Physiology, of which all the newer institutes were off shoots."

[23] Erna Lesky, *The Vienna Medical School of the 19th Century* [Baltimore, MD: Johns Hopkins University Press, 1976], 219.

[24] Erna Lesky, 220. In German: *Grundzüge der pathologischen Histologie*, 1855.

[25] Erna Lesky, 102.

[26] Arleen Marcia Tuchman, *Science, Medicine, and the State of Germany: The Case of Baden, 1815–1871* [New York: Oxford University Press, 1993], 76. German universities took the lead in introducing microscopy in the medical curriculum. "Between 1845 and 1855 fifteen medical faculties also began including microscopical demonstrations in their courses on pathology, histology, semiotics, and diagnostics." Arleen Marcia Tuchman, *Science, Medicine, and the State of Germany: The Case of Baden, 1815–1871* [New York: Oxford University Press, 1993], 82–83. By mid-century, the microscope had become for the symbol of excellence in teaching and research. In 1845, students in the University of Heidelberg held a torchlight parade in honor of Jacob Henle, a former assistant of Johann Müller, as a champion of microscopy in teaching and research, and "as a thinker and scientist who campaigns unremittingly and without stop at the head of those who are struggling and fighting against a desolate empiricism in our science."

[27] Erna Lesky, 221.

[28] Owen H. Wangensteen and Sarah D. Wangensteen, *The Rise of Surgery: From Empiric Craft to Scientific Discipline* [Minneapolis, MN: University of Minnesota Press, 1978], 440.

[29] Rickman John Godlee, *Lord Lister* [Oxford: Clarendon Press, 1924], 54–55. Earlier in the day Rokitansky spent over 3 h showing the Lister and other visitors specimens in the Vienna Pathological Museum.

[30] Rickman John Godlee, 55: "The medical school at Vienna was the largest and most important he had yet seen. It provided much of general interest; (quoting Joseph Lister) 'and best of all as yet, Professor Rokitansky, the most eminent pathologist in the world spend three hours and a quarter the other day, in going over his wonderfully rich museum of preparations of diseases, to me and some other visitors.' Rokitansky was extremely hospitable; he had dined at Upton fourteen years before, and had been much impressed with Lister's two sisters, though he had no recollection of the young surgeon, who, he said was 'nothing in those days.'"

[31] Rickman John Godlee, 22–23. Joseph Lister wrote two papers on microscopy, both published in the Quarterly Journal of Microscopical Science in 1853. The first dealt with muscular tissue of the iris of the eye. Joseph Lister, *Quarterly Journal of Microscopical Science* 1853;1:8. The second involved observations on the involuntary muscular fibers of the skin. Joseph Lister, *Quarterly Journal of Microscopical Science* 1853;1:262.

[32] Not only did Rokitansky engage in scholarly debates with Rudolph Virchow in the medical literature, at least on one occasion – November 10, 1853 – he wrote a formal letter to Virchow commenting on the latter's "discovery of subependymal corpora

theory of 1855 – *omnis cellula a cellula* [all cells from other cells] – into a theory "that all disease was a disease of cells."[33] Virchow "transformed pathology" in 1858 with the publication of *Cellularpathologie*.[34]

Each of these events may well have contributed to Rokitansky's decision in 1859 to permit Virchow's lectures on cellular pathology to be taught in the Department of Pathology at the University of Vienna. "In the winter semester of 1859–60…Klob, Rokitansky's assistant in Vienna, posted on his blackboard the following notice: 'From Thursday on, lectures on pathological anatomy will be delivered according to the cell doctrine of Virchow.'"[35] Furthermore, by the late 1850s there was mounting pressure at the University of Vienna, to go much further than importing just one German physiologist to integrate the German "experimental-physiological" approach of Johannes Müller and his school into pathological anatomy and other departments to make the classification of disease more precise.[36]

amylacea of the brain ventricle," adding his own observations on the subject. This letter was written in immediate response to Rokitansky receiving the "first issue of volume 6 of your Archives." See Christian Andree and Roland Sedivy, "Discovery of a letter from Rokitansky to Virchow about subependymal corpora amylacea," *Virchow's Archive* 2005;446:177–180. "Subependymal means beneath the ependyma (the cellular membrane lining the central canal of the spinal cord and the brain ventricles) and corpora amylacea means (one of a number of small ovoid or rounded, sometimes laminated, bodies resembling a grain of starch and found in nervous tissue, in the prostate, and in pulmonary alveoli; of little pathological significance, and apparently derived from degenerated cells or proteinaceous secretions." *Illustrated Stedman's Medical Dictionary,* 24th ed. [Baltimore, MD: Williams & Wilkins, 1982], 323, 473. Rokitansky's letter to Virchow was found by Christian Andree at the Berlin-Brandenburg Academy of Sciences. Professor Sedivy sent the author an autographed reprint.

In the first pages of volume 6 of his journal, Virchow "unexpectedly praised Rokitansky's work and the Vienna School of Medicine." Rudolph Virchow, Uber eine im Gehirn und Ruckenmark des Menchen aufgefundene Substanz mit der chemischen Reaction der Cellulose. Arch Path Anat u Physiol u Klin Med 1854;6:135–138. Shortly thereafter in the very pages of Virchow's Journal, Rokitansky found an article on subependymal corpora amylacea (CA) written by Virchow that prompted a letter to Virchow from Rokitansky, the only known correspondence between the two men. This episode reveals that not only did Rokitansky faithfully read Virchow's journal, but also that he must have been pleased to read the unexpected praise for his own work and that of the Second Vienna School of Medicine; words of praise from his old critic. Andree and Sedivy noted that "Virchow mentioned in the addendum to his article that Rokitansky and Kolliker had seen CA in the N. opticus and retina, respectively. When mentioning Rokitansky, Virchow used the passive voice, indicating that he was not sure whether Rokitansky really had observed them." From this observation, Andree and Sedivy speculated "that this fact was the background behind his letter to Virchow." See Christian Andree and Roland Sedivy, "Discovery of a letter from Rokitansky to Virchow abut subependymal corpora amylacea," *Virchow's Archive* 2005;446:177–180.

To this may be added the further speculation that Rokitansky's friendly, though formal letter to Virchow may have been possible in the first place because Virchow's unexpected praise helped heal an old wound that Rokitansky had sustained in 1846. See Rudolph Virchow, *Rokitansky, Handbuch der allgemeinen pathologischen Anatomie,* Literarische Beilage, Preussische Medicinal-Zeitung 1846;XV:237–238, 243–244. Perhaps this rapprochement between the doyen of German pathology and the doyen of Austrian Pathology in 1854 may have contributed to Rokitansky's greater interest in microscopy and histology that, further stimulated by the publication of Virchow's *Cellular Pathology* in 1858, led Rokitansky to inaugurate Virchow's lectures on pathology in his department in 1859.

[33] 7. E. M. Tansey, "From the Germ Theory to 1945," in *Western Medicine,* ed. Irvine Loudon [Oxford: Oxford University Press, 1997], 102.

[34] Paul Strathern, A Brief History of Medicine from Hippocrates to Gene Therapy [New York: Carroll & Graf, 2005], 211–212. Henry E. Sigerist, Man and Medicine: An Introduction to Medical Knowledge [New York: WW Norton & Company, 1932], 124. Referring to Virchow's *Cellular Pathology* of 1858, the medical historian Henry Sigerist opined that "Virchow placed the microscope into the hands of pathologists. This only made it possible to see the minuter changes and to undertake a more exact classification of disease. The microscope alone gave us the opportunity of observing other processes of disease, inflammation for instance." The dominance of naked-eye macromorphology gave way to micropathology as the first major step in the long process of reductionism that led to ultramicroscopic pathologic investigation and molecular biology in the twentieth century.

[35] Fielding H. Garrison, *Contributions to The History of Medicine.* [New York: Hafner Publishing Company, 1966], 190. "In the winter semester of 1859–60…Klob, Rokitansky's assistant in Vienna, posted on his blackboard the following notice: 'From Thursday on, lectures on pathological anatomy will be delivered according to the cell doctrine of Virchow.'" Erna Lesky, *The Vienna Medical School of the 19th Century* [Baltimore, MD: Johns Hopkins University Press, 1976], 172. By the late 1850s, cellular pathology was taught in Vienna and "even in Rokitansky's own institute." Lesky, p. 112. "Rokitansky was not a professional microscopist. The task that his time posed before him was of a macromorphological nature and as a macromorphopathologist he fulfilled it. From the very beginning, however, he considered it to be the task of pathological anatomy to raise pathology to physiological pathology. This comprehensive concept as held by Rokitansky makes it possible to understand why he, being a genuine macromorphologist, not only encouraged the development of medical chemistry, and pathological histology, but also that of experimental pathology, and why he acquainted his school with these methods of research when he had exhausted his own method. This took place in the middle of the fifties. The year 1858 marked the beginning of the epoch of cellular pathology."

[36] Erna Lesky, *The Vienna Medical School of the 19th Century* [Baltimore, MD: Johns Hopkins University Press, 1976], 145.

The rise of surgery constituted another factor that contributed to the obsolescence of macroscopic morbid pathological anatomy. Influenced by Rokitansky and Skoda, Franz Schuh (1804–1865) elevated surgery to a science at the University of Vienna.[37] Schuh implemented the methods of microscopic and chemical research established by Johannes Müller for research into benign and malignant growths.[38] On January 27, 1847, he introduced ether anesthesia in Vienna.[39] The availability of surgical anesthesia, chemical testing, and microscopic histopathology for research combined to increase the importance and prestige of the department of surgery.[40] In 1867, on the initiative of Rokitansky and several other professors, Theodor Billroth (1829–1894) was appointed professor of surgery, 1 year after the disastrous Austro-Prussian War of 1866.[41] Having trained under Rudolf Wagner, Johannes Müller, Schonlein, Romberg, Traube, and von Langenbeck; Billroth "embodied all those tendencies which had made German medicine great since the middle of the nineteenth century."[42]

Once Rokitansky had completed his *Handbook* and, sensing the inevitability of microscopic histopathology, an aging master macroscopic pathologist made the decision to use microscopy to study the histopathology of select benign lesions. This step was a necessary precursor to the discovery of endometriosis. In sum, taking Rokitansky at his word – that he relied on his own experience – we can accept that the references to microscopy in the 1846 publication were based on his own, albeit, limited personal experience. Armed with his Brunner microscope, he had begun experimenting with the histopathology of malignancy only 4 years before Virchow devastated his hematohumoral theory of disease. Gradually Rokitansky accepted Virchow's theory of cellular pathology and found it compatible with his own localistic pathology. Finally, he changed a lifelong habit and began to use the microscope to study the histopathology of interesting benign lesions. In the final analysis, Virchow's influence was decisive.

Sigerist opined that "Upon the shoulders of Virchow rests the whole structure of modern pathology. Much preparatory work had been done macroscopically, especially by the Viennese, Rokitansky, but Virchow placed the microscope into the hands of pathologists. This only made it possible to see the minuter changes and to undertake a more exact classification of disease."[43] With those words the German physician-medical historian Henry Sigerist recognized Virchow's influence on Rokitansky. For the microscope was crucial not only for Rokitansky's entrée to the histopathology of malignant disease; the microscope was also the instrument and histopathology the technique necessary for Rokitansky's identification of benign uterine and extrauterine endometriosis.

1860: Discovery of Two New Diseases – Endometriosis and Adenomyosis

> Sarcoma and carcinoma…Kindred new growths, important from their frequency no less than from the question arising, in every concrete case, as to their innocency or malignancy. We have selected the term **sarcoma** to designate the **benign growths**, not because of any especial analogy with muscle-flesh, but in order to fix and define a name familiarized by long usage, and also by no little abuse. [Italics added] The malignant we shall leave in possession of their ancient characteristic appellation *cancer,-carcinoma.*
> Carl Rokitansky[44]

After observing thousands of benign uterine fibroids, benign hemorrhagic ovarian cysts and benign uterine polyps macroscopically, what specimen so riveted

[37] Erna Lesky, 168.

[38] Erna Lesky, 171.

[39] Erna Lesky, 173.

[40] Erna Lesky, 197. After Rokitansky's retirement in 1874, the advent of Lister's antisepsis would elevate surgery under Billroth to leadership in the University of Vienna. Billroth adopted antisepsis.

[41] Erna Lesky, 293. Very high Austrian battle casualties were caused by the Prussian breech loading rifle in the Austro-Prussian War of 1866. The Prussian soldiers were able to fire and reload in the prone position which reduced their silhouette and vulnerability considerably. In contrast the Austrian soldiers had to stand upright when they reloaded their muzzle loading muskets which made them prime targets. "When the Medical Faculty submitted a proposal for a successor to Schuh in 1867, it demanded, on the initiative of Arlt, Brücke, Hebra, and Rokitansky, that the ministry appoint 'a man to be professor of surgery of whom the greatest promotion of science may be expected, a man who is not only famous in the field of practical surgery, but also in areas of physiological and pathological research who has demonstrated a special genius as teacher, surgeon and writer, who is still in the prime of life, from whom it may be expected that he will represent the most modern trends in surgery in its relation to physiology and pathological anatomy, and who is able to establish a surgical school in Vienna which will bring fame to the university and the greatest benefit to the country.'" Erna Lesky, *The Vienna Medical School of the 19th Century* [Baltimore, MD: Johns Hopkins University Press, 1976], 261. To get some idea of the importance of this appointment, consider the words of Billroth: "…it almost seems a fairy tale that I am appointed Imperial Royal professor of the First

Rokitansky's attention in 1860 that he examined it microscopically?[45] It was a *fresh* surgical specimen! A *fresh* "fist sized uterine polyp" from a live patient![46] That specimen, once examined microscopically, led to further investigation of autopsy specimens and specimens preserved in "wine-spirits."[47] What is the evidence for this assumption? We must contrast the brilliant internist Adolph Kussmaul's recollection of Rokitansky's taciturn nature[48] with Rokitansky's exclamation that he examined a *fresh* specimen. The invitation to examine a rare fresh specimen microscopically must have proved irresistible. Careful microscopic examination then led to the identification and description of endometriosis in several other specimens. The discovery of endometriosis was merely one of many pathologic lesions detected by his discerning gaze, but an incident of transcendent importance to the history of endometriosis.[49]

In 1860 Rokitansky described three phenotypes of endometriosis containing endometrial stroma and glands: one invaded the uterine muscular wall (*Sarcoma adenoids uterinum* and the cystic variety: *Cystosarcoma adenoids uterinum*) accompanied by myometrial hypertrophy, the second invaded the endometrial cavity forming a polyp (*Cystosarcoma adenoids uterinum polyposum*), and the third invaded the ovary (*Ein Ovarial-Cystosarcom).*[50] Rokitansky gave the three phenotypes descriptive Latin names following common practice at mid-nineteenth century. He selected the term *sarcoma* to designate a *benign* growth. At mid-nineteenth century, Rokitansky defined sarcoma and carcinoma:

Department of Surgery and the first Director of the Postgraduate Institute of surgery; appointed by His Apostolic Majesty, the Emperor of Austria..."

[42] Erna Lesky, 274. With ready acceptance in Europe of Lister's principles and practice of antisepsis combined with painless surgery afforded by general anesthesia, general surgery and gynecologic surgery assumed academic prominence over pathologic anatomy. Erna Lesky, *The Vienna Medical School of the 19th Century* [Baltimore, MD: Johns Hopkins University Press, 1976], 394. Europeans respected the impressive surgical results that the Englishman Spencer Wells (1818–1897) achieved in his operations for removal of ovarian tumors; surgical results supported by "objective statistical analysis." There occurred a gradual shift from operating dead patients in the morgue to operating live patients in surgery, patients who now survived surgery in increasing numbers. This, in turn, generated need for examination of surgical specimens which led the transition from morbid to microscopic surgical pathology near the end of the century.

[43] Henry E. Sigerist, *Man and Medicine: An Introduction to Medical Knowledge* [New York: WW Norton & Company, 1932], 124.

[44] Carl Rokitansky, *A Manual of Pathological Anatomy*, Volume I. *General Pathological Anatomy* trans. William Edward Swaine [Philadelphia, PA: Blanchard & Lea, 1855], 189, 190.

[45] Klemperer P. Notes on Carl von Rokitansky's autobiography and inaugural address. *Bulletin History Medicine* 1961:374–380:378. In his professorial inaugural address of 1844, Rokitansky revealed the philosophical basis of his actions. "It is the painstaking study with all methods available to anatomic investigations of morphologic alterations according to tangible physical criteria; because soundest knowledge of morbid phenomena is gained by sensual perception of material appearances."

[46] Carl Rokitansky, Ueber Uterusdrüsen-Neubildung in Uterus- und Ovarial-Sarcomen. Zeitschift Gesellschaft der Aerzte in Wien. 1860;16:577–581. "Of the existing connective tissue tumors of the uterus, the round fibroids are to be differentiated from the so called fibrous polyps of the uterus in which glandular tubules are found. These are connective tissue tumors rooted in the basal stroma of the uterus and cannot be shelled out (Paget's continuous growth) in contrast to the well circumscribe fibrous tumors." Carl Rokitansky, Ueber Uterusdrüsen-Neubildung in Uterus- und Ovarial-Sarcomen. Zeitschift Gesellschaft der Aerzte in Wien. 1860;16:577–581. Carl Rokitansky, *A Manual of Pathological Anatomy*, Volume II. *The Abdominal Viscera.* trans. Edward Sieveking [Philadelphia, PA: Blanchard & Lea, 1855], ix. Editor's Preface. Of the difficulties connected with the translation, I will only say that they are much increased by the figurative style of the author. He constantly uses terms in a sense peculiar to himself, and his total disregard for the ordinary rules of composition is an additional and frequent course of obscurity." Translation of Rokitansky's 1860 article was equally difficult.

[47] Given that Rokitansky emphasized the *fresh* specimen, it is a reasonable to assume that the *fresh* surgical specimen caught Rokitansky's attention and not one of the surgical specimens preserved in wine alcohol, nor any of the autopsy specimens.

[48] Owen H. Wangensteen and Sarah D. Wangensteen, *The Rise of Surgery: From Empiric Craft to Scientific Discipline* [Minneapolis, MN: University of Minnesota Press, 1978], 440. Kussmaul spent 4 months assisting Rokitansky in his morgue. "During all that time the only words Rokitansky spoke to him occurred during an interruption of work while the two stood together for a few minutes in the doorway on a fine autumn morning. Rokitansky said: 'Today we have beautiful weather.' The astounded Kussmaul pulled himself together and replied, 'Yes, it is truly a beautiful day.'" Robert Meyer, *Autobiography of Dr. Robert Meyer (1864–1947): A Short Abstract of a Long Life* [New York: Henry Schuman, 1949], 16–17. Meyer recalled his teacher, Adolph Kussmaul. "The most brilliant teacher was the internist, Adolf Kussmaul, known among the gynecologists for his book *The Malformations of the Uterus*. His diagnoses were not far from infallible, so that when he retired in 1887, von Recklinghausen at a banquet could say of him that he had not once been able to reverse a diagnosis after dissecting one of his patients. It was always astonishing how carefully he examined his patients in order to arrive at a diagnosis."

[49] Roland Sedivy, 200 Jahre Rokitansky – sein Vermachtnis fur die heutige Pathologie Wiener Klinische Wochenschrift 2004;116/23:779–787: Table 1, page 780. Histopathology for benign disease never became a routine in Rokitansky's autopsy house.

[50] Carl Rokitansky, Ueber Uterusdrüsen-Neubildung in Uterus- und Ovarial-Sarcomen. Zeitschift Gesellschaft der Aerzte in Wien. 1860;16:577–581.

> Sarcoma and carcinoma…Kindred new growths, important from their frequency no less than from the question arising, in every concrete case, as to their innocency or malignancy. We have selected the term *sarcoma* to designate the benign growths, not because of any especial analogy with muscle-flesh, but in order to fix and define a name familiarized by long usage, and also by no little abuse. The malignant we shall leave in possession of their ancient characteristic appellation *cancer,-carcinoma.*[51]

Rokitansky was well aware that both cellular atypia and invasion were required to diagnose carcinoma (cancer).[52]

From the beginning of their history, endometriosis and adenomyosis have been characterized as benign invasive diseases. Regarding adenomyosis (internal endometriosis), Rokitansky described the "wedge" of benign basal endometrium composed of endometrial glands and stroma that invaded the underlying muscle of the uterine wall.[53]

> On rare occasions the elongation of the uterine glands extend in both directions, towards the uterine cavity as well as into the parenchyma. In this case the incumbent bulge acts as a plug of parallel fibers driven into the uterus. Such a picture was encountered in the thick walled uterus of an older woman. Below the left tubal opening was a club-shaped, smooth polyp, about 1" 2'" long, with a 1 ½'" diameter in the neck, and enlarging to 4–5'" at the free end. A cut through the entire mass showed that the neck penetrated in a wedge-shaped fashion into the uterus to a depth of 4'". The cut surface appears as thready-fibers in its entire length and can be unraveled in that direction. This arrangement is provided by extremely long glandular tubules kept together by a nuclei rich connective tissue.[54]

Rokitansky also distinguished between *benign* solid tumors of the uterus – fibroids and adenomyomas. Adenomyomas composed of endometrial glands and stroma without an outer fibrous capsule invaded deeply within the uterine muscle making their removal difficult. To this benign lesion he gave the descriptive name "*Sarcoma adenoids uterinum*," or in modern terminology, adenomyosis.[55] If this benign lesion degenerated and became cystic, Rokitansky called it "*Cystosarcoma adenoids uterinum*." It cannot be emphasized often enough that Rokitansky defined sarcoma as a *benign* lesion. For other benign glandular tumors that projected into the cavity of the uterus, Rokitansky retained the old name: "Polyp, Uteruspolyp would be distinguished from the round fibroids prolapsed into the uterine cavity."[56] Rokitansky credited prior authorities as having described uterine polyps: H. Müller[57] of Würzburg (1854) [58] and Paget's "continuous growth," the latter descriptive of adenomatous uterine polyps.[59]

Rokitansky also described external endometriosis, a *benign* ovarian endometrioma as an "*ovarian cystosarcoma*."[60]

> d) *An Ovarian – Cystosarcoma.* The autopsy performed on 2, March 1859 on a 68 years old, malnourished female yielded the following: the body is small and thin; both lungs for the most part are adherent, in the right upper lobe there is a walnut sized cavity with extensive, indurated desiccation of the tissue and an incorporated yellow, cheesy nodules. In the lung there are numerous thickened, airless areas infiltrated by tenacious, yellow – brownish pus. The ventricles of the heart contain loose fibrin clots.

---

[51] Carl Rokitansky, *A Manual of Pathological Anatomy*, Volume I. 189, 190.

[52] Carl Rokitansky, *A Manual of Pathological Anatomy*, Volume I. *General Pathological Anatomy.* trans. William Edward Swaine [Philadelphia, PA: Blanchard & Lea, 1855], 189, 190. See also Robert Meyer, *Autobiography of Dr. Robert Meyer (1864–1947): A Short Abstract of a Long Life* [New York: Henry Schuman, 1949], 34. Meyer "stressed the fact that the infiltrative proliferation alone does not necessarily mean malignancy (1903)."

[53] Carl Rokitansky, 1860;16:577–581. See also Emge LA. The elusive adenomyosis of the uterus: its historical past and its present state of recognition. *Am J Obstet Gynecol* 1962;83:1541–1563:1542. "It is just one hundred years ago that there appeared in the *Transactions of the Vienna Medical Society* a report describing unusual proliferative qualities of the endometrial stroma and glands. Its author, the eminent pathologist Carl Rokitansky." Though published in 1962, Ludwig A. Emge delivered the Eleventh Joseph L. Baer Lecture of the Chicago Gynecological Society on 21 October 1960, the 100th anniversary year of the discovery of endometriosis.

[54] Carl Rokitansky, 1860;16:577–581.

[55] Sarcoma adenoids uterinum of Rokitansky is equivalent to adenomyoma of von Recklinghausen which is equivalent to diffuse adenomyoma of Cullen and equivalent to the term internal endometriosis.

[56] Carl Rokitansky, Ueber Uterusdrüsen-Neubildung in Uterus- und Ovarial-Sarcomen. Zeitschift Gesellschaft der Aerzte in Wien. 1860;16:577–581.

[57] This was not Johannes Peter Müller (1801–1858).

[58] Carl Rokitansky, 1860;16:577–581. His reference to Müller reads: "The mucosa hypertrophies in one or more circumscribed places accompanied by elongation of glands producing the bulge." (H. Müller: Verhandl. D. Phys. Med. Gesellschaft in Würzburg, 4.1854.)

[59] Carl Rokitansky, Ueber Uterusdrüsen-Neubildung in Uterus- und Ovarial-Sarcomen. Zeitschift Gesellschaft der Aerzte in Wien. 1860;16:577–581. Rokitansky's reference to Paget reads: "Of the existing connective tissue tumors of the uterus, the round fibroids are to be differentiated from the so called fibrous polyps of the uterus in which glandular tubules are found. These are connective tissue tumors rooted in the basal stroma of the uterus and cannot be shelled out (Paget's continuous growth) in contrast to

The liver is enlarged and fatty, the spleen s small, the stomach, bowels and kidneys are pale; in the capsule of the left kidney there is a white fibroid node and the bladder is empty. A small, retroflexed uterus is situated in the left recto-vaginal space whereas its fundus is wedged between the cervix and the left ovarian tumor. The latter is degenerated to a fist sized tumor, the right half presents as a dense, fibrous mass, whereas the left half consists of an aggregate of serous cysts. The largest of the cysts partially protruded into a cavity of the fibrous mass. The remaining small cysts were adherent to the rest of the surface. The entire tumor was twisted by its sheltered position so that the cystic portion pointed to the right. The tube was somewhat stretched over the tumor and fixed to it up to its fimbriated end. The right ovary was dense, atrophied and contained a bean sized cyst which protruded through the surface. Closer examination of the fibrous part of the tumor disclosed on cross-section, especially around the cysts, a glandular appearance with scattered, delicate vesicles and grainy nodules. In addition, it contained individual mucous containing cysts of millet – hemp corn size. The microscopic examination revealed numerous tubular, epithelial lined structures within a thick, connective tissue layer. On cross section of these tubular structures, individual slit-like, lacunar clefts were evident into which papillary excrescences of connective tissue intruded.

Rokitansky drew conclusions from his observations: Conclusions 1–4 related to *sarcoma adenoides uterinum* and *cystosarcoma adenoides uterinum.* Conclusion 5 relates to the degenerated left ovary and Conclusion 6 relates to the right ovary as well as the left ovary.

5. Sarcoma tissue in the form of papillary excrescences grow into the space of the cyst-like, degenerated tubules. The slit-like, lacunar clefts scattered within the sarcoma produce on cross section a granular appearance. The circumscribed nodes, which can be shelled out, and appear incorporated in the sarcoma mass doubtless originate from the filling of the greater cyst spaces by intruding tumor tissue – A common appearance, which is especially pronounced in cystosarcoma adenoides mammarium.

6. A sarcoma, containing uterine glandular tubules is also found in the ovaries and some cystic structures of the ovaries, therefore become a *Cystosarcoma adenoides uterinum.*

Recall once more that Rokitansky defined the term sarcoma as a *benign* lesion. "We have selected the term *sarcoma* to designate the benign growths, not because of any especial analogy with muscle-flesh, but in order to fix and define a name familiarized by long usage, and also by no little abuse."[61]

With a few strokes of his pen, Rokitansky described several phenotypes of benign endometriosis. He established the objective diagnostic criteria for adenomyosis and endometriosis, the presence of endometrial glands and stroma by which endometriotic diseases have been defined ever since. The very definition of endometriosis – the microscopic identification of *excess* endometrial glands and stroma located in ectopic locations – is based on Rokitansky's research. By the same strokes of his pen, Rokitansky established pathology as the premier basic science for gynecology and for endometriosis research for the next 100 years.

In 1861, Rokitansky discussed adenomyomas in the third volume of his Textbook of Pathological Anatomy.[62] He observed several types of "*omas*" (benign tumors), which he classified as distinct phenotypes of endometriosis: benign solid and cystic intramural uterine adenomy*omas*, benign solid intracavitary uterine aden*omas*, and a benign cystic ovarian endometri*oma.* All were composed of excess müllerian tissue acquired after birth. Rokitansky set a precedent when he used the descriptive suffix "oma," meaning a tumor or neoplasm, to denote the appearance of endometriotic lesions, both uterine and extrauterine. All investigators, from Rokitansky until Sampson's pathbreaking research in

the well circumscribed fibrous tumors. They commonly develop within or form the submucosal stratum and grow into the uterine cavity as so called polyps of various shapes (cylindric-, pear – or club shaped) and are covered by an adherent uterine mucosa. The various changes in its texture may appear identical to the changes seen as a result of chronic inflammation. In contrast to the easily removable fibrous tumors, we commonly consider these connective tissue tumors as *sarcoma,* here specifically as *uterus sarcoma.* These tumors growing into a mucosal cavity generally retain their old name of *polyp* and *uterus polyp* and, according to the discussion above, would be distinguished from the round fibroids prolapse into the uterine cavity."

[60] Carl Rokitansky, Ueber Uterusdrüsen-Neubildung in Uterus- und Ovarial-Sarcomen. Zeitschift Gesellschaft der Aerzte in Wien. 1860;16:577–581. "A sarcoma containing uterine glandular tubules is also found in the ovaries and some cystic structures of the ovaries, therefore become *Cystosarcoma adenoids uterinum.*"

[61] Carl Rokitansky, *A Manual of Pathological Anatomy*, Volume I. *General Pathological Anatomy* trans. William Edward Swaine [Philadelphia, PA: Blanchard & Lea, 1855], 189, 190.

[62] Carl Rokitansky, *Lehrbuch der pathologischen Anatomie* [Wien: Braumüller, 1861], III: 475–490.

the 1920s, saw only solid and cystic endometriotic "oma" tumors. Until Sampson, pathologists and surgeons saw only the "oma search image" that Rokitansky had prepared them to see.[63]

The story leading up to Rokitansky's discovery has chronicled his extensive experience, his educated medical gaze and exacting observation and his prepared mind. Commencing with his criticism of 1846, Rudolph Virchow influenced Rokitansky over the next decade and a half. Virchow reinforced the importance of microscopic cellular pathology as the key to the discovery and histological definition of endometriosis. From the start, technology influenced the emergence of knowledge regarding endometriosis and all benign müllerian diseases.

Rokitansky identified and described uterine and extrauterine endometriosis two decades before refrigeration systems were installed in European morgues to retard decomposition.[64] Even then the state of decay must have varied in direct proportion to the length of time between death and autopsy. Such were the conditions that in all probability long delayed the differentiation of uterine endometriosis from degenerated uterine fibroids and cancer, [65] and ovarian endometriomas from non-endometriotic chocolate cysts.[66] Regarding simple ovarian cysts, Rokitansky observed in 1846 that they may contain "an opaque chocolate-colored or inky fluid."[67] Undoubtedly, some of them were ovarian endometriomas, ovarian cysts lined by ectopic endometrial glands and stroma containing old menstrual blood.

Rokitansky's magnificent *Handbook of Pathological Anatomy* and his report of the new diseases endometriosis and adenomyosis in 1860 was based on dissections performed in "miserable quarters" of the old Leichenhaus, the University of Vienna autopsy house.[68] Considering the protocol for rapid evisceration of corpses under such circumstances, combined with limited light making it difficult to see into the depths of the pelvis, it is not surprising that Rokitansky first identified endometriosis in visceral organs – uterus and ovary – *after* removal from the pelvis. Extrauterine endometriosis in the deep pelvis awaited detection until the end of the nineteenth century when asepsis permitted safer surgery and surgical pathology afforded clinical pathological correlation. In sum, Rokitansky not only described adenomyosis and endometriosis microscopically – detailing the presence of endometrial glands and stroma; he differentiated uterine endometriosis (adenomyomas) from uterine fibroids, described ovarian endometriosis, gave the disease descriptive Latin names, and suggested chronic inflammation as possibly

---

63 Colin Tudge with Josh Young, *The Link: Uncovering Our Earliest Ancestor* [New York: Little, Brown and Company, 2009], 192, 193.

64 Vanessa R. Schwarz, *Spectacular Realities: Early Mass Culture in Fin-de-Siecle Paris* [Berkeley, CA: University of California Press, 1999], 49, 58. The first morgue in Paris was built in 1718. In 1864, 3 years after Rokitansky identified and described uterine endometriosis, a new Paris Morgue was built behind Notre-Dame on the quai de l'Archeveche. This morgue "can be seen in the context of growing state interest in and responsibility for the dead and as part of an ever-increasing reliance on the 'expert knowledge' of a professionalized corps of doctors of forensic medicine." But it was not until 1882 that "the administration installed a system for the refrigeration of the corpses-a system that slowed their decay and thus extended display time…The new refrigeration system, modeled on one developed for the transport of meat to markets, 'has served as a model for all the large European cities.'"

65 Carl Rokitansky, *A Manual of Pathological Anatomy*, Volume I. *General Pathological Anatomy* trans. William Edward Swaine [Philadelphia, PA: Blanchard & Lea, 1855]. "In an extended sense, the collective term *fibroid texture* may be made to comprise all fibrous tissues, the development of which has been already delineated, and the occurrence of which as a more or less essential component of various new growths, it becomes our business to discuss." "Nowhere is the insufficiency of a mere anatomical principle more felt than here - a principle which would need occasion us to class side by side, the most heterogeneous new growths, for example, fibro-carcinoma and the perfectly benign fibroid tumor."

66 Carl Rokitansky, *A Manual of Pathological Anatomy*, Volume I. *General Pathological Anatomy* trans. William Edward Swaine [Philadelphia, PA: Blanchard & Lea, 1855], 168. "Let us begin with the results of an examination with the naked eye of perfect cysts, and in particular of the exquisite specimens so frequently met with in the ovaries…We have the simple (unicancellated) and the compound cyst (Müller's compound cystoid)." Carl Rokitansky, *A Manual of Pathological Anatomy*, Volume I. *General Pathological Anatomy.* trans. William Edward Swaine [Philadelphia, PA: Blanchard & Lea, 1855], 34. [Author's] Introduction. "The female sex greatly favors the occurrence, in the sexual system, of cystoids, of cystosarcoma, of the majority of cancerous growths."

67 Carl Rokitansky, *A Manual of Pathological Anatomy*, Volume II. *The Abdominal Viscera.* trans. Edward Sieveking [Philadelphia, PA: Blanchard & Lea, 1855], 248, 249. Chapter III. Abnormalities of the Female Sexual Organs.

68 Roswell Park, *An Epitome of the History of Medicine*, 2nd ed. [Philadelphia: FA Davis Company, 1908], 250–1. One year later a magnificent new Institute of Pathological Anatomy was erected specially for him, a building Rokitansky had demanded for years. Erna Lesky published illustrations of

the pathogenesis of *Sarcoma adenoids uterinum*, *Cystosarcoma adenoids uterinum*, *Cystosarcoma adenoids uterinum polyposum*, and *Ein Ovarial-Cystosarcom.*[69]

Two New Diseases with Descriptive Names

What is the importance of a name? Based on ontological theory of specific diseases, a descriptive name for an entity such as "*Sarcoma adenoids uterinum*,"[70] establishes a new disease, separate and distinct from other diseases, thereby focusing the attention of other physicians and investigators to identify similar cases.[71] Equally important to discovering and naming a new disease is the professional stature of the author. Rokitansky possessed an international reputation when he described adenomyomas in 1860, which was an important reason for general acceptance of his findings. Endometriosis was a nameless disease before Rokitansky.[72]

What did physicians perceive before Rokitansky diagnosed endometriosis? We have information in only one instance. One physician perceived and removed a uterine polyp, the fresh specimen that caught Rokitansky's attention. What were the patient's complaints before Rokitansky examined specimens that had been removed from their bodies at autopsy and diagnosed endometriosis? There is no record. However, from clinical experience, the author can be reasonably certain that one patient experienced "labor pains" as she delivered a fist-sized uterine polyp. Once named in 1860, the study of endometriosis took on a life of its own. But it was not until 1896 that Freund of Strassburg – and some years later Cullen of Baltimore – described patient's complaints and the physical signs of uterine endometriosis detectable by physicians.

In support of Rokitansky as discover of endometriosis and adenomyosis, the author's interpretation of the criteria of the eminent surgeon Owen H. Wangensteen may be applied: "(1) who showed the way; (2) continuance of the practice; (3) influence of the discovery on contemporary and current practice."[73] In other words: (1) who discovered endometriosis, gave a detailed description, published the findings, and was cited and acknowledged as the discoverer by subsequent investigators;[74] (2) did other pathologists continued to diagnose uterine endometriosis by the same techniques as Rokitansky: macroscopic

Rokitansky's postmortem rooms from his student days until 1862 and of his new institute. Author's note: Thus we are reassured by Erna Lesky that Rokitansky identified uterine and extrauterine endometriosis in his old "primitive" Leichenhaus described by Roswell Park. Erna Lesky, *The Vienna Medical School of the 19th Century* [Baltimore, MD: Johns Hopkins University Press, 1976], 262. "Rokitansky received an institute of pathological anatomy in 1862, something he had demanded persistently for thirty-years; in 1868 laboratory space for experimental pathology also was made available in this building. In 1874 a separate institute was founded for medical chemistry, and in 1873 one for embryology." Erna Lesky, *The Vienna Medical School of the 19th Century* [Baltimore, MD: Johns Hopkins University Press, 1976], Illustration 20. "Rokitansky's post-mortem rooms." Illustration 21. Rokitansky's new Institute of Pathological Anatomy. Both illustrations are at the back of the book.

[69] Carl Rokitansky, Ueber Uterusdrüsen-Neubildung in Uterus- und Ovarial-Sarcomen. Zeitschift Gesellschaft der Aerzte in Wien. 1860;16:577–581. "The various changes in its texture may appear identical to the changes seen as a result of chronic inflammation…In view of the above discussion, it is important to recognize the changes occurring in the mucosa and the submucosal stratum of the uterus as consequences of chronic inflammation…7. The ones in question and the mucosa lined uterine polyps as a whole undergo changes in their texture which similarly occur in the uterine mucosa in the course or as the end result of chronic inflammation." For many years the eminent gynecologic pathologist, Robert Meyer, would also believe chronic inflammation the pathogenesis for uterine endometriosis; eventually he changed his opinion.

[70] Carl Rokitansky, 1860;16:577–581.

[71] Knud Faber, *Nosography in Modern Internal Medicine* [New York: Paul B. Hoeber, Inc., 1923], 8–15, 37–39, 45, 53–54.

[72] Ziporyn, Terra. *Nameless Diseases*. New Brunswick, NJ: Rutgers University Press, 1992:36–39. A disease remains nameless until recognized, described, and named by a medical scientist or medical practitioner. Similarly, in clinical practice a disease in the patient remains nameless until correctly diagnosed by her medical practitioner.

[73] Owen H. Wangensteen and Sarah D. Wangensteen, *The Rise of Surgery: From Empiric Craft to Scientific Discipline* [Minneapolis, MN: University of Minnesota Press, 1978], 438. "In 1969 the senior author outlined three criteria to decide the role of discover: (1) who first showed the way; (2) continuance of the practice; (3) influence of the discovery upon contemporary and current practice."

[74] Emge LA. The elusive adenomyosis of the uterus: its historical past and its present state of recognition. *Am J Obstet Gynecol* 1962;83:1541–1563. Although Rokitansky only gave internal endometriosis a descriptive name, "*cystosarcoma adenoids uterinum*," and not a proper name such as adenomyosis, Emge – a life-time student of adenomyosis – contended: "the honor of having rendered the first detailed description of adenomyosis, or internal endometriosis, rightly goes to him."

description and histopathology?[75] (3) Taking influence on practice to mean treatment of patients, did Rokitansky's discovery influence clinical practice?[76]

Rokitansky met the criteria of Wangensteen. First, Rokitansky discovered and described uterine endometriosis (adenomyoma, adenomyosis) and extrauterine endometriosis (ovarian endometriosis) and his priority has been acknowledged into the twenty-first century.[77] Second, innumerable pathologists have identified internal endometriosis – adenomyosis – using the diagnostic criteria established by Rokitansky. His former assistant Hans Chiari described tubal endometriosis (salpingitis isthmica nodosa). Third, through Chiari, Rokitansky influenced the eminent German pathologist von Recklinghausen and the German gynecologist Wilhelm A. Freund; the latter wrote the first clinical description of the disease uterine adenomyoma in 1896, a description that empowered physicians to make a presumptive diagnosis of uterine adenomyoma in the office. In evidence, von Recklinghausen cited: "Rokitansky's Cystosarcoma adenoides uterinum" in 1893[78]; Rokitansky's "Lehrbuch der pathology. Anatomie. 1861. III. 475 u. 490" and "H. Chiari, Zur pathology. Anatomie d. Eileiterkatarrhs. Prager Zeitschr. F. Heilkunde. 1887. VIII. 457" in 1896.[79]

Then the personal criteria of Robert Scully, the doyen of gynecologic pathology, may be considered. Scully held identification of two cases of a disease to be both necessary and sufficient proof to establish a new disease entity.[80] By Scully's criteria, Rokitansky did not establish new disease entities in 1860. Rokitansky described one case of uterine endometriosis (adenomyosis) and one case of extrauterine endometriosis (bilateral ovarian endometriomas) as well as several cases of uterine polyps.

Henry Sigerist noted that pathology, like anatomy and physiology, is a natural science that "describes natural phenomena, arranges them in systems and inquires into their origin." Viewed from the perspective of the social historian, Sigerist, there are four levels of pathological investigation embracing three analytic questions and one synthetic question. With respect to the disease endometriosis, Rokitansky might have asked three analytic questions: (1) what is its etiology, (2) its pathological anatomy, and (3) its pathologic physiology; and one synthetic question: what is its pathogenesis?[81] Rokitansky did not enquire into etiology or pathologic physiology, but he did describe macroscopic and microscopic pathological anatomy and he speculated on an inflammatory pathogenesis for adenomyosis. See Appendix II for the full translation of Carl Rokitansky's *New Growth of Uterine Glands in Sarcomas of the Uterus and Ovaries*.[82]

In 2011, Benagiano and Brosens offered what they believed would be two "uncontroversial criteria" upon which to attribute the discovery of endometriosis and adenomyosis. "We believe that the identification of the pathology we today distinguish in peritoneal, deep, and ovarian endometriosis and in adenomyosis must be based on two objective criteria: the observation of the presence of endometrial glands and stroma outside the uterine cavity and the specification that this invasion was 'benign' (non-neoplastic) in nature."[83]

---

[75] Emge LA. The elusive adenomyosis of the uterus: its historical past and its present state of recognition. *Am J Obstet Gynecol* 1962;83:1541–1563:1542. According to Emge, Virchow did identify stromal endometriosis in 1864, 3 years after Rokitansky identified adenomyosis. Emge did not give a reference to Virchow's contribution.

[76] Owen H. Wangensteen and Sarah D. Wangensteen, *The Rise of Surgery: From Empiric Craft to Scientific Discipline* [Minneapolis, MN: University of Minnesota Press, 1978], 438.

[77] Hudelist G, Keckstein J, Wright JT. The migrating adenomyoma: past views on the etiology of adenomyosis ad endometriosis. *Fertil Steril* 2009;92:1536–43.

[78] Recklinghausen F. Uber die Adenocysten der Uterustumoren und Ueberreste des Wolff'schen Organs. Deutsche Medicinische Wochenschrift 1893;xix:825–826.

[79] Friedrich v. Recklinghausen, Die Adenomyome und Cystadenome der Uterus- und Tubenwandung ihre Abkunft von Resten des Wolff'schen Korpers. Im Anhang: Von W. A. Freund, Klinische Notizen zu den voluminosen Adenomyomen des Uterus [Berlin: Verlag von August Hirschwald, 1896.]

[80] Juan Rosai, A tribute to Robert E. Scully on his 80th Birthday. Seminars in Diagnostic Pathology. 2001;18:151–154. "Sometimes the question arises as to how many cases of an undescribed entity somebody needs to see before concluding that one is dealing with something 'new.'" Dr. Scully, known to the world at large as "Mr. Gynecologic Pathology… gave me once the answer as it applies to himself when joking about the fact that he keeps a box of slides (he did not say whether in his office or in his head), each of them from a case that he thinks represents an undescribed entity, and he is simply waiting for the second case to come along and prove it."

[81] Henry E. Sigerist, *Man and Medicine: An Introduction to Medical Knowledge* [New York: WW Norton & Company, 1932], 127.

[82] Carl Rokitansky, Ueber Uterusdrüsen-Neubildung in Uterus- und Ovarial-Sarcomen. Zeitschift Gesellschaft der Aerzte in Wien. 1860;16:577–581.

[83] Benagiano G, Brosens I. Who identified endometriosis? *Fertil Steril* 2011;95:13–16.

Benagiano and Brosens' objective criterion one – "the observation of the presence of endometrial glands and stroma outside the uterine cavity"[84] – was fulfilled for adenomyosis in 1860 by Rokitansky, which disease he named *sarcoma adenoides uterinum* and cysto*sarcoma adenoides uterinum.*

> On rare occasions the elongation of the uterine glands extend in both directions, towards the uterine cavity as well as into the parenchyma. In this case the incumbent bulge acts as a plug of parallel fibers driven into the uterus. Such a picture was encountered in the thick walled uterus of an older woman. Below the left tubal opening was a club-shaped, smooth polyp, about 1ii 2iii long, with a 1 ½"' diameter in the neck, and enlarging to 4–5"' at the free end. A cut through the entire mass showed that the neck penetrated in a wedge-shaped fashion into the uterus to a depth of 4"'. The cut surface appears as thready-fibers in its entire length and can be unraveled in that direction. This arrangement is provided by extremely long glandular tubules kept together by a nuclei rich connective tissue.[85]

In 2006, Benagiano and Brosens accepted Rokitansky's discovery and histologic description of adenomyosis (adenomyoma) and his name for the disease: cysto*sarcoma adenoides uterinum*: "…the first description of the condition initially named 'adenomyoma' was that provided in 1860 by the German pathologist Carl von Rokitansky, who found endometrial glands in the myometrium and designated this finding as 'cystosarcoma adenoids uterinum.'"[86]

Benagiano and Brosens' objective criterion one also was fulfilled for (ovarian) endometriosis in 1860 by Rokitansky, which disease he named *Ovarial-Sarcomen* and *Ovarial-Cystosarcom.*[87] Recall that Rokitansky described external endometriosis and ovarian endometrioma as an "*ovarian cystosarcoma*."

> d) *An Ovarian – Cystosarcoma.* The autopsy performed on 2, March 1859 on a 68 years old, malnourished female yielded the following: the body is small and thin; both lungs for the most part are adherent, in the right upper lobe there is a walnut sized cavity with extensive, indurated desiccation of the tissue and an incorporated yellow, cheesy nodules. In the lung there are numerous thickened, airless areas infiltrated by tenacious, yellow – brownish pus. The ventricles of the heart contain loose fibrin clots. The liver is enlarged and fatty, the spleen s small, the stomach, bowels and kidneys are pale; in the capsule of the left kidney there is a white fibroid node and the bladder is empty. A small, retroflexed uterus is situated in the left recto-vaginal space whereas its fundus is wedged between the cervix and the left ovarian tumor. The latter is degenerated to a fist sized tumor, the right half presents as a dense, fibrous mass, whereas the left half consists of an aggregate of serous cysts. The largest of the cysts partially protruded into a cavity of the fibrous mass. The remaining small cysts were adherent to the rest of the surface. The entire tumor was twisted by its sheltered position so that the cystic portion pointed to the right. The tube was somewhat stretched over the tumor and fixed to it up to its fimbriated end. The right ovary was dense, atrophied and contained a bean sized cyst which protruded through the surface. Closer examination of the fibrous part of the tumor disclosed on cross-section, especially around the cysts, a glandular appearance with scattered, delicate vesicles and grainy nodules. In addition, it contained individual mucous containing cysts of millet – hemp corn size. The microscopic examination revealed numerous tubular, epithelial lined structures within a thick, connective tissue layer. On cross section of these tubular structures, individual slit-like, lacunar clefts were evident into which papillary excrescences of connective tissue intruded.[88]

Rokitansky drew conclusions from his observations: Conclusion 6 relates to the right ovary as well as the left ovary.

> 6. A sarcoma, containing uterine glandular tubules is also found in the ovaries and some cystic structures of the ovaries, therefore become a *Cystosarcoma adenoides uterinum.*[89]

Note that Rokitansky equated the histology of the "uterine glandular tubules" found in the ovaries to the uterine glandular tubules of adenomyosis in the uterus: *Cystosarcoma adenoides uterinum.* In other words, both adenomyosis and ovarian endometriosis exhibited the same histologic structure.

Benagiano and Brosens' objective criterion two – "the specification that this invasion was 'benign' (non-neoplastic) in nature"[90] – was fulfilled for adenomyosis

[84] Benagiano G, Brosens I. Who identified endometriosis? *Fertil Steril* 2011;95:13–16.

[85] Carl Rokitansky, Ueber Uterusdrüsen-Neubildung in Uterus- und Ovarial-Sarcomen. Zeitschift Gesellschaft der Aerzte in Wien. 1860;16:577–581.

[86] Benagiano G, Brosens I. History of adenomyosis. *Best Pract Res Clin Obstet Gynecol* 2006;20:449–63.

[87] Carl Rokitansky, Ueber Uterusdrüsen-Neubildung in Uterus- und Ovarial-Sarcomen. Zeitschift Gesellschaft der Aerzte in Wien. 1860;16:577–581.

[88] Carl Rokitansky, Ueber Uterusdrüsen-Neubildung in Uterus- und Ovarial-Sarcomen. Zeitschift Gesellschaft der Aerzte in Wien. 1860;16:577–581. "A sarcoma containing uterine glandular tubules is also found in the ovaries and some cystic structures of the ovaries, therefore become *Cystosarcoma adenoids uterinum*."

[89] Carl Rokitansky, Ueber Uterusdrüsen-Neubildung in Uterus- und Ovarial-Sarcomen. Zeitschift Gesellschaft der Aerzte in Wien. 1860;16:577–581.

[90] Benagiano G, Brosens I. Who identified endometriosis? *Fertil Steril* 2011;95:13–16.

in 1860 by Rokitansky; he named this disease *sarcoma adenoides uterinum* and cysto*sarcoma adenoides uterinum*. Benagiano and Brosens' objective criterion two also was fulfilled for endometriosis, which disease Rokitansky named *ovarian cystosarcoma*. Rokitansky was well aware that both cellular atypia and invasion were required to diagnose carcinoma (cancer).[91] Rokitansky was repeatedly influenced by Virchow, so much so, that in 1859 he permitted Virchow's lectures on cellular pathology to be taught in his Department of Pathology at the University of Vienna. "In the winter semester of 1859–60…Klob, Rokitansky's assistant in Vienna, posted on his blackboard the following notice: 'From Thursday on, lectures on pathological anatomy will be delivered according to the cell doctrine of Virchow.'"[92] Furthermore, Rokitansky, the first full-time professor of pathology defined sarcoma as "benign growths" and carcinoma as "malignant" at mid-nineteenth century:

> Sarcoma and carcinoma…Kindred new growths, important from their frequency no less than from the question arising, in every concrete case, as to their innocency or malignancy. We have selected the term *sarcoma* to designate the benign growths, not because of any especial analogy with muscle-flesh, but in order to fix and define a name familiarized by long usage, and also by no little abuse. The malignant we shall leave in possession of their ancient characteristic appellation *cancer,-carcinoma.*[93]

This English translation from Rokitansky's *A Manual of Pathological Anatomy*, Volume I was published by the prestigious Sydenham Society in 1855, just 5 years before Rokitansky discovered and described adenomyosis and ovarian endometriosis.

Rokitansky deserves full credit for the discovery of endometriosis and adenomyosis as well as for establishing them as new disease entities. His prodigious reputation was responsible for their recognition as new diseases and his publications of 1860 and 1861 were the printed medium for its dissemination.[94] Considering the long interval of observation required of the gifted Rokitansky to discover adenomyosis and endometriosis, a persuasive argument may be mounted that it is unlikely that anyone in the generation immediately preceding him or in more remote generations discovered either disease and fulfilled the criteria of discovery of Wangensteen, Sigerist, or Benagiano and Brosens. Several authorities credit Rokitansky for the discovery of adenomyosis (*sarcoma adenoides uterinum* and *cystosarcoma adenoides uterinum*): von Recklinghausen,[95] Cullen,[96] Emge,[97] Benagiano and Brosens,[98] and Hudelist, Keckstein, and Wright.[99] Other authorities credit Rokitansky for the

---

[91] Carl Rokitansky, *A Manual of Pathological Anatomy*, Volume I. *General Pathological Anatomy* trans. William Edward Swaine [Philadelphia, PA: Blanchard & Lea, 1855], 189, 190. See also Robert Meyer, *Autobiography of Dr. Robert Meyer (1864–1947): A Short Abstract of a Long Life* [New York: Henry Schuman, 1949], 34. Meyer "stressed the fact that the infiltrative proliferation alone does not necessarily mean malignancy (1903)."

[92] Fielding H. Garrison, *Contributions to The History of Medicine.* [New York: Hafner Publishing Company, 1966], 190. "In the winter semester of 1859–60…Klob, Rokitansky's assistant in Vienna, posted on his blackboard the following notice: 'From Thursday on, lectures on pathological anatomy will be delivered according to the cell doctrine of Virchow.'" Erna Lesky, *The Vienna Medical School of the 19th Century* [Baltimore, MD: Johns Hopkins University Press, 1976], 172. By the late 1850s, cellular pathology was taught in Vienna and "even in Rokitansky's own institute." Lesky, p. 112. "Rokitansky was not a professional microscopist. The task that his time posed before him was of a macromorphological nature and as a macromorphopathologist he fulfilled it. From the very beginning, however, he considered it to be the task of pathological anatomy to raise pathology to physiological pathology. This comprehensive concept as held by Rokitansky makes it possible to understand why he, being a genuine macromorphologist, not only encouraged the development of medical chemistry, and pathological histology, but also that of experimental pathology, and why he acquainted his school with these methods of research when he had exhausted his own method. This took place in the middle of the fifties. The year 1858 marked the beginning of the epoch of cellular pathology."

[93] Carl Rokitansky, *A Manual of Pathological Anatomy*, Volume I. *General Pathological Anatomy.* trans.

William Edward Swaine [Philadelphia, PA: Blanchard & Lea, 1855], 189, 190.

[94] Carl Rokitansky, Ueber Uterusdrüsen-Neubildung in Uterus- und Ovarial-Sarcomen. Zeitschift Gesellschaft der Aerzte in Wien. 1860;16:577–581. Carl Rokitansky, Lehrbuch der Pathologischen Anatomie III. Auflage 1855–1861. III. Band p. 488–491.

[95] Recklinghausen F. Uber die Adenocysten der Uterustumoren und Ueberreste des Wolff'schen Organs. Deutsche Medicinische Wochenschrift 1893;xix:825–826. See also: Friedrich v. Recklinghausen, *Die Adenomyome und Cystadenome der Uterus- und Tubenwandung ihre Abkunft von Resten des Wolff'schen Korpers. Im Anhang:* Von W. A. Freund, *Klinische Notizen zu den voluminosen Adenomyomen des Uterus* [Berlin: Verlag von August Hirschwald, 1896.]

[96] Cullen, Thomas S. Adeno-myoma uteri diffusum benignum. Johns Hopkins Hospital Reports, 1897, vol. vi, p. 133. Cullen, Thomas Stephen. *Cancer of the Uterus: Its Pathology, Symptomatology, Diagnosis, and Treatment. Also the Pathology of Diseases of the Endometrium.* New York: D. Appleton and Company, 1900: 535–536. Rokitansky is mentioned in the text, but not in the index. Cullen, Thomas Stephen. *Adenomyoma of the Uterus.* Philadelphia: WB

discovery of ovarian endometriosis: Pick, [100] Sampson,[101] and Hudelist, Keckstein, and Wright.[102]

In fact, Sampson noted in 1925: "When these endometrial hematomas or cysts were described by me in 1921, I was not aware that they had been previously recognized and described. Three years later I found that Pick had described them in 1905 and had designated them adenoma or cystoma endometroides ovarii. Pick suggest that these cysts may be the same as Rokitansky's cystosarcoma adenoides ovarii uterinum, described by the latter in his textbook of pathologic anatomy published in 1861. Should anyone's name be attached to these ovarian cysts, it should be Pick's or Rokitansky's, not mine."[103]

However, some authors such as Ridley[104] and Knapp[105] disagree. Ridley was the gynecologist who demonstrated experimentally that shed human endometrium could be transplanted into the patient's abdominal wall to cause external endometriosis.[106] In his 1968 review of the histogenesis of endometriosis, Ridley stated that he reviewed the writings and references in a "pamphlet" of Breus[107] and found "several references" that antedated Rokitansky's 1860 description of an adenomyoma.[108] Breus was concerned with the developmental pathology and embryology of the female reproductive organs and with cystic uterine fibroids and adenomyomas, some of huge proportions.[109] He described two of great size,[110] one the size

Saunders Company, 1908. Cullen, Thomas Stephen. *Cancer of the Uterus: Its Pathology, Symptomatology, Diagnosis, and Treatment. Also the Pathology of Diseases of the Endometrium.* Philadelphia: WB Saunders Company, 1909: 535–536. The 1909 edition seems to be a reprint of the 1900 edition, with minor changes, but with a different publisher. A minor change: Rokitansky is mentioned in the text *and* in the index.

[97] Emge LA. The elusive adenomyosis of the uterus: its historical past and its present state of recognition. Am J Obstet Gynecol 1962;83:1541–1563. Although Rokitansky only gave internal endometriosis a descriptive name, "*cystosarcoma adenoids uterinum*," and not a proper name such as adenomyosis, Emge – a lifetime student of adenomyosis – contended: "the honor of having rendered the first detailed description of adenomyosis, or internal endometriosis, rightly goes to him."

[98] Benagiano G, Brosens I. History of adenomyosis. *Best Pract Res Clin Obstet Gynecol* 2006;20:449–63. Interestingly, the same authors in 1991 do not mention Rokitansky. See: Benagiano G, Brosens I. The history of endometriosis: Identifying the disease. *Hum Reprod* 1991;6:963–8.

[99] Hudelist G, Keckstein J, Wright JT. The migrating adenomyoma: past views on the etiology of adenomyosis and endometriosis. *Fertil Steril* 2009;92:1536–43.

[100] Pick L. Ueber Neubildungen am Genitale bei Zwittern nebst Beitragen zur Lehre von den Adenomen des Hodens und Eierstockes. Arch f Gynaek 1905;lxxvi:251–275. On page 262, Pick cites Rokitansky: "1) Vielleicht ist diese Geschwulstform identisch mid dem alten Rokitansky-schen Cystosarcoma adeoides ovarii uterinum. (Lehrb. D. pathology. Anatom. III. Aufl. Bd.III. 1861. Wien. S. 423, 431).

[101] Sampson JA. Heterotopic or misplaced endometrial tissue. *Am J Obstet Gynecol* 1925;10:649–664:655.

[102] Hudelist G, Keckstein J, Wright JT. The migrating adenomyoma: past views on the etiology of adenomyosis and endometriosis. *Fertil Steril* 2009;92:1536–43.

[103] Sampson JA. Heterotopic or misplaced endometrial tissue. *Am J Obstet Gynecol* 1925;10:649–664:655.

[104] John H. Ridley, The histogenesis of endometriosis: A review of facts and fancies. *Obstetrical and Gynecological Survey* 1968;23:1–35.

[105] Knapp VJ. How old is endometriosis? Late 17th- and 18-century European descriptions of the disease. *Fertility Sterility* 1999;72:10–14.

[106] John H. Ridley, The validity of Sampson's theory of endometriosis. *American Journal Obstetrics Gynecology* 1961;82:777–82.

[107] C. Breus, Pamphlets-Liepzig und Wien-Pamphlet Vol. 4054 - Army Med. Library, Washington, DC While in Washington, DC, I attempted to get this pamphlet [Ridley's reference number 10] but was unsuccessful. However I was successful in obtaining a pamphlet by C. Breus [Ridley's reference number 9] that fits the description and which I believe is the same publication that Ridley refers to in his reference number 10. In short, I believe that Pamphlet Vol. 4054 by Breus and the 1894 pamphlet by Breus are one and the same publication. Carl Breus, *Uber Wahre Epithel Führende Cystenbildung in Uterusmyomen* [Leipzig und Wien: Franz Deuticke, 1894], 1–36. Appended are 25 pages of advertisements, a good source for contemporary books and data. In 1894, Breus was Privatdocent in Obstetrics and Gynecology at the University of Vienna. Appropriately, this small pamphlet on developmental pathology was dedicated to the memory of Hans Kundrat, former assistant to Rokitansky who was the second pathologist to succeed to Rokitansky's chair as professor of pathological anatomy in Vienna. This volume was borrowed from The John Crerar Library in Chicago. Breus mentioned Kiwisch, Klinische Vortrage. II. Auflage. 1852. 1. Abtheilung, p. 389. The author was unable to obtain this document.

[108] John H. Ridley, The histogenesis of endometriosis: A review of facts and fancies. *Obstetrical and Gynecological Survey* 1968;23:1–35.

[109] Carl Breus, *Uber Wahre Epithel Führende Cystenbildung in Uterusmyomen* [Leipzig und Wien: Franz Deuticke,1894]. On pages 20, 21, Breus discussed congenital anomalies, embryonic rests; on pages 19, 23, 24 vestiges of the Gartner, Wolffian, and Müllerian ducts with an illustration on page 25.

[110] Carl Breus, 26, figure 7. Cuthbert Lockyer, *Fibroids and Allied Tumours (Myoma and Adenomyoma): Their Pathology, Clinical Features and Surgical Treatment* [London: Macmillan and Company, 1918], 266. Lockyer, like Breus before him, illustrated some cystic and cavernous adenomyomas that stretch the imagination of the modern viewer accustomed to imaging

of a child's head, the other containing 7 L of fluid.[111] Some communicating cystic uterine adenomyomas grew laterally between the leaves of the broad ligament; other submucosal cystic uterine myomas or "polypoid cystic myomas" grew into the uterine cavity.[112] Breus speaks of cystic myomas and fibromas lined with "Flimmerepithelium," glimmering or sparkling columnar epithelium.[113] In the case described by Pfannenstiel, the "Flimmerepithelium" was associated with metastases from another organ, possibly the left ovary.[114] Breus also cited Rokitansky (1861) as having described similar lesions in conjunction with cystic carcinoma of the ovaries and vegetations of the peritoneum.[115] Referring to the copy of Breus that the author read, Ridley stated: "Breus[116] (1894) described a typical 'chocolate cyst' using that term, of the uterus and cul-de-sac of Douglas. On page 15 of the pamphlet there is reference to a 'chokoladebraunes' secretion that filled a cyst. Since Breus not only had worked with Kolisko, a student of Kundrat,[117] but also dedicated his pamphlet to Kundrat,[118] one of Rokitansky's last assistants, surely Breus should have known of Rokitansky's contributions on endometriosis. One might expect that Breus would have referred to adenomyomas by the Latin descriptive name assigned by Rokitansky, as von Recklinghausen did in his article of 1893.

In short, Ridley believed that documents Breus cited contained evidence that Rokitansky was not the first to describe endometriosis. However, none before Rokitansky fulfilled the aforementioned criteria of discover.[119] Applying the cardinal principle of genealogy to the history of disease, the researcher must be able to trace *backward* from the known to the unknown – generation by generation. To skip a generation is tantamount to pure speculation, yielding to wistful yearnings to extend the legacy, as if so doing increases legitimacy and stature of the disease. For some the temptation is irresistible. Everything from furniture to family pedigree gains a patina that comes only with age; the same might be said for diseases. Endometriosis may have existed for a very long time; millennia may be too short a time frame, considering that endometriosis is intimately related to a woman's biology and sexuality, to her reproductive organs and more directly to the biologic phenomenon of menstruation. Despite the speculations of Ridley, there appears to be no documentation of endometriotic disease before mid-nineteenth century.[120]

So said, Vincent J. Knapp, professor of History at Potsdam College, State University of New York launched a serious study of 12 manuscripts, 1 from 1690 and 11 dating from 1739 to 1797 that he found in the National Library of Medicine in Bethesda,

---

techniques that would have detected them before they could reach such bizarre configurations and size.

[111] Carl Breus, 27.

[112] Carl Breus, 27, 29. See also Cuthbert Lockyer, *Fibroids and Allied Tumours (Myoma and Adenomyoma): Their Pathology, Clinical Features and Surgical Treatment* [London: Macmillan and Company, 1918], 266. "Breus records a case of a voluminous tumour which contained 7 liters of fluid, and on section presented many cysts lined by ciliated epithelium. The general structure was that of a myoma which had spread out into the broad ligament. There was a second growth, the size of a child's head, in the posterior wall of the uterus, and this communicated with the cavity of the uterus by a canal."

[113] Carl Breus, 29, 33.

[114] Carl Breus, 33, 34.

[115] Rokitansky, *Lehrbuch* III. Auflage 1861. III. Band p. 488.

[116] Carl Breus, *Uber Wahre Epithel Führende Cystenbildung in Uterusmyomen* [Leipzig und Wien, 1894], 1–36. [Ridley's reference number 9]

[117] Erna Lesky, *The Vienna Medical School of the 19th Century* [Baltimore, MD: Johns Hopkins University Press, 1976], 424, 516. Karl Breus, an associate professor of gynecology and Alexander Kolisko (1857–1918), a student of Kundrat and a professor of forensic medicine wrote "the standard work *Die Pathologischen Beckenformen (Pathological Forms of the Pelvis) (Vienna and Leipzig.* 1900–1912."

[118] Carl Breus, 1–36 plus 25 pages of advertisement. In 1894, Breus was Privatdocent in Obstetrics and Gynecology at the University of Vienna. Appropriately, this small monograph on developmental pathology was dedicated to the memory of Hans Kundrat, former assistant to Rokitansky who was the second of Rokitansky's assistants to succeed to Rokitansky's chair as professor of pathological anatomy in Vienna. This volume was borrowed from The John Crerar Library in Chicago.

[119] John H. Ridley, The histogenesis of endometriosis: A review of facts and fancies. *Obstetrical and Gynecological Survey* 1968;23:1–35:2. For example, Ridley specified that Breus cited Kiwisch (1852) (The author has not been able to identify Kiwisch or find his work) and "Cruveilhier who in 1835 referred in his textbook of human anatomy to the existence of cysts of the adnexa, uterus, and vagina, forming along the course of the Wolffian (mesonephric) and Mullerian (paramesonephric) remnants." (Jean Cruveilhier, *Anatomie Pathologique du Corps Humain*. Livraison XIII, Planche IV, Paris, 1835.) Then Ridley issued a disclaimer: "Although, here lacking are accurate descriptions, both gross and microscopic, it is plausible to think that such "cysts" were probably of an endometrial nature." Parenthetically, it should be noted that Rokitansky had noted similar cystic formations about female internal reproductive organs in the 1846 edition of his Manual of Pathological Anatomy, translated by the Sydenham Society in 1855. (Carl Rokitansky, *A Manual of Pathological Anatomy*, Volume II. *The*

Maryland.[121] Knapp emphasized the 1690 manuscript of the German physician, Daniel Shroen. Key descriptive words that Knapp abstracted from the 12 manuscripts and translated into English included "ulcers, sores, inflammations, pus-filled, abscesses, loss of consciousness, convulsions, adhesions, one ovarian cyst, suppuration, developing abscess, ulceration, danger of gangrene, life threatening gangrene, pain"; and phrases: "these ulcers of the bladder could penetrate the rectum, where they could produce rectal-intestinal inflammations; the ovaries seemed to be the least damaged organ." Knapp's summation is not convincing: "To ask that European physicians, struggling to identify endometriosis in the late 17th and 18th centuries, [to] come up with tissue samples to distinguish the disease would be to write the present back into the past. Such histologic knowledge simply did not exist for them. However, given the plethora of organic damage that they recognized and recorded, along with identification of numerous constitutional symptoms, most of which today can be found repeated over and over again in medical and biologic journals and even in self-help books, one can come to a conclusion about their investigative efforts. They not only recognized the impact of endometriosis, albeit not in its entirety, but then perceptively and analytically linked together the disease case's greater and lesser symptoms and quickly understood that there was a pathologic syndrome at work."[122]

Two letters were sent to the editor of Fertility and Sterility in response to Knapp's provocative article. In the first letter, Brosens and Steno of Leuven, Belgium located one of five manuscripts that Knapp thought originated from the University of Leuven in Belgium, that of Jacobus Josephus Henry of August 10, 1796.

Abdominal Viscera trans. Edward Sieveking [Philadelphia, PA: Blanchard & Lea, 1855], 248, 249. Chapter III. Abnormalities of the Female Sexual Organs. "In no part of the body are cysts so frequent, or so various as in the ovary, in the peritoneum, in the neighborhood of the internal sexual organs, or in the subperitoneal cellular tissue; as, for instance, between the laminae of the broad ligaments, and at the fimbriated extremities of the tubes. Moreover, the size attained by the ovarian cysts is extraordinary."

[120] King, Helen. *The Disease of Virgins: Green Sickness, Chlorosis, and the Problems of Puberty.* New York: Routledge, 2004, Helen King, *The Disease of Virgins: Green sickness, chlorosis, and the problems of puberty* [New York: Routledge, 2004], 30. Originally, amenorrhea or the absence of menstruation had been the defining characteristic of the disease of virgins. Helen King, *The Disease of Virgins: Green sickness, chlorosis, and the problems of puberty* [New York: Routledge, 2004], 24. Parenthetically, by the eighteenth century, diversion of menstruation or vicarious menstruation from various body orifices and tissues was considered by some physicians as disease; however there was nothing to suggest the clinical signs and symptoms of endometriosis. Helen King, *The Disease of Virgins: Green sickness, chlorosis, and the problems of puberty* [New York: Routledge, 2004], 30. By mid-nineteenth century, the focus on the disease of virgins changed from amenorrhea to the green color of the skin – green sickness or chlorosis. Helen King, *The Disease of Virgins:* 33. In reality, the skin color was not green, but pale or white, perhaps with a greenish hue. Helen King, *The Disease of Virgins: Green sickness, chlorosis, and the problems of puberty* [New York: Routledge, 2004], 116. Finally, "By the end of the nineteenth century, chlorosis had been reinvented yet again, this time as a blood disorder: hypochromic [iron deficiency] anaemia. In its earlier incarnation as the disease of virgins, blood was responsible for the symptoms because it was too thick and sticky to pass through a virgin's narrow channels into the womb; its thickness could be due to a faulty diet." King's entire treatise resolves around iron deficiency anemia with none of the signs or symptoms of endometriosis. Several years ago, before publication of her book, the author spoke to Helen King at a meeting of the American Association of the History of Medicine when she spoke on this subject. At first hearing I thought the disease of virgins might be endometriosis, but when I read the book, it was obviously not. Jacalyn Duffin, *History of Medicine: A Scandalously Short Introduction* [Toronto: University of Toronto Press, 2000], 181–2. "Andral was the first to suggest that anemia could occur if red cells were destroyed (hemolysis), and he described anemia as a decrease in the number of red cells. He associated anemia with pregnancy and with chlorosis. Once called the 'green sickness of virgins' for the peculiar cast it gave to the complexion, chlorosis had been described in the sixteenth century by Johannes Lange, who recommended marriage as therapy. It has come to be synonymous with what we would now call iron-deficiency anemia, although it also resembles anorexia nervosa. Andral was the first to observe the small size of red cells in chlorosis."

[121] Knapp VJ. How old is endometriosis? Late 17th- and 18-century European descriptions of the disease. *Fertil Steril* 1999;72:10–14. Knapp thanked Jerome F. Strauss, III, MD and Celso-Ramon Garcia, MD, the latter an authority on endometriosis from the University of Pennsylvania, "for encouraging this study throughout." Knapp also thanked Marc Laufer, MD of Harvard University, an authority on adolescent endometriosis, "for suggesting refinements in the text." Knapp had published a book on disease in 1989: Vincent J. Knapp, *Disease and Its Impact on Modern European History* [Lewiston, NY: Mellon E. Press, 1989]. This treatise dealt with infectious diseases: plague, syphilis, smallpox, typhus and cholera, tuberculosis, and influenza and their demographic and sociological consequences. In addressing the possible early recognition of endometriosis, Knapp dealt with a chronic disease. Nevertheless, this was not his first venture into history of disease.

[122] Knapp VJ. How old is endometriosis? Late 17th- and 18-century European descriptions of the disease. *Fertil Steril* 1999;72:10–14:13–14.

On examination, Brosens and Steno concluded: "The article under discussion appeared to be about infection and without symptoms suggesting endometriosis or adenomyosis...From our reading of the documents in hand we must conclude that there is no evidence that endometriosis was an endemic or even a recognized disease in the eighteenth century in Belgium."[123] Subsequently, Brosens and Benagiano reported they had read the original manuscripts of 3 of the 12 theses examined by Knapp. They concluded: "We could not find any description that would make us believe the lesions reported were in any way similar to endometriosis, adenomyoma or adenomyosis."[124]

The second letter to the editor of Fertility and Sterility, written by the author, noted that the manuscripts were written during the medical enlightenment of the eighteenth century. The author asked Knapp to clarify some clinical issues.[125] The observations of Brosens and Steeno and questions raised by the author went unanswered because unfortunately Professor Knapp died in the interim. Considering that the master macropathologist Rokitansky had not identified endometriosis in over 30 years of prodigious work, combined with the observations put forth by Brosens and his colleagues that none of the "lesions reported [by Knapp] were in any way similar to endometriosis, adenomyoma or adenomyosis," the author has reached the conclusion that the isolated and scattered observations found by Knapp in the seventeenth- and eighteenth-century literature do not constitute a viable claim for the discovery of endometriosis.[126] In 2011, Benagiano and Brosens argued persuasively that the lesions reported by Knapp were not endometriosis.[127]

In sum, this discussion has been as much about demonstrating the difficulty of recognizing and defining a new benign chronic disease in the interior of the human body in the middle third of the nineteenth century as it has been about granting Rokitansky "the honor of having rendered the first detailed description of adenomyosis, or internal endometriosis"[128] and ovarian endometriosis.

---

123 Brosens I, Steeno O. A compass for understanding endometriosis. *Fertil Steril* 2000;73:179–180. Brosens and Steeno recommended the reading of the manuscript of Daniel Schroen [note different spelling] published by Krebs in Jena in 1690. Ivo Brosens, the doyen of Belgian gynecology, is an internationally recognized scholar and authority on endometriosis and adenomyosis.

124 Benagiano G, Brosens I. History of adenomyosis. *Best Pract Res Clin Obstet Gynaecol* 2006;20:449–63: 450.

125 Ronald E. Batt. A compass for understanding endometriosis. *Fertil Steril* 2000;73:179. Questions asked of Professor Knapp: "What were the ages at menarche and at autopsy? Under what circumstances did these women come to autopsy? Were they 'executed criminals or recently deceased indigents'? Absence of endometriotic lesions in Douglas' pouch is unusual, because this is a common site for peritoneal endometriosis. Were the observations made in situ at autopsy or after removal of the reproductive organs from the body? Were the 17th and 18th century authors physician-professors and surgeons as described by Roger? Did the authors perform the autopsies? [Professor Knapp stated: 'What is remarkable about this epistemology is that virtually every published investigator of the time said exactly the same thing.'] Did they make reference to each other? Did they make reference to even earlier authors?"

126 This conclusion is drawn from evidence in the literature, but with the caveat that at some time in the future all the "Knapp manuscripts" should be examined by a team consisting of eighteenth-century scholars and linguists as well authorities on endometriosis in order to establish a definitive judgment.

127 Benagiano G, Brosens I. Who identified endometriosis? *Fertil Steril* 2011;95:13–16.

128 Emge LA. The elusive adenomyosis of the uterus: its historical past and its present state of recognition. Am J Obstet Gynecol 1962;83:1541–1563. Ludwig A. Emge spent his professional life time studying adenomyosis, beginning shortly after Cullen published *Adenomyoma of the Uterus* in 1908. On the occasion of the 100th anniversary of Rokitansky's description of adenomyosis, Emge presented his lifelong experience with the disease and recounted its history and pathogenesis and etiology at the eleventh Joseph L. Baer Lecture of the Chicago Gynecological Society in 1960 at which time he discussed both its pathogenesis and etiology. Even appendicitis was an unsolved problem at this time. Rickman John Godlee, *Lord Lister* [Oxford: Clarendon Press, 1924], 123. For the history of the recognition of appendicitis, see Smith DC. A historical overview of the recognition of appendicitis – Part I. *NY State J Med* 1986;86:571–83. Smith DC. A historical overview of the recognition of appendicitis – Part II. *NY State J Med* 1986;86:639–47. Smith DC. Appendicitis, appendectomy, and the surgeon. *Bull Hist Med* 1996;70: 414–41.

From von Rokitansky to von Recklinghausen to Cullen

4

Rokitansky's Interest in Developmental Pathology

At the top of the hierarchy of the Vienna Medical School in the 1860s, Rokitansky was aware of the growing academic sentiment that macroscopic morbid pathological anatomy was no longer at the cutting edge of medical research.[1] By mid-nineteenth century, the precision, control, and reproducibility of experimental science "had greatly increased scientists' understanding of the laws governing chemical, physiological, and physical processes...For this reason physicians viewed experimental physiology, more than pathological anatomy or the clinical sciences, as the cornerstone of scientific medicine."[2] Publication of Virchow's *Cellularpathologie* in 1858 had opened the era of physiologic pathology and sounded the death knell of macroscopic pathologic anatomy.[3] Though he did not embrace experimentation or routine microscopic examinations of tissues in his own research, in his ministerial position at the University, Rokitansky had prepared himself, his department, and the University for this important transition.[4]

Then, in 1861, came a call from within the University of Vienna, a demand for a paradigm shift in academic pathology from the "morphologically-organicistically" French school approach that Rokitansky had "deepened and perfected" to the German "experimental–physiological" approach. This was a more fundamental change than a call for microscopic analysis of pathological specimens. Together, experimental medicine and cellular pathology represented a "shift in the center of gravity of European medicine" toward "therapy as the ultimate purpose of the entire medical science."[5] Rokitansky found himself and his department in a position not unlike that of anatomy in 1786 when Emperor Joseph II demoted the department to a position inferior to physiology. Shortly after he discovered uterine and ovarian endometriosis, Rokitansky turned his attention to developmental pathology. Despite the assertion that his macromorphologic approach to anatomy was obsolete, Rokitansky still had much to contribute using this approach for developmental pathology.

[1] Erna Lesky, *The Vienna Medical School of the 19th Century* [Baltimore, MD: Johns Hopkins University Press, 1976], 274, 397: According to Erna Lesky, historian of the Second Vienna Medical School, "Around 1860...the idea gained ground ... that the potentialities of the anatomical-diagnostic trend of the Rokitansky and Skoda school had been exhausted."

[2] Arleen Marcia Tuchman, Science, Medicine, and the State of Germany: The Case of Baden, 1815–1871 [New York: Oxford University Press, 1993], 10.

[3] Erna Lesky, 112.

[4] Erna Lesky, 264. "The fact than an associate professorship for experimental pathology was created in 1868, and that it was raised to the rank of a chair in 1873, is related to the close contact of this subject and its representative, Salomon Stricker, with the pathological anatomist and ministerial consultant Rokitansky." Lesky, 349. "The first edition of Moriz Rosenthal's *Klinik der Nervenkrankheiten* (*Clinical Aspects of Nervous Diseases*) appeared in 1870, and a completely new edition was published in 1875. The book was dedicated to Carl von Rokitansky, and in its solid pathological basis as well as in the careful and surprisingly complete review of the results of contemporary research in neurophysiology and neuropathology, it demonstrates the work of an indefatigable scientist who could rightly be called a student of Rokitansky and of Türck." The same may be said of several other books by Rosenthal.

[5] Erna Lesky, 145.

R.E. Batt, *A History of Endometriosis*,
DOI 10.1007/978-0-85729-585-9_4,

Years earlier, following a debate with Virchow on the development of neoplasms, the "importance of ontogenetic development for the understanding of congenital malformations became increasingly clear" to Rokitansky.[6] Stemming from his early work on vaginal agenesis, Rokitansky generated a decided interest in developmental biology in his later years, an interest focused on the study of midline organs of mesodermal origin. He published on cardiovascular malformations, "Persistence of the Ductus arteriosus" and "The Defects of the Septa of the Heart."[7] Undoubtedly, this work in developmental pathology, late in his career, not only motivated his assistant, Hans Kundrat (1845–1893),[8] to concentrate in this field but also contributed to Rokitansky's reputation and the naming of partial müllerian agenesis as the Rokitansky Syndrome.

Kundrat not only mastered morbid macroscopic anatomical pathology but also took a keen interest in developmental pathology. Rokitansky, nearing the end of his own career, actively promoted Kundrat's rapid academic advancement. Kundrat had graduated from medical school in 1868 and immediately became Rokitansky's assistant. He was promoted to lecturer in 1873, titular associate professor in 1875, and in 1877 to full professor to succeed Heschl in the Chair of Pathology at Graz, Austria. In 1882, Kundrat was called to Rokitansky's Chair of Pathological Anatomy in Vienna on the death of Richard Heschl (1824–1881).[9]

A colleague and friend of Kundrat from student days described the characteristics that had attracted the attention of Rokitansky. "Kundrat was without doubt a great and important morphologist. His formative concepts of observation were most extraordinary. He visualized the very complicated processes of developmental history so exactly and explained the disturbances of these processes so easily, that this in itself made him the most outstanding expert in the field of congenital malformations."[10]

In effect, Rokitansky had reinvented himself in the last decade and a half of his career, but apparently not without a cost to his department. William Osler studied in Vienna for the first 5 months of 1874 and observed the deteriorated state of medicine and pathology relative to surgery, obstetrics, and dermatology.[11] In a letter dated March 1, 1874, Allgemeines Krankenhaus, Osler wrote: "Altogether, midwifery and skin diseases are specialties in Vienna, while in general medicine and pathology it is infinitely below Berlin…After having seen Virchow it is absolutely painful to attend postmortems here, they are performed in so slovenly a manner, and so little use is made of the material."[12] Such was the state of pathologic anatomy on Rokitansky's retirement in 1874, seen from the perspective of a Canadian physician.[13]

The near simultaneous observations of William Osler in Vienna make a telling comparison with those of William Welch in Strassburg. According to Welch, when he visited Strassburg in 1876, von Recklinghausen

[6] Erna Lesky, 112–113.

[7] Erna Lesky, 112–113.

[8] "Kundrat's interest was a direct continuation of the developmental trend of research of Rokitansky's late period; it was concerned with malformations due to arrested development, and had found its expression in the last work *Die Defecte der Scheidewande des Herzens* (Defects of the Inter-Ventricular Septa) (Vienna, 1875)." Kundrat included etiology in his theories of congenital malformations. Erna Lesky, *The Vienna Medical School of the 19th Century* [Baltimore, MD: Johns Hopkins University Press, 1976], 516. Edward Albert, a friend and colleague of Kundrat from his student days, "characterized the main field of interest of Kundrat…'Kundrat was without doubt a great and important morphologist. His formative concepts of observation were most extraordinary. He visualized the very complicated processes of developmental history so exactly and explained the disturbances of these processes so easily, that this in itself made him the most outstanding expert in the field of congenital malformations.'"

[9] Erna Lesky, 515.

[10] Erna Lesky, 516. "Kundrat's interest was a direct continuation of the developmental trend of research of Rokitansky's late period."

[11] Harvey Cushing, *The Life of Sir William Osler* [Oxford, UK: Clarendon Press, 1926], 113–114. In a letter dated "March 1st, 1874. Allgemeines Krankenhaus," Osler wrote "Altogether, midwifery and skin diseases are specialties in Vienna, while in general medicine and pathology it is infinitely below Berlin… After having seen Virchow it is absolutely painful to attend postmortems here, they are performed in so slovenly a manner, and so little use is made of the material."

[12] Harvey Cushing, 113–114.

[13] Harvey Cushing, 114. Osler explained. "Carl Rokitansky, at his best merely a descriptive pathologist, was at this time near the end of his career, and indeed the group of other Bohemians, the great masters who had made the 'new Vienna School' and turned the eyes of the medical world towards Austria, had most of them, with the exception of Billroth, been born in the first decade of the century. The Berlin School, with Virchow as its chief figure, represented a group fifteen years younger." Michael Bliss. *William Osler: A Life in Medicine* [Oxford, UK: Oxford University Press, 1999], 78.

was "perhaps the most celebrated teacher of pathology in Germany."[14] Welch was astonished at the volume of pathological material available. Because he did not know normal tissue histology, Welch was not able to take von Recklinghausen's pathological histology course. However, he did attend von Recklinghausen's demonstration course in gross pathology and found it "unsurpassed" by anything he had seen.[15] Welch observed that autopsies – postmortem examinations –conducted by German medical students were "thorough beyond anything I have ever seen."[16] Welch's observation of the high level of the academic practice of pathology in Strassburg in 1876 contrasted sharply with Osler's observation of the poor state of pathological anatomy in Vienna in 1874, at the time of the celebration of Rokitansky's seventieth birthday. Among the differences, von Recklinghausen was a master microscopic pathologist and Rokitansky was not; furthermore, von Recklinghausen was 43 years old and entering the peak years of his career in 1876, while von Rokitansky was an infirm 70-year-old man on the threshold of retirement.[17]

Rokitansky's Legacy

Nosographic Classification of Human Disease Based on Pathologic Anatomy

Carl Freiherr von Rokitansky, the founder of modern anatomic pathology, devoted his entire professional life to the specialty of anatomic pathology to the exclusion of all other medical practice.[18] In 1875, Rokitansky wrote of his career and his academic legacy: "In accordance with a pressing need of my time…I have pursued pathological anatomy first of all in the sprit of investigation fruitful for clinical medicine."[19] Two powerful examples of his success were his collaboration with the internist Skoda and his influence on the remarkable career of the internist Kussmaul as well as the hundreds of students from foreign countries he attracted to his dissecting table.[20] A quotation from Rokitansky's final lecture sums up his thinking. "Pathological Anatomy is the essential basis for pathological physiology, to be supplemented further by pathological histology, chemical pathology, and experimental pathology."[21]

While Virchow had severely criticized the hematohumoral theory of Rokitansky contained in the first volume of the first edition of his three-volume magnum opus published in 1846, he lauded Rokitansky as the Linne of anatomical pathology for the second edition – expunged of the discredited theory – published in 1855.[22] Ironically, 1855 marked the year of publication of the *second* German edition of Rokitansky's Handbook as well as publication of the Sydenham Society's honorific English translation of the *first* [1846] edition.[23] Due, largely, to this unfortunate coincidence, Rokitansky's reputation suffered in the eyes of some historians who read only the English translation of the first edition [1855] and not the revised second German edition [1855]. Some chose the fluent English in the Sydenham Society's translation of the first edition of the *Handbook of Pathological Anatomy*

[14] Simon Flexner and James Thomas Flexner, *William Henry Welch and the Heroic Age of American Medicine* [Baltimore, MD: Johns Hopkins University Press, 1993], 78.

[15] Simon Flexner and James Thomas Flexner, *William Henry Welch and the Heroic Age of American Medicine* [Baltimore, MD: Johns Hopkins University Press, 1993], 78.

[16] Simon Flexner and James Thomas Flexner, 78.

[17] Robert Joseph Miciotto, "Carl Rokitansky: Nineteenth-Century Pathologist and Leader of the New Vienna School" [PhD dissertation.] The Johns Hopkins University, 1979], 273–274.

[18] Schaller, Anton. Reflexionen des Frauenarztes der Gegenwart auf das pathologisch-anatomische Lebenswerk Carl Freiherr v. Rokitanskys. Wien Med Wochenschr 2004;154:477–481. (Reflections of a present –day gynaecologist on the work of Carl Freiherr v. Rokitansky in the fields of pathology and anatomy).

[19] R.J. Rather, Eva R. Rohl. An English Translation of the Hitherto Untranslated Part of Rokitansky's *Einleitung* to volume 1 of the *Handbuch der allgemeinen Pathologie* (1846), with a Bibliography of Rokitansky's Published Works. Clio medica 1972;7:215–227:216. Rather and Rohl quoted from Rokitansky's farewell address: Carl von Rokitansky, *Abschiedsrede des Professors Carl Freiherr von Rokitansky* [Vienna, 1875].

[20] R.J. Rather, Eva R. Rohl. An English Translation of the Hitherto Untranslated Part of Rokitansky's *Einleitung* to volume 1 of the *Handbuch der allgemeinen Pathologie* (1846), with a Bibliography of Rokitansky's Published Works. Clio medica 1972;7:215–227:216.

[21] Venita Jay, "The legacy of Karl Rokitansky," Arch Pathol Lab Med 2000;124:345–346. See also: Erna Lesky, *The Vienna Medical School of the 19th Century* [Baltimore, MD: Johns Hopkins University Press, 1976], 498–499. "In professional circles in Germany, the old master of pathological anatomy, Carl von Rokitansky, caused quite a stir when he established a separate Chair for General and Experimental Pathology in Vienna in 1873." He himself had stated, as early as 1846, in the introduction to

rather than coping with the Rokitansky's idiosyncratic German in the revised and more praiseworthy second edition.[24] Those readers of the English translation who judged Rokitansky unfavorably based their judgment on the discredited hematohumoral theory, thereby giving Rokitansky virtually no credit for his life's work organizing and categorizing anatomical pathology.[25]

The German physician–historian, Karl Sudhoff, came to Rokitansky's defense. "From the past of our science, modern investigation may take its guide-posts, while, on the other hand, the most recent scientific findings will shed light upon the scientific life of the past, thus enabling us better to understand and more justly estimate the significance of the mental struggles and honest endeavors of seekers after truth in bygone days. Thus, today one might ask: 'The great Rokitansky, the real creator of modern pathological anatomy in its essential parts as well as in its total conception, was he in his doctrine of crases [hematohumoral theory] nothing more than a victim of atavistic notions, which he could not get rid of, an impractical dreamer, in comparison with whom the sober-sided localistic clinician gained all the more admiration?' Just for this reason, perhaps, we may learn to admire Rokitansky's genial, far-seeing vision; he did not want to throw overboard the intuitive conclusions of the past because they had begun to seem improbable by comparison with the ever-advancing triumphs of the localistic gospel, of which he was the most successful standard-bearer himself. And we are bound to admire him all the more in that the unparalleled successes in one trend of investigation did not prevent him from envisaging basic pathological problems that could get no satisfactory answer from 'localistic' doctrine."[26]

The American historian, Robert Miciotto, also defended Rokitansky by explaining the ideas of prominent scientists who influenced the formulation of his rather extreme theory of disease. "…as late as 1853 (seven years after the review, and two years prior to *omnis cellula a cellula*), Virchow himself was still expressing the belief in intracellular blastemas as a productive source of cellular contents. In fact, one of the ironies of Virchow's depiction of many of Rokitansky's ideas as outmoded and unproven occurs in his negative

---

Volume 1 of his manual: "pathological anatomy should be the basis not only of medical knowledge but also of medical practice, and it should include all the knowledge and fundamentals of the science and practice in medicine. Subsequently, however, Rokitansky…was [un]able to incorporate in pathological anatomy the microscopic and experimental methods which had developed so vigorously from the forties. In Vienna these methods were employed and developed outside the realm of pathological anatomy: microscopy in the laboratories of Brücke and Wedl, and animal experiments in Carl Ludwig's laboratory."

[22] Erna Lesky, *The Vienna Medical School of the 19th Century* [Baltimore, MD: Johns Hopkins University Press, 1976], 107–108. Referring to Virchow, Lesky wrote: "No one was able to evaluate this achievement better than the man who continued to work on the basis thereof. Rudolph Virchow (1821–1902) referred to Rokitansky as the Linne of pathological anatomy." Lesky cited: Rudolph Virchow, WMW 5, 417 (1855). Owsei Temkin, *The Double Face of Janus and Other Essays in the History of Medicine* [Baltimore and London: Johns Hopkins University Press, 1977], 273. Temkin noted that 1855 marked the year that Virchow published his article entitled "Cellular Pathology," in which he enunciated his "famous formula, *omnis cellula a cellula*." See Rudolph Virchow, Zellular-Pathologie. Virchows Archiv 1855;8:23.

[23] Carl Rokitansky, *A Manual of Pathological Anatomy*, Volume II. *The Abdominal Viscera.* trans. Edward Sieveking [Philadelphia, PA: Blanchard & Lea, 1855], ix. Editor's Preface. "The fact of the Work having been selected for translating by the Council of the Sydenham Society, is in itself a proof that it is deserving of the high estimation in which it has been held by all pathologists acquainted with continental literature; but it may not be superfluous to state that the value of the Professor's remarks is enhanced by his being entirely unfettered by preconceived notions or prejudiced views, as to the disease of the individual brought to the dead-house for examination." Carl Rokitansky, *A Manual of Pathological Anatomy*, Volume I. *General Pathological Anatomy.* trans. William Edward Swaine [Philadelphia, PA: Blanchard & Lea, 1855]. American Publisher's Notice, Philadelphia, August 1855. "The world-wide reputation of the author and of his work render eulogy superfluous, while the appearance of the translation under the auspices of the Sydenham Society is a guarantee of its fidelity."

[24] Carl Rokitansky, *A Manual of Pathological Anatomy*, Volume II. vii–ix. Editor's Preface. "Owing to the acknowledged difficulty of the author's style, it has however been thought advisable to divide the translation into four volumes, each of which is entrusted to a different editor." "Of the difficulties connected with the translation, I will only say that they are much increased by the figurative style of the author. He constantly uses terms in a sense peculiar to himself, and his total disregard for the ordinary rules of composition is an additional and frequent source or obscurity."

[25] Robert J. Miciotto, "Carl Rokitansky: A Reassessment of the Hematohumoral Theory of Disease," *Bulletin of the History of Medicine* 53, no. 2 [Summer 1978]: 183. Rokitansky's reputation gradually declined, undeservedly tarnished by his hematohumoral theory of disease, which compared unfavorably to Virchow's theory of cellular pathology, especially when the latter evolved into molecular biology.

response to the Rokitansky suggestion that an alternative method of cellular production may be, 'The propagation of nuclei and cells…within a parent cell.' It is a concept which the father of cellular pathology derides as having been concluded 'by means of the most arbitrary playing with facts and explanations…'"[27]

Many knowledgeable physicians, who were contemporaries of Rokitansky, attested to his legacy as scientist and educator. When Carl Wunderlich (1815–1877), whose seminal treatise on the relation of disease and body heat became the basis for the use of the thermometer in clinical medicine, visited the University of Vienna autopsy house in 1840, he wrote that Rokitansky labored on the cutting edge of medical science.[28] In 1878, the year of Rokitansky's death, Klebs expressed appreciation for Rokitansky's teaching: "[He] taught us to think anatomically at the bedside and to weave at the autopsy table the individual phases of the morbid process into the pattern of the clinical progress."[29] Based on his immense experience in the autopsy house, Rokitansky taught clinicians to analyze the morbid finding and to reconstruct the evolution of the pathological process. This enabled clinicians to analyze the patient's symptoms and signs and detect disease patterns, thus leading to earlier and more accurate diagnosis in the living.[30] It was the constant feedback from pathology laboratory to clinic, from autopsy to hospital that developed diagnostic skills. Robert Meyer recalled that his "most brilliant teacher" was the internist, Adolf Kussmaul, who had been instructed in pathology by Rokitansky. Meyer related that Kussmaul's "diagnoses were not far from infallible." At a retirement banquet for Kussmaul in 1887, von Recklinghausen said "that he had not once been able to reverse a diagnosis after dissecting one of his patients." Meyer continued, "It was always astonishing how carefully [Kussmaul] examined his patients in order to arrive at a diagnosis."[31]

In 1895, 40 years after its second edition, Virchow spoke of Rokitansky's Handbook as the "unsurpassed treatise of pathological anatomy."[32] At the turn of the century, Virchow credited Rokitansky for helping to "emancipate" pathological anatomy in the German-speaking lands and for having brought pathological anatomy into closer harmony with clinical medicine.[33] The American Roswell Park, considered "Baron von Rokitansky…one of the most famous men in modern times."[34] By 1933, Sigerist opined that Rokitansky's great contributions had become the common property of medicine; his contributions had become timeless and thus "nameless."[35] Commenting on Rokitansky's Autobiography and Inaugural Address, Paul Klemperer contributed a mid-twentieth century assessment of Rokitansky's legacy. Klemperer noted that "for many a pathologist of today [1961] Rokitansky might appear as an almost legendary figure reminiscent of a period referred to euphemistically as classical but appraised as outmoded in terms of modern pathology."[36] Reference to classical has more currency among musicians and historians than physicians and scientists, as Klemperer asserted.

---

[26] Karl Sudhoff, "What is history of medicine?" in *Essays in the History of Medicine* trans. by various hands and ed. Fielding H. Garrison [New York: Medical Life Press, 1926], 71, 72.

[27] Robert J. Miciotto, "Carl Rokitansky: A Reassessment of the Hematohumoral Theory of Disease," *Bulletin of the History of Medicine* 53, no. 2 [Summer 1978]: 183–199: 185–186.

[28] Paul Klemperer, Notes on Carl von Rokitansky's Autobiography and Inaugural Address. Bulletin History of Medicine 1961;35:364–380:376–377. Klemperer quoted Wunderlich: "Wunderlich, an enthusiastic visitor in 1840, wrote: 'The Vienna Institute no more counts the number of autopsies in the hundreds, and Rokitansky can consult thousands of protocols in reference to more than one disease.' I do not believe that any other institute can match this proportion."

[29] Paul Klemperer, Notes on Carl von Rokitansky's Autobiography and Inaugural Address. Bulletin History of Medicine 1961;35:364–380:379.

[30] Paul Klemperer, 1961;35:364–380:379.

[31] Robert Meyer, *Autobiography of Dr. Robert Meyer (1864–1947): A Short Abstract of a Long Life* [New York: Henry Schuman, 1949], 17.

[32] Paul Klemperer, 1961;35:364–380:379. Klemperer cited Rudolph Virchow, *Hundred Jahre allgemeiner Pathologie* [Berlin: August Hirschwald, 1895].

[33] R.J. Rather, Eva R. Rohl. An English Translation of the Hitherto Untranslated Part of Rokitansky's *Einleitung* to volume 1 of the *Handbuch der allgemeinen Pathologie* (1846), with a Bibliography of Rokitansky's Published Works. Clio medica 1972;7:215–227: 216. Rather and Rohl quoted from : Rudolph Virchow, "Ein alter Berichte ueber die Gestaltung der pathologischen Anatomie in Deutschland, wie sie is und wie sie widen muss," Virchows Archiv 1900;159:24–39.

[34] Park, Roswell. *An Epitome of the History of Medicine.* 2nd Ed. Philadelphia: FA Davis Company, 1908: 250.

[35] Paul Klemperer, Notes on Carl von Rokitansky's Autobiography and Inaugural Address. Bulletin History of Medicine 1961;35:364–380:379. Klemperer quoted Sigerist from: Henry E. Sigerist, *Grosse Aerzte* [Muenchen: J.F. Lehmann, 1933].

[36] Paul Klemperer, 1961;35:364–380:376, 379. Referring to Rokitansky's Handbook of Pathological Anatomy, Klemperer, a pathologist, stated in 1961: "Today its contents are inadequate for the second year medical student."

Historians, such as Roy Porter, assess Rokitansky and his department from an entirely different perspective. "Rokitansky had a superb mastery of anatomy and pathological science, and left notable studies of congenital malformations and reports on numerous conditions, including pneumonia, peptic ulcer, and valvular heart disease."[37] Porter, nonetheless, as virtually every other historian of medicine and science, did not include endometriosis among conditions Rokitansky reported, undoubtedly because Rokitansky did not give the disease a proper name. Nor have historians included endometriosis or adenomyosis in their historical compendiums of disease.

Developmental Pathology to Evolutionary Developmental Biology

From Rokitansky though Kundrat and his students, one stream of scientific investigation flowed and blended with similar streams and eventually with the field of evolutionary biology. Only in the 1990s did the field of evolutionary biology evolve into the interdisciplinary field of evolutionary developmental biology, a field that has given new direction to the study and history of endometriosis.[38]

Mayer-Rokitansky-Küster-Hauser Syndrome and Developmental Pathology

In the late stage of his career, Rokitansky developed a special interest in developmental pathology of the genitourinary and cardiovascular systems, two midline organ systems of mesodermal origin. In medical school, his interest in embryology had been ignited by the works of Johan Friedrich Meckel (1781–1833),[39] and by actually holding in his hands the specimen jar containing the anomalous "sexual organs of the 60-year-old Magdalena Fischer" from the Vienna pathology museum.[40] One has only to recall the stifling lectures and rote memorization of Rokitansky's student days to appreciate the experience of visualizing a pathological specimen and thinking of its embryological development and how it affected the life of the very woman whose identify had been preserved with her anomalous body parts. This interest was stoked by Müller's treatise on embryology in 1830,[41] and first reported in 1838 as a case series: "Concerning the so-called duplication of the uterus."[42] Furthermore, Paris hospital medicine informed Rokitansky's clinicopathologic perspective: physicians and pathologists no longer thought in terms of sick individuals; "they saw diseases," diseases they could study at autopsy.[43]

A physician never forgets an observation early in his career that so captures his interest that he publishes the case in the medical literature.[44] Rokitansky's description of those specimens added to the importance and recognition of uterovaginal malformations.[45] Rokitansky must have had an intense interest in malformations because he imparted this interest to Kussmaul, an internist, who later published a book entitled *The Malformations of the Uterus.*[46] Rokitansky's report of 1838 has resounded into the twenty-first century as an integral part of the Mayer-Rokitansky-Küster-Hauser syndrome.[47] The very name of the syndrome embodies

---

[37] Roy Porter, "Medical Science," in *The Cambridge Illustrated History of Medicine,* ed. Roy Porter [Cambridge: Cambridge University Press, 1996], 154–201:177.

[38] Brosens IA, Brosens JJ. Endometriosis. Eur J Obstet Gynecol Reprod Biol 2000;414:105–112. Ronald E. Batt, Smith RA, Buck Louis GM, Martin DC, Chapron C, Koninckx PR, Yeh J. Müllerianosis. Histol Histopathol 2007;22:1161–1166. Bloom MS, Buck Louis GM, Schisterman EF, Liu A, Kostyniak PJ. Maternal serum polychlorinated biphenyl concentrations across critical windows of human development. Environ Health Perspect 2007; 115:1320–1324. Buck Louis GM, Hediger ML, Pena JB. Intrauterine exposures and risk of endometriosis. Hum Reprod 2007;22:3232–3236. Buck Louis GM, Gray LE Jr, Marcus M, Ojeda SR, Pescovitz OH, Witchel SF, Sippell W, Abbott DH, Soto A, Tyl RW, Bourguignon JP, Skakkeback NE, Swan SH, Golub MS, Wabitsch M, Toppari J, Euling SY. Environmental factors and puberty timing: expert panel research needs. Pediatrics 2008;121 Suppl 3:S192-207.

[39] Venita Jay, "The legacy of Karl Rokitansky," Arch Pathol Lab Med 2000;124:345–346. "Rokitansky was profoundly influenced…by the concepts of comparative anatomy and embryology" of Johan Friedrich Meckel. Meckel published *Handbuch der pathologischen Anatomie* (1812–1816) and *System der vergleichenden* [comparative] *Anatomie* (1821–1831).

[40] See specimen one [Magdalena Fischer], first seen by Rokitansky in 1828 and described in 1838 in: Von Prof. Dr. Rokitansky, Uber die sogenannten Verdoppelungen des Uterus. Medicinische Jahrbucher des kaiserl. konigl osterreichischen Staates 1838;26:S39-S77:40.

[41] Johannes Müller, Bildungsgeschichte der Genitalien aus anatomischen Untersuchungen an Embryonen des Menschen and der Thiere, nebst einem Anhang über die chirurgische Behandlung der Hypospadia. [Düsseldorf, 1830]. Goethe, the poet-scientist, inspired Johannes Müller to a lifetime of meticulous basic science research and teaching that in turn motivated investigators in the German speaking world. In that scientific atmosphere, Rokitansky investigated müllerian anomalies.

[42] Von Prof. Dr. Rokitansky, Uber die sogenannten Verdoppelungen des Uterus. Medicinische Jahrbucher des kaiserl. konigl osterreichischen Staates 1838;26:S39-S77.

the sense of scientific continuity, of a community of scholars who influenced one another in the search for pathogenesis, etiology, diagnosis, and treatment.[48]

In sum, being steeped in embryology, Rokitansky's early publications on uterovaginal anomalies (Mayer-Rokitansky-Küster-Hauser syndrome) made him more conscious of midline developmental abnormalities. This interest led, in later years, to Rokitansky's intensive study of the cardiovascular[49] and genitourinary systems,[50] and in the interim, may have been one more factor in his recognition of endometriosis. Rokitansky published lasting contributions not only to the understanding of diseases characterized by *excessive* müllerian tissue, such as endometriosis and adenomyosis,[51] but also to the congenital anomaly characterized by *deficient* müllerian tissue, partial müllerian aplasia.[52] The Mayer-Rokitansky-Küster-Hauser syndrome illustrates precisely the author's argument that gynecologic diseases apparent on the body surface or on cursory examination of the body interior were diagnosed much earlier than more subtle chronic diseases – like endometriosis and adenomyosis – in the body interior.

From Rokitansky to von Recklinghausen

> "Conflicts in theories are common and can be settled satisfactorily only by experiment and critical observations rather than by speculative thinking. And yet, the latter approach has been the common one because the human brain craves understanding and aims at bringing everything under a single system of laws for the sake of making prediction safer and easier…This common pitfall is well demonstrated by the history of the evolution of theories aiming to explain the etiology of adenomyosis."
> Emge[53]

According to the Austrian gynecologist Carl Breus – who dedicated his pamphlet on cystic adenomyomas to Hans Kundrat, assistant to Rokitansky and second

---

[43] Ann La Berge and Caroline Hannaway, "Paris Medicine: Perspectives Past and Present," in *Constructing Paris Medicine,* ed. Caroline Hannaway and Ann La Berge [Amsterdam, NL: Editions Rodopi B. V., 1998], 1–69:5.

[44] The author is referring to the 1828 case of partial müllerian agenesis that was retrieved in a specimen jar on 30 July 1838. See: Von Prof. Dr. Rokitansky, Uber die sogenannten Verdoppelungen des Uterus. Medicinische Jahrbucher des kaiserl. konigl osterreichischen Staates 1838;26:S39–S77. For the importance of case reports in medicine, see Owsei Temkin, "The Scientific Approach to Disease: Specific Entity and Individual Sickness," in *The Double Face of Janus and Other Essays in the History of Medicine* [Baltimore, MD: Johns Hopkins University Press, 1977], 441–455:452–453. Temkin notes: "It is not immediately clear why the anatomical interpretation of disease had to follow the road from case histories to disease entities….The role of the case history in a particular phase of medical development elucidates further the notion of the abnormal in medicine…The case history is the form in which the physician links the science, which does not deal with the unique directly, and the patient, who requires attention as an individual."

[45] Ghirardini G, Popp LW. The Mayer-von Rokitansky-Küster-Hauser syndrome (uterus bipartitus solidus rudimentarius cum vagina solida): the development of gynecology through the history of a name. Clin Exp Obstet Gynecol 1995;22:86–91.

[46] Robert Meyer, *Autobiography of Dr. Robert Meyer (1864–1947): A Short Abstract of a Long Life.* With a Memoir of Dr. Meyer by Emil Novak, MD. [New York: Henry Schuman, 1949], 16–17.

[47] Roland Sedivy, "200 Jahre Rokitansky – sein Vermachtnis fur die heutige Pathologie," *Wiener Klinische Wochenschrift* 2004;116/23: 779–787. This article contains a bust and a photograph of Rokitansky executed in 1874 on the occasion of his retirement at age 70. In February 2004, Roland Sedivy conducted a PubMed search of "Rokitansky"; 238 citations (47%) were in reference to the Mayer-Rokitansky-Küster-Hauser syndrome, the next nearest citation, 138 (27%), was in reference to history. Table 1 gives a list of seventeen of Rokitansky's discoveries by surname or scientific name. Item 7 in the list is: "Endometriose." See also: Ottokar Rokitansky, "Carl Freiherr von Rokitansky – zum 200, Geburtstag: Eine Jubilaumsgedenkschrift, *Wiener Klinische Wochenschrift* 2004;116/23: 773–788.

[48] Ghirardini G, Popp LW. The Mayer-von Rokitansky-Küster-Hauser syndrome (uterus bipartitus solidus rudimentarius cum vagina solida): the development of gynecology through the history of a name. Clin Exp Obstet Gynecol 1995;22:86–91.

[49] Venita Jay, "The legacy of Karl Rokitansky," Arch Pathol Lab Med 2000;124:345–346. Rokitansky published *On some of the Most important Diseases of the Arteries* (1852) and *The Defects in the Septum of the Heart* (1875). See also: Davies MK, Hollman A. Karl Freiherr von Rokitansky (1804–1878). Heart 1997;78(5):425.

[50] Park, Roswell. *An Epitome of the History of Medicine.* 2nd Ed. Philadelphia: FA Davis Company, 1908:250–251. Roswell Park wrote: "for fourteen years he studied the defects of the septum of the heart and the comparative anatomy of the uterus and genito-urinary organs."

[51] Rokitansky C. Ueber Uterusdrüsen-Neubildung in Uterus- und Ovarial-Sarcomen. Zeitschift Gesellschaft der Aerzte in Wien. 1860;16:577–581. See also: Simpson JL. Genetics of the female reproductive ducts. Am J Med Genet 1999;89:224–239. Simpson reports two cases of a rare condition of excessive müllerian tissue: true duplication of the müllerian ducts: "affected women must have two separate uteri, each of which can have two fallopian tubes." Simpson believes it may result from division of one or both müllerian ducts early in embryogenesis. Recall the spectacular case of true duplication with two vaginas, two uteri each with two fallopian tubes, in which the woman conceived and carried a normal male child until a therapeutic abortion had to be performed to preserve the life of the mother due to deficient pelvic capacity to carry the child further.

[52] Von Prof. Dr. Rokitansky, Uber die sogenannten Verdoppelungen des Uterus. Medicinische Jahrbucher des kaiserl. konigl osterreichischen Staates 1838;26:S39–S77. Partial müllerian agenesis, the Mayer-Rokitansky-Küster-Hauser syndrome.

successor to his chair of pathological anatomy in Vienna – Carl Schroeder, Herr, and Grosskopf had by 1884 collected more than 100 references to adenomyomata from the medical literature for a dissertation.[54] At the end of World War I, Cuthbert Lockyer, a reliable English authority on the subject of adenomyomas accepted the authenticity of the 100 references.[55] In 1924 a third authority, the Englishman K. Vernon Bailey writing primarily on extrauterine adenomyomas, did not reference any literature before the 1880s.[56] In 1962 a fourth authority Ludwig Emge, an American with a life-long interest in uterine adenomyosis, stated endometrial stromatosis "was first described by Virchow." This was in 1863, just 3 years after Rokitansky's initial report on uterine adenomyosis.[57] However, Emge had been unable to locate the "some hundred cases [that] had been collected by Carl Schroeder, Herr (sic), and Grosskopf."[58]

How to explain the discrepancy? What circumstances would explain the loss of interest in the more than 100 cases of cystic adenomyomas described by Breus in 1884?[59] Lockyer offered an explanation: "until the year 1894 (sic) there [were] very few reliable records of myomas containing cysts lined by epithelium."[60] Lockyer attributed to Babes (1882) the first description of an adenomyoma – in a 91-year-old woman – a hazelnut size intramural myoma lying in the fundus of the uterus [which] contained cysts lined with low cuboidal epithelium "derived from embryonic germs."[61] This also appears to be the first mention in the literature of the theory of embryonic (congenital) müllerian rests proposed for the pathogenesis of uterine adenomyomas. According to Lockyer, "Up to 1896 the *müllerian* origin of adenomyoma had been generally accepted. The supporters of this view included Diesterweg, Schroeder, C. Ruge, Babes, Schottlander,

[53] Emge LA. The elusive adenomyosis of the uterus: its historical past and its present state of recognition. Am J Obstet Gynecol 1962;83:1541–1563.

[54] Carl Breus, *Uber Wahre Epithel Führende Cystenbildung in Uterusmyomen* [Leipzig und Wien: Franz Deuticke, 1894], 6. "Oskar Schroeder, O. Heer und C. Grosskopf haben die Mühe nicht gescheut, in ihren Dissertationsschriften alle in der Literatur mitgetheilten Falle von solchen Cystomyomen zu sammeln und haben so bis 1884 über 100 derselben zusammengestellt." See also Breus, page 10, where he cites the 1860 article of Rokitansky. See: Erna Lesky, *The Vienna Medical School of the 19th Century* [Baltimore, MD: Johns Hopkins University Press, 1976], 424. Carl Breus (1852–1914) and the pathologist Alexander Kolisko, a student of Kundrat – second successor to Rokitansky's chair of pathological anatomy in Vienna, wrote the classical book *Pathological Shapes of the Pelvis* (3 Vols. Vienna, 1900–1912). Leopold G. Koss and Philip H. Lieberman, "Surgical Pathology at Memorial Sloan-Kettering Cancer Center," in *Guiding the Surgeon's Hand: The History of American Surgical Pathology*, ed. Juan Rosai [Washington, DC: Armed Forces Institute of Pathology, 1997], 66. Alexander Kolisko, Carl Breus's coauthor, was the third successor to Rokitansky's chair of pathological anatomy in Vienna. See also: Thomas Stephen Cullen, *Adenomyoma of the Uterus* [Philadelphia: WB Saunders, 1908], 1. Thomas Cullen, who was conversant with the Austrian and German literature, also recorded that Breus had credited Schroeder, Herr, and Grosskopf with having collected 100 cases of myomata containing glandular elements up to the year 1884.

[55] Cuthbert Lockyer, *Fibroids and Allied Tumours (Myoma and Adenomyoma): Their Pathology, Clinical Features and Surgical Treatment* [London: Macmillan and Company, 1918], 265. Lockyer did not refer to the original report of Breus of 1884. Instead, he cited Cullen and gave the incorrect year. Lockyer wrote: "Cullen mentions that about one hundred had been recorded under various titles up to 1896."

[56] Bailey KV. The etiology, classification, and life history of tumors of the ovary and other female pelvic organs containing aberrant müllerian elements, with suggested nomenclature. J Obstet Gynaecol Brit Emp 1924;xxxi:539–573:540. Bailey made only passing reference to the first two authorities, Cullen and Lockyer.

[57] Emge LA. The elusive adenomyosis of the uterus: its historical past and its present state of recognition. Am J Obstet Gynecol 1962;83:1541–1563:1554. Emge may have stated the date incorrectly when he wrote: "stromatosis was first described by Virchow in 1864." Additionally, Emge did not cite the reference to Virchow; he was probably recalling a reference he had read years before. However, von Recklinghausen did reference Virchow in 1863, not 1864. See: Friedrich v. Recklinghausen, *Die Adenomyome und Cystadenome der Uterus- und Tubenwandung ihre Abkunft von Resten des Wolff'schen Korpers. Im Anhang: Von W. A. Freund, Klinische Notizen zu den voluminosen Adenomyomen des Uterus* [Berlin: Verlag von August Hirschwald, 1896.], 96. Referring to Virchow's description of endometrial stromatosis, von Recklinghausen stated: "So by the first look under the microscope at the simple construction of the histology of this organoid tumor of Virchow we arrive at the conviction that we must separate this special tumor from the usual spherical myoma." See: Reference 60: R. Virchow, Die krankhaften Geschwulste. 1863. I. 263–286, III. 150. (The pathological tumors)

[58] Emge LA. 1962;83:1541–1563:1542. It is possible that the dissertation to which Breus referred was located in a university library or archive in Austria. That might explain Emge's failure to find it.

[59] Erna Lesky, *The Vienna Medical School of the 19th Century* [Baltimore, MD: Johns Hopkins University Press, 1976], 424. Breus was a reliable authority who was promoted to associate professor in 1894.

[60] Cuthbert Lockyer, *Fibroids and Allied Tumours (Myoma and Adenomyoma): Their Pathology, Clinical Features and Surgical Treatment* [London: Macmillan and Company, 1918], 265. "1894" Instead of 1884 in all probability represents a typographic or type-setting error. Lockyer states that "Cullen mentions that about one hundred [myomas containing cysts lined by epithelium] had been recorded under various titles up to 1896,

Hauser, Strauss, Orloff, Ricker (for the uterus), and A. Martin, Orthmann, Chiari, Baraban, Pilliet (for the tube)."[62] Significantly, the German pathologist Friedrich von Recklinghausen in his monograph of 1896 made no reference to adenomyomas before 1882, other than references to Rokitansky (1860 and 1861) and Virchow (1863).[63] Von Recklinghausen's first reference was also to Babes in 1882. From this, we may conclude there was nothing of significance in the medical literature on adenomyomas before 1882, other than the works of Rokitansky and Virchow.[64] In sum, Friedrich Daniel von Recklinghausen remains the decisive authority on what constitutes the significant literature on adenomyomas between 1860 and 1896.[65]

What happened in the 1880s to make that literature memorable? It was then, as we have seen in the article by Babes that investigators began to postulate the pathogenesis of tumors from embryonic rests.[66] As early as 1854, Robert Remak, a student of Johannes Müller, suggested that tumors might originate "at an early developmental stage of the human embryo." Remak anticipated the hypothesis of Julius Cohenheim that tumors originated from embryonic rests.[67] In the first edition of his book *Vorlesungen* published in 1877, Cohenheim, a student of Virchow,[68] put forth the idea that "the growth as well as the structure of tumors might be accounted for on the assumption of an origin from embryonal cells...from residual embryonal rudiments [rests]."[69]

The search for pathogenesis and etiology was stimulated further when, after meticulous experimentation, Robert Koch announced to a select audience in Berlin in 1882 that he had discovered the bacillus that caused human tuberculosis.[70] Using tuberculosis as the model, Michael Worboys described the evolution of *theories of disease* in the nineteenth century as developing in

---

but only a few of the most important need here be given [in Lockyer's monograph of 1918]."

[61] Cuthbert Lockyer, 265. Babes G. Uber epitheliale Geschwulste in Uterusmyomen Allgem. Wiener med Ztschr 1882;27:36–48. Lockyer never mentioned the contributions of Rokitansky. 1882 was the year that Koch announced his discovery of the tuberculosis bacillus which stimulated investigators to search for the cause of disease. For chronic diseases, the search began for pathogenesis, for an explanation of the pathway taken by the disease process.

[62] Cuthbert Lockyer, 274–275.

[63] Friedrich v. Recklinghausen, *Die Adenomyome und Cystadenome der Uterus- und Tubenwandung ihre Abkunft von Resten des Wolff'schen Korpers. Im Anhang: Von W. A. Freund, Klinische Notizen zu den voluminosen Adenomyomen des Uterus* [Berlin: Verlag von August Hirschwald, 1896.] Von Recklinghausen most certainly was aware of the entire German and Austrian literature on the subject of adenomyomas as well as contributions from England and the other countries on the Continent of Europe.

[64] Von Recklinghausen, Cullen, and Lockyer all picked Babes (1882) as the first reliable reference to "myomas containing cysts lined by epithelium."

[65] Friedrich v. Recklinghausen, *Die Adenomyome und Cystadenome der Uterus- und Tubenwandung ihre Abkunft von Resten des Wolff'schen Korpers. Im Anhang: Von W. A. Freund, Klinische Notizen zu den voluminosen Adenomyomen des Uterus* [Berlin: Verlag von August Hirschwald, 1896.] Bailey KV. The etiology, classification and life history of tumours of the ovary and other female pelvic organs containing aberrant müllerian elements, with suggested nomenclature. J Obstet Gynaecol Brit Emp 1924;xxxi:539–573:540. Writing two decades after von Recklinghausen, Bailey considered articles on the pathology of adenomyomas by Breus, Chiari, Martin, Orthmann, Werth, and Schauta worthy of mention.

[66] *Illustrated Stedman's Medical Dictionary*. 24th ed. [Baltimore, MD: Williams & Wilkins, 1982], 1224. Embryonic rest: "[From the Latin *restare,* to remain]. A group of cells or a portion of fetal tissue that has become displaced and lies embedded in tissue of another character."

[67] LJ Rather, *The Genesis of Cancer: A Study in the History of Ideas* [Baltimore, MD: Johns Hopkins University Press, 1978], 122.

[68] Owsei Temkin, "Basic Science, Medicine, and the Romantic Era," in *The Double Face of Janus and Other Essays in the History of Medicine* [Baltimore, MD: Johns Hopkins University Press, 1977], 257.

[69] LJ Rather, *The Genesis of Cancer*, 170–171. See also: David Cantor, "Cancer." In *Companion Encyclopedia of the History of Medicine.* Vol. 1. ed. W. F. Bynum and Roy Porter [London: Routledge, 1997], 537–561:540–544. David Cantor, "Cancer." In *Companion Encyclopedia of the History of Medicine.* Vol. 1. ed. W. F. Bynum and Roy Porter [London: Routledge, 1997], 537–561:540–542. The search for the cause of malignant as well as benign tumors constitutes an interesting chapter in the history of science and medicine. Until Bichat argued at the turn of the nineteenth century that for the seat of cancer in body tissues, "the history of cancer was part of a broader history of inflammation." Subsequently Laennec distinguished between gangrene and cancer. David Cantor, 542. In the late 1830s, Johannes Müller integrated Schwann's cell theory into the genesis of cancer. Müller believed that "both normal and pathological cells were structured aggregates of transformed cells, developed for the most part *de novo* from an amorphous blastema ultimately derived from circulating blood." Later, "Virchow believed that tumour cells developed from 'embryonic' cells, scattered throughout the omnipresent connective tissue." Cantor, 543. In 1867, Wilhelm Waldeyer argued that "normal epithelium was the sole source of epithelial cells contained in a given carcinoma. The sole mechanism of local spread was the active or passive movement of cancer cells into adjacent tissue, while the sole mechanism of metastatic spread was through the transport of

three stages. Worboys contended "at its simplest [theories of disease] can be seen as moving from defining diseases by their symptoms and results to defining them in terms of processes and causes."[71] [Stage I] In the early nineteenth century, the disease was known as consumption, or *phthisis*, from the Greek word for "wasting." This characterization was based on a holistic view of the *symptoms* and results; patients wasted away as their body literally consumed itself. [Stage II] "In the first half of the nineteenth century, the term 'tuberculosis' came to be used, referring to the localized pathological process of tubercle (nodule) formation in the lungs. Thus the disease was defined by *process* and results, but these were now described at the tissue and cellular level." [Stage III] "However, the identification and acceptance of the *Tubercule bacillus* in the 1880s as the essential cause, over an extended period it must be said, led to the creation of an *aetiological* definition of the disease."[72]

Uterine and ovarian endometriosis were defined by Rokitansky in 1860 by the second-stage theory of disease, as a localized pathological process in the uterus and ovary. Rokitansky offered a theory of inflammatory pathogenesis. K. Codell Carter's observation is pertinent: "While the medical profession accepted new discoveries only as evidence was forthcoming, everyone was open to the idea that universal necessary causes could be found even for non-bacterial diseases."[73] For the next 7 decades, investigators offered other theories of pathogenesis, but were not able to identify the aetiology, the universal necessary cause of endometriosis, a chronic disease with many characteristics of cancer.

Greaves summarized the complexity of cancer causation, a summary directly applicable to the pathogenesis and etiology of endometriosis. "The composite and probabilistic nature of risk for cancer, plus its extended time frame of evolutionary development, poses the major intellectual obstacle in understanding causation for the public and professionals alike. The ingredients and pattern of the composite are different for each type of cancer and, even for a single type of cancer, risk factors can vary in weight or importance. This is not intuitively easy to grasp given past false assumptions about disease causality. There is often a tacit assumption that not only can and should causation in cancer be formally and indisputably provable but that singular causes must exist and these are both necessary and sufficient for the disease. This is simplistic and it is wrong. Causation can be inferred as 'the most probable explanation' but it is extraordinarily difficult, if not impossible, to prove culpability beyond doubt. Moreover, since all cancers are multifactorial in origin and can arise via alternative causal mechanism, the necessary and sufficient criterion is entirely inappropriate for cancer – as it is for the causation of most of our aliments."[74]

The Austrian gynecologist Breus published a pamphlet in 1883 in which he documented a 7-L cystic uterine myoma lined with ciliated epithelium.[75] Lockyer noted that in 1883, Diesterweg described two polypoid lesions located on the posterior uterine wall that contained blood-filled cysts lined with ciliated epithelium.[76] And, 2 years later, Diesterweg removed a fist-sized cystic tumor lined by ciliated epithelium from the same patient.[77] Diesterweg theorized the pathogenesis of uterine adenomyomas resulted from

cancer cells to the metastatic sites via the blood, lymph, or other body fluids." Cantor, 544. In the twentieth-century, the cause of cancer has shifted between two polarities "explanations favouring the action of exogenous factors such as viruses, parasites, environmental chemicals, or physical agents such as radiation; and those favouring endogenous factors such as genetic mutation." Alexander Berglas, *Cancer: Nature, Cause, and Cure* [Paris: Institute Pasteur, 1957] 6–7. Berglas from the Pasteur Institute compared cancer to a "runaway healing attempt." Once the cancer cells dedifferentiates to a functionally more primitive cell, "control mechanisms of the body no longer have any influence on the constantly dividing 'malignant' cells; they no longer submit to the regulatory processes of the organism."

[70] K. Codell Carter, *The Rise of Causal Concepts of Disease: Case Histories* [Burlington, VT: Ashgate, 2003], 134. Carter quotes Paul Ehrlich's recollection of that meeting: "all who were present were deeply moved and that evening has remained my greatest experience in science."

[71] Michael Worboys, *Spreading Germs: Disease Theories and Medical Practice in Britain, 1865–1900.* [Cambridge, UK: Cambridge University Press, 2000], 4.

[72] Michael Worboys, 4.

[73] K. Codell Carter, *The Rise of Causal Concepts of Disease: Case Histories* [Burlington, VT: Ashgate, 2003], 143.

[74] Mel Greaves, "Finale: Cause, Complexity, and the Evolutionary Rub," in *Cancer: The Evolutionary Legacy* [Oxford: Oxford University Press, 2000], 213–220:213.

[75] Carl Breus, *Uber Wahre Epithel Führende Cystenbildung in Uterusmyomen* [Leipzig und Wien, Franz Deuticke, 1894], 1–36

[76] Diesterweg B. Ein Fall von Cystofibrom uteri verum Zeitschr f Geb 1883:9:191.

[77] Cuthbert Lockyer, *Fibroids and Allied Tumours (Myoma and Adenomyoma): Their Pathology, Clinical Features and Surgical Treatment* [London: Macmillan and Company, 1918], 265–266.

invasive idiopathic stromal hyperplasia, a theory supported by "Carl Ruge (1889), Carl Schroeder (1892), and Hauser (1893)."[78] In 1887, Hans Chiari described the inflammatory pathogenesis of salpingitis isthmica nodosa, i.e., invasion of the muscular wall of the fallopian tube by its mucosal lining.[79] Lockyer explained Chiari's reasoning based on observations of postmortem specimens of thickened fallopian tubes: "these swellings were the outcome of a chronic salpingitis, which he explained by stating that during an acute inflammation there was sufficient intratubal tension to force portions of the mucous membrane into the oedematous muscle-wall. The extruded portions of mucosa at first retain their communication with the lumen of the tube, but later on they become isolated, and form the gland-spaces which are found in the wall of the tube. These 'adenomas,' by setting up irritation, produce hypertrophy and hyperplasia of the muscle-tissue; and to this inflammatory *histoid* node the name *Salpingitis isthmica nodosa* was given by Chiari."[80]

Chiari's *Salpingitis isthmica nodosa* (tubal adenomyosis) was directly analogous to uterine adenomyosis; invasion of the muscular wall of the uterus by its mucosal lining that was described by Chiari's mentor Rokitansky in 1860. Neither uterus nor fallopian tube has a submucosa to retard invasion, such as the bowel possesses. Interestingly, Chiari and Rokitansky attributed mucosal invasion of the tube and uterus, respectively, to an inflammatory process. Chiari's inflammatory theory of pathogenesis of tubal adenomyosis did not go unchallenged.

Von Recklinghausen postulated a different theory of pathogenesis of cystic uterine adenomyomas in a one and a quarter page note published in 1893. He believed they originated from "Ueberresten der Wolff'schen Canale," that is, from embryonic rests of the Wolffian duct. The fact that von Recklinghausen specifically cited "Rokitansky's Cystosarcoma adenoids uterinum" by name in his 1893 article indicates that he was familiar with the literature on uterine adenomyomas and the chronological limits of the literature dating back to Rokitansky's original article in 1860.[81] Other authors cited by von Recklinghausen included Babes, Diesterweg, and Hauser. In 1895, von Recklinghausen published a short but illuminating note entitled "Concerning the adenomyomas of the uterus and tube."[82] Therein, he described microscopic pseudoglomeruli that resembled the glomeruli of the kidney; the basis for his theory of mesonephric embryonic rests – Wolffian rests.

After reviewing the literature on adenomyomas, Von Recklinghausen wrote a monograph on the subject in 1896 entitled: *Adenomyomas and Cystadenomyomas of the Uterus and Fallopian tubes and Their Origin from the Wolffian Body*.[83] In 1918, two decades after its publication, the English surgeon Cuthbert Lockyer, a contemporary of von Recklinghausen, evaluated the medical and historical importance of von Recklinghausen's monograph. "It was in the year 1896 that full interest in the subject [adenomyoma] was aroused by the publication of Friedrich von Recklinghausen's magnificent work, *Die Adenomyome und Cystadenomyome der Uterus und Tubenwandung*."[84] According to Lockyer, the American investigator Rabinovitz recorded that von Recklinghausen "attempted completely to overthrow the inflammatory theory [of Chiari], and enunciated the *congenital* origin of *salpingitis nodosa*."[85] Recall that there were three theories of pathogenesis of uterine adenomy-

[78] Emge LA. The elusive adenomyosis of the uterus: its historical past and its present state of recognition. Am J Obstet Gynecol 1962;83:1541–1563:1543.

[79] Chiari H. Zur pathologischen Anatomie des Eileiter-Catarrhs. Pager Ztschr. Heilkunde 1887;8:457–473. That same year, Martin reported cases similar to Chiari. Martin. Uber Tubenkrankung. Zeitschr für Geb und Gynak 1887;13. S. 299. Martin cited by: Cuthbert Lockyer, *Fibroids and Allied Tumours (Myoma and Adenomyoma): Their Pathology, Clinical Features and Surgical Treatment* [London: Macmillan and Company, 1918], 284.

[80] Cuthbert Lockyer, *Fibroids and Allied Tumours (Myoma and Adenomyoma): Their Pathology, Clinical Features and Surgical Treatment* [London: Macmillan and Company, 1918], 307.

[81] Von Recklinghausen F. Ueber die Adenocysten der Uterustumoren und Ueberreste des Wolff'schen Organs. Deutsche Medicinische Wochenschrift 1893;xix:325–326.

[82] Von Recklinghausen F. Ueber die Adenomyome des Uterus und der Tuba. Wiener Klinische Wochenschrift 1895;29:530.

[83] Friedrich v. Recklinghausen, *Die Adenomyome und Cystadenome der Uterus- und Tubenwandung ihre Abkunft von Resten des Wolff'schen Korpers. Im Anhang: Von W. A. Freund, Klinische Notizen zu den voluminosen Adenomyomen des Uterus* [Berlin: Verlag von August Hirschwald, 1896].

[84] Cuthbert Lockyer, *Fibroids and Allied Tumours (Myoma and Adenomyoma): Their Pathology, Clinical Features and Surgical Treatment* [London: Macmillan and Company, 1918], 266. Cuthbert Lockyer, MD, BS, FRCP, FRCS was Vice-President Obstetrical and Gynaecological Section, Royal Society of Medicine; Corresponding member of the Societe d'Obstetrique Belge; Surgeon to In-Patients, Samaritan Hospital for Women; Obstetric Physician to Out-Patients Charing Cross Hospital; Joint-Lecturer on gynaecology and Obstetrics, Charing Cross

omas at this time; the 1860 Rokitansky hypothesis of chronic inflammation,[86] the 1854–1877–1882 Remak-Cohenheim-Babes theory of embryonic rests,[87] and the 1883 Diesterweg theory of hyperplastic endometrial invasion of the uterus.[88] In the introduction to his article, Rabinovitz stated that the subject of "salpingitis nodosa" (or as he preferred "adenomyosalpingitis") was subject to "copious, and at times, even acrimonious debate" among proponents of three conflicting views of the pathogenesis of the disease: inflammatory, congenital, or some compromise between the two.[89] This statement of Rabinovitz goes to the heart of von Recklinghausen's motivation for studying adenomyomas in the first place.

Recall that von Recklinghausen's interest in the pathogenesis of uterine and tubal adenomyomas began in 1893, when he published his first short note on the subject. If Rabinovitz was correct, then one might conclude, as did Lockyer, that von Recklinghausen's major work on the pathogenesis of adenomyomas of the uterus and fallopian tubes was undertaken to disprove the inflammatory hypothesis of Chiari, a former assistant of Rokitansky.[90] Thus, one may trace intellectual continuity from Rokitansky through Chiari to von Recklinghausen.

However, there appears to be more to the story. In 1883, Diesterweg had hypothesized the pathogenesis of uterine adenomyomas resulted from invasive idiopathic stromal hyperplasia; Diesterweg's hypothesis was supported by others.[91] As Lockyer pointed out, in 1894 Pilliet expressed "the view that cysts and glands of adenomyoma were of mucosal origin."[92] The articles by Diesterweg and Pilliet may have alerted von Recklinghausen to the idea of mucosal origin, for he cited both among the 107 references in his 1896 monograph.[93] But far more importantly, Pilliet's article of 1889 may also have been the source for von Recklinghausen's theory that the vast majority of uterine and tubal adenomyomas were derived

Hospital Medical School; Examiner to the Royal College of Physicians and Surgeons; Late Examiner in Midwifery and Diseases of Women to the University of London.

[85] Cuthbert Lockyer, 307–308. The theories of pathogenesis and etiology of cancer and endometriosis have been discussed earlier in this chapter.

[86] Carl Rokitansky, Ueber Uterusdrüsen-Neubildung in Uterus- und Ovarial-Sarcomen. Zeitschift Gesellschaft der Aerzte in Wien. 1860;16:577–581. "Of the existing connective tissue tumors of the uterus, the round fibroids are to be differentiated from the so called fibrous polyps of the uterus in which glandular tubules are found. These are connective tissue tumors rooted in the basal stroma of the uterus and cannot be shelled out (Paget's continuous growth) in contrast to the well circumscribed fibrous tumors. They commonly develop within or from the submucosal stratum and grow into the uterine cavity as so called polyps of various shapes (cylindric, pear-club shaped) and are covered by an adherent uterine mucosa. The various changes in its texture may appear identical to the changes seen as a result of *chronic inflammation.* [Italics added]. In contrast to the easily removable fibrous tumors, we commonly consider these connective tissue tumors as *sarcoma* [benign], here specifically as *uterus sarcoma.* These tumors growing into a mucosal cavity generally retain their old name of *polyp* and *uterus polyp* and, according to the discussion above, would be distinguished from the round fibroids prolapsed into the uterine cavity. As round fibroids may develop within the inner tissue layers of the uterus, so can sarcomas on rare occasion develop from a mucosal-free outer layer. In view of the above discussion, it is important to recognize the changes occurring in the mucosa and the submucosal stratum of the uterus as consequences of *chronic inflammation.*" [Italics added]. When Rokitansky stated: "As round fibroids may develop within the inner tissue layers of the uterus, so can sarcomas on rare occasion develop from a mucosal-free outer layer," did he anticipate Iwanoff's serosal theory of metaplasia of 1898?

[87] LJ Rather, *The Genesis of Cancer: A Study in the History of Ideas* [Baltimore, MD: Johns Hopkins University Press, 1978], 122. As early as 1854, Robert Remak, a student of Johannes Müller, suggested that tumors might originate "at an early developmental stage of the human embryo." Remak anticipated the hypothesis of Julius Cohenheim that tumors originated from embryonic rests.

[88] Emge LA. The elusive adenomyosis of the uterus: its historical past and its present state of recognition. Am J Obstet Gynecol 1962;83:1541–1563:1543. Diesterweg theorized the pathogenesis of uterine adenomyomas resulted from invasive idiopathic stromal hyperplasia, a theory supported by "Carl Ruge (1889), Carl Schroeder (1892), and Hauser (1893)."

[89] Rabinovitz M. The pathogenesis of adenomyosalpingitis (salpingitis nodosa): report of ten cases. American Journal of Obstetrics and Diseases of Women and Children 1913; lxviii;711–752.

[90] Erna Lesky, *The Vienna Medical School of the 19th Century* [Baltimore, MD: Johns Hopkins University Press, 1976], 115, 558.

[91] Emge LA. The elusive adenomyosis of the uterus: its historical past and its present state of recognition. Am J Obstet Gynecol 1962;83:1541–1563:1543. Diesterweg theorized the pathogenesis of uterine adenomyomas resulted from invasive idiopathic stromal hyperplasia, a theory supported by "Carl Ruge (1889), Carl Schroeder (1892), and Hauser (1893)."

[92] A. Pilliet. Fibromyome de la trompe uterine. Bull de la Soc Anat de Paris 1894:554. Cited by Cuthbert Lockyer, *Fibroids and Allied Tumours (Myoma and Adenomyoma): Their Pathology, Clinical Features and Surgical Treatment* [London: Macmillan and Company, 1918], 284. Sampson, JA. Ovarian hematomas of endometrial type (perforating hemorrhagic cysts of the ovary) and implantation adenomas of endometrial type. Boston Medical and Surgical Journal 1922;186:445–456. Sampson wrote, without direct citation, "In 1894, Pilliet took the view that the cysts and glands of adenomyoma were of mucosal origin." Undoubtedly, Sampson's information came from Lockyer whom he acknowledged in the opening sentence of this paper.

from Wolffian rests.[94] Like Bichat, Rokitansky, and Virchow before him, von Recklinghausen read widely in the medical literature when formulating his theory.[95] In this case, he was searching for alternatives to the inflammatory theory postulated by Chiari. In his 1896 monograph, Von Recklinghausen postulated that adenomyomas were organoid tumours derived from Wolffian rests originating from the mesonephros – Wolffian body – as he had first postulated in 1893.[96] He divided uterine adenomyomas into two classes, those arising peripherally in the uterus and fallopian tube from Wolffian remnants and the rare central lesions arising from the endometrium.[97] Lockyer transcribed von Recklinghausen's classification of uterine adenomyomas by morphology into four varieties:

1. *Hard*, in which the muscle tissue is in excess of the gland elements
2. *Cystic*, with spaces visible to the naked eye, possessing gland tissue and muscle in equal amounts
3. *Soft*, in which the gland tissue appears microscopically as islands and is the predominating feature
4. *Telangiectatic*, soft, very vascular growths, which are almost devoid of cysts[98]

This first pathological classification of uterine adenomyomas was important because it had diagnostic significance for pathologists and for any surgeon sufficiently curious to incise and examine a growth in situ or after its removal.

Von Recklinghausen's colleague, the gynecologist Wilhelm A. Freund, wrote an afterward to von Recklinghausen's monograph in which he attempted to define the clinical signs and symptoms by which uterine adenomyomas could be diagnosed. Viewed from the perspective of the twenty-first century, the critical clinical features were profuse and painful periods, pelvic peritonitis, and severe anemia.[99] Lockyer presented the full clinical picture presented by Freund. "There was a history of debilitated childhood. Menstruation appeared late; puberty was postponed. The periods were profuse and painful. Irregular haemorrhage was common; there was pelvic peritonitis and marked anaemia. Body-functions were impaired, and the growth led eventually to complete incapacity for work. Objectively there were signs of general hypoplasia and infantilism. The tumour had its situation in the dorsal wall of the uterus. Pelvic peritonitis and fixation of the pelvic organs was a marked feature. The site of election was the *cornu uteri,* from whence the growth spread downwards towards the cervix."[100] Freund's "clinical picture" was considered too general to make

93 Friedrich v. Recklinghausen, *Die Adenomyome und Cystadenome der Uterus- und Tubenwandung ihre Abkunft von Resten des Wolff'schen Korpers. Im Anhang: Von W. A. Freund, Klinische Notizen zu den voluminosen Adenomyomen des Uterus* [Berlin: Verlag von August Hirschwald, 1896.] Ref. No. 19.

94 A. Pilliet, Les debris du corps de Wolff et leur role dans la pathogenie des tumours. Tribune medicale. 1889. See: Friedrich v. Recklinghausen, *Die Adenomyome und Cystadenome der Uterus- und Tubenwandung ihre Abkunft von Resten des Wolff'schen Korpers. Im Anhang: Von W. A. Freund, Klinische Notizen zu den voluminosen Adenomyomen des Uterus* [Berlin: Verlag von August Hirschwald, 1896.]: Ref. No 20.

95 Erwin H. Ackerknecht, *A Short History of Medicine* [New York: Ronald Press, 1968], 166. Bichat and Virchow were fortunate, their theories endured. But Ackerknecht's assessment of Rokitansky would apply to von Recklinghausen: "But unfortunately his factual foundation was insufficient."

96 Harold Speert, *Obstetric & Gynecologic Milestones: Illustrated* [New York: Parthenon Publishing Group, 1996], 89. "The female genital tact, from the ovary to the hymen, contains a mine of embryonic remnants, vestiges of the primitive urogenital system, which provides a yield of never-ending interest to the clinical gynecologist as well as the student of embryology." The mesonephros – the primitive vertebrate kidney – comprises two elongated masses in the early vertebrate embryo. The mesonephros was named the Wolffian body to honor Caspar Wolff who discovered these primitive kidneys in 1759. A Wolffian rest represents a group of cells or a portion of the mesonephros (Wolffian body) that has become displaced and lies embedded in tissue of another character that persists as an embryonic remnant in the adult.

97 Cuthbert Lockyer, *Fibroids and Allied Tumours (Myoma and Adenomyoma): Their Pathology, Clinical Features and Surgical Treatment* [London: Macmillan and Company, 1918], 266. Von Recklinghausen's four varieties of adenoma are taken directly from Lockyer. See: Friedrich v. Recklinghausen, *Die Adenomyome und Cystadenome der Uterus- und Tubenwandung ihre Abkunft von Resten des Wolff'schen Korpers. Im Anhang: Von W. A. Freund, Klinische Notizen zu den voluminosen Adenomyomen des Uterus* [Berlin: Verlag von August Hirschwald, 1896]. My copy of this monograph obtained online from the Center for Research Libraries, Identifier: m-r-000252-f3, Scan Date: September 26, 2007 contained only text, no illustrations.

98 Cuthbert Lockyer, *Fibroids and Allied Tumours* (*Myoma and Adenomyoma*): *Their Pathology, Clinical Features and Surgical Treatment* [London: Macmillan and Company, 1918], 267–268.

99 Friedrich v. Recklinghausen, *Die Adenomyome und Cystadenome der Uterus- und Tubenwandung ihre Abkunft von Resten des Wolff'schen Korpers. Im Anhang: Von W. A. Freund, Klinische Notizen zu den voluminosen Adenomyomen des Uterus* [Berlin: Verlag von August Hirschwald, 1896].

100 Cuthbert Lockyer, *Fibroids and Allied Tumours* (*Myoma and Adenomyoma*): *Their Pathology, Clinical Features and Surgical Treatment* [London: Macmillan and Company, 1918], 437.

an exact preoperative diagnosis of uterine adenomyomas. The aforementioned symptoms and objective signs were contested by many investigators and were found wanting to differentiate uterine adenomyomas from uterine fibroids. Investigators concluded that only a tentative preoperative diagnosis was possible; positive diagnosis could only be made at surgery and many times only by histologic examination.[101]

Notwithstanding, von Recklinghausen's macro-, micro-morphologic classification of adenomyomas combined with Freund's description of symptoms and signs was a major first effort to establish clinical–pathological correlation and give adenomyomas a name and nosographic significance for clinicians and pathologists. Von Recklinghausen's prestige guaranteed that the monograph would be influential and widely read. Recall that most investigators had accepted the theory of müllerian rests to explain the origin of pelvic adenomyomas until 1896. After 1896, von Recklinghausen's theory of mesonephric origin of adenomyomas from Wolffian rests displaced the müllerian theory.[102] Von Recklinghausen's challenge to the older müllerian theory started a "*Streitfrage*,"[103] a great controversy in Europe over the pathogenesis of uterine and tubal adenomyomata. When von Recklinghausen's monograph crossed the Atlantic Ocean in 1896 to North America, it ignited a *mini-Streitfrage* at Johns Hopkins Hospital.

From von Recklinghausen to Cullen

At the time that Friedrich von Recklinghausen, the first and most brilliant assistant of Rudolf Virchow, published his brief note on uterine adenomyoma on May 19, 1893,[104] Thomas Cullen was studying at the Pathological Institute of the University of Göttingen under Johannes Orth.[105] Under Orth's direction, Cullen became thoroughly indoctrinated in German Scientific methods and the concept of *Wissenschaft*, self-directed scholarship and research.[106] Cullen studied under Orth while waiting to begin a residency in gynecologic surgery under Howard A. Kelly at Johns Hopkins Hospital in Baltimore, Maryland. Cullen was befriended by Orth who taught him the "root fact" of teaching: "You can't teach a man anything worth knowing. You can only show him what there is to learn."[107] Cullen made Orth's aphorism his own; it shaped Cullen's method of teaching gynecologic pathology and surgery.[108] In Göttingen, Cullen became a Germanophile.[109]

When Cullen returned to Baltimore in October 1893, the residency position Kelly had promised him had been reclaimed by William W. Russell. Inspired, Howard Kelly arranged for Cullen to be given charge of gynecological pathology. As if endowed with foresight, Cullen had returned from Germany with his own microscope.[110] A small room was set aside for gyneco-

[101] Cuthbert Lockyer, 438–439.

[102] Cuthbert Lockyer, 274–275. Lockyer named the supporters of the Müllerian origin of adenomyomas as: "Diesterweg, Schroeder, C. Ruge, Babes, Schottlander, Hauser, Strauss, Orloff, Ricker (for the uterus), and A. Martin, Orthmann, Chiari, Baraban, Pilliet (for the tube)." Müllerian rest: The paired müllerian tubes – primitive vertebrate fallopian tubes, uterus, cervix, and upper vagina – comprise two elongated masses in the early vertebrae embryo. A müllerian rest represents a group of cells or a portion of the müllerian anlage that has become displaced and lies embedded in tissue of another character that persists as an embryonic remnant in the adult. Wolffian rest: The mesonephros – the primitive vertebrate kidney – comprises two elongated masses in the early vertebrate embryo. A Wolffian rest represents a group of cells or a portion of the mesonephros (Wolffian body) that has become displaced and lies embedded in tissue of another character that persists as an embryonic remnant in the adult.

[103] Cuthbert Lockyer, 281.

[104] Von Recklinghausen F. Ueber die Adenocysten der Uterustumoren und Ueberreste des Wolff'schen Organs. Deutsche Medicinische Wochenschrift 1893;xix:325–326.

[105] Judith Robinson, *Tom Cullen of Baltimore* [London, Toronto, New York: Oxford University Press, 1949], 106. Orth was Virchow's favorite assistant and future successor to his chair.

[106] Andreas W. Daum, "*Wissenschaft* and knowledge," in *The Short Oxford History of Germany: Germany 1800–1870* [Oxford: Oxford University Press, 2004], 137–161:137. Daum equated the German term *Wissenschaft* with scholarship and research, which included "the sciences, social sciences, and humanities." See Martzloff KH. Thomas Stephen Cullen. Am J Obstet Gynecol 1960;80:833–843:835: Cullen spent 6 months in the laboratory of Johannes Orth. The tradition of *Wissenschaft* was strong in the laboratory of Johannes Orth; it was based on an intellectual genealogy directly traceable to Goethe himself. Goethe profoundly influenced Johannes Müller who, in turn, became the great German medical educator of the nineteenth century. Müller trained Virchow, who trained Orth who directly influenced Cullen in his early and formative 6 months spent in Orth's pathology laboratory.

[107] Judith Robinson, *Tom Cullen of Baltimore,* 108–109.

[108] Judith Robinson, *Tom Cullen of Baltimore* [London, Toronto, New York: Oxford University Press, 1949], 404–411.

[109] Judith Robinson, 216. Soon after he returned to Johns Hopkins Hospital, Cullen began a lifelong friendship with Max Broedel, Howard Kelly's master medical illustrator. The two made a pact; Broedel would write and converse with Cullen in English and Cullen would reciprocate in German. To his biographer, Cullen recalled: "All his life I don't think I spoke two hours of English to him, or wrote fifty

logic pathology, one floor below Welch's pathological anatomy laboratory, referred to as the Pathological. There, Cullen, the assistant of Howard Kelly, stayed for 3 years studying and examining fresh surgical specimens under the influence of William H. Welch and Simon Flexner, Welch's assistant.[111] Unlike German laboratories where the professor assigned a subject for investigation, at the Pathological, each person was free to choose the subject.[112] Thus, Cullen's opportunity for independent research on a subject of his own choosing was made possible by Welch's liberal philosophy of research. Welch came to the "Hopkins eager to establish the German system of laboratory education there, but the result was very different. In Germany, a laboratory entered on the investigation of a large subject which presented a variety of separate problems that were parceled out among the advanced students, the professor keeping the many threads in his own hands. The nature and comprehensiveness of the general subject reflected the inventiveness, fertility, and technical skill of the professor, which also determined the results achieved. This was not Welch's way. He never devoted his laboratory to the investigation of any single subject, nor did he show any special fertility in the choice of problems for himself or others; his own choices...were determined by fortuitous circumstances, not any plan. And he never set a student to work on a concrete problem, seeming rather to avoid any such commitment; he held that men do not work well on assigned tasks."[113] In September 1895, after just 2 years in charge of gynecological pathology, Cullen sent reprints of his first publications to Welch, who responded with a note of encouragement to the young investigator.[114] Cullen recalled many years later that his experience in pathology under Welch was "priceless."[115]

In 1893, the same year Cullen started research in pathology under Welch, Frederick Jackson Turner read a paper before the American Historical Association entitled "The Significance of the Frontier in American History."[116] According to Turner, the 1890s marked the end of an era in American history when the Superintendent of the United States Census declared the American Frontier closed.[117] Turner argued persuasively the grand concept of American exceptionalism; a hypothesis that Americans were shaped by the harsh environment of the frontier into self-reliant, rugged individuals. The quick actions of Howard Kelly and William Welch to found gynecologic pathology at Johns Hopkins Hospital and the equally quick action of Thomas Cullen to respond – thus

words that were not German." See also Judith Robinson, *Tom Cullen of Baltimore* [London, Toronto, New York: Oxford University Press, 1949], 168. This practice facilitated Cullen's lectures in Germany and his communication with von Recklinghausen.

110 Judith Robinson, 113.

111 Judith Robinson, 113, 117.

112 Judith Robinson, 118. Simon Flexner & James Flexner, *William Henry Welch and the Heroic Age of American Medicine* [Baltimore: Johns Hopkins University Press, 1993], 163. See also: Kenneth M. Ludmerer, *Learning to Heal: The Development of American Medical Education* [New York: Basic Books, 1985], *41*. William H. Welch maintained in 1886 that medicine had become a model of experimental research and that if a university wished to achieve creditability as a research university, it had to accommodate scientific medicine.

113 Simon Flexner & James Flexner, *William Henry Welch and the Heroic Age of American Medicine* [Baltimore: Johns Hopkins University Press, 1993], 163.

114 Simon Flexner & James Flexner, *William Henry Welch and the Heroic Age of American Medicine* [Baltimore: Johns Hopkins University Press, 1993], 245. "You are to be congratulated upon the excellent way in which you have written up and discussed these interesting cases. The drawings are works of art and make everything clear. You are taking the right way to build up a scientific reputation." See also: Judith Robinson, *Tom Cullen of Baltimore* [London, Toronto, New York: Oxford University Press, 1949], 119.

115 Judith Robinson, 113. Howard A. Kelly was so impressed with Cullen's foundation in gynecological pathology that, after his residency in gynecologic surgery, he took Cullen as his assistant with the rank of Instructor in Gynecology in the Johns Hopkins University and Assistant Resident Gynecologist in the Johns Hopkins Hospital. Kelly had recognized that Cullen's talents in gynecological pathology complemented his own extraordinary talents as a gynecological surgeon; they made a good team for research and teaching. Furthermore, subsequent to Cullen's experience, Kelly made a year of gynecologic pathology requisite before beginning the residency in gynecologic surgery. Judith Robinson, 136. Howard Kelly later remarked to Cullen that "he would give fifty thousand dollars to have had [Cullen's] experience in pathology." Judith Robinson, 113.

116 Frederick Jackson Turner, "The Significance of the Frontier in American History," in *The Early Writings of Frederick Jackson Turner*, ed. Frederick Jackson Turner [Madison WI, [1893] 1938], 185–229. The essence of Turner's Frontier Thesis is contained in the last sentence of the first paragraph of his famous 1893 essay: "The existence of an area of free land, its continuous recession, and the advance of American settlement westward explain American development." Turner was one of the first American professional historians; he trained at Johns Hopkins University.

117 There was no territory within the United States that had fewer than two inhabitants per square mile.

becoming the first gynecologic pathologist in North America – represent nothing less than actions of self-reliant individuals; exemplars of American – and Canadian – exceptionalism.

And their decisiveness paid off handsomely.[118] On October 31, 1894, during his second year in the laboratory, Cullen received an unusual *fresh* surgical specimen that piqued his curiosity[119] – a scene reminiscent of the *fresh* surgical specimen that caught the attention of Rokitansky 34 years earlier in the old Leichenhaus in Vienna. Cullen examined a "uniformly enlarged uterus about four times normal size…caused by a diffuse thickening of the whole anterior wall." Unsure how to process the specimen, Cullen walked upstairs for a consultation with Dr. Welch. Welch, too, had never seen anything like it. He recommended that histologic sections be cut through the full thickness of the anterior wall of the uterus.[120] Cullen followed Welch's advice and cut giant serial sections with a microtome. "Examination of these sections showed that the increase in thickness was due to the presence of a diffuse myomatous tumor occupying the inner portion of the uterine wall, and that the uterine mucosa was at many points flowing into the diffuse myomatous tissue." In March 1895, Cullen reported this case to a meeting of the Johns Hopkins Medical Society.[121] On April 6, 1895, Cullen received his second specimen, an adenomyoma that involved the posterior uterine wall. He duly processed the second specimen as he had the first. And there the matter rested until 1896.

In 1896, Friedrich von Recklinghausen published a monograph entitled: *Die Adenomyome und Cystadenome der Uterus- und Tubenwandung ihre Abkunft von Resten des Wolff'schen Korpers*; Adenomyomas and Cystadenomas of the Uterus and Tubal Wall, their Origin from Embryonic Rests of the Wolffian body.[122] *Die Adenomyome und Cystadenome der Uterus- und Tubenwandung*[123] fully documented von Recklinghausen's theory of the pathogenesis of adenomyomas from remnants of the Wolffian body; only in the Anhang or appendix did the author include one case whose pathogenesis he attributed to mucosal invasion. With the publication of von Recklinghausen's monograph, the disease "adenomyoma uteri," virtually leapt over the Atlantic Ocean – from the German University of Strassburg in Alsace to the German – oriented Johns Hopkins University in Baltimore, Maryland; from the laboratory of Friedrich Daniel von Recklinghausen (1833–1910)[124] to the laboratory of William Henry Welch (1850–1934), who had studied under von Recklinghausen.[125] Or more poetically, the European experience with adenomyomas was transferred from von Rokitansky to Chiari to von Recklinghausen to Cullen.

When the 27-year-old Johns Hopkins' instructor in gynecologic pathology, Thomas Stephen Cullen, read von Recklinghausen's monograph, he experi-

[118] Thomas Stephen Cullen, *Adenomyoma of the Uterus* [Philadelphia: WB Saunders, 1908], v. Cullen recounted the story of his first encounter with an adenomyoma in the opening paragraph of the preface. Ironically, the first case that Cullen encountered was the less common variety, an adenomyoma of the anterior wall of the uterus; the more common site being the posterior wall.

[119] Cullen discovered his first case of diffuse uterine adenomyomas in October 1894 while engaged in a study of uterine myomata with his surgical mentor, Howard A. Kelly. He had just returned from Europe where he spent 6 months in the pathology laboratory of Carl Orth in Berlin. See: Howard A. Kelly and Thomas S. Cullen, *Myomata of the Uterus* [Philadelphia: WB Saunders, 1909], v. "In 1894 we commenced a careful study of uterine myomata and contemplated publishing the results of our findings. A year later, however, the work was temporarily laid aside, as it was deemed wiser to take up the subject of carcinoma of the uterus. After the publication of that work in 1900 we again turned our attention to uterine myomata, and since that time we have been continually gathering data on that subject."

[120] Thomas Stephen Cullen, *Adenomyoma of the Uterus* [Philadelphia: WB Saunders, 1908], v. Judith Robinson, *Tom Cullen of Baltimore* [London, Toronto, New York: Oxford University Press, 1949], 195.

[121] Thomas Stephen Cullen, *Adenomyoma of the Uterus* [Philadelphia: WB Saunders, 1908], v.

[122] Friedrich v. Recklinghausen, *Die Adenomyome und Cystadenome der Uterus- und Tubenwandung ihre Abkunft von Resten des Wolff'schen Korpers. Im Anhang: Von W. A. Freund, Klinische Notizen zu den voluminosen Adenomyomen des Uterus* [Berlin: Verlag von August Hirschwald, 1896].

[123] Friedrich v. Recklinghausen, *Die Adenomyome und Cystadenome der Uterus.*

[124] In 1862, 2 years after Rokitansky's description of endometriosis, von Recklinghausen described lymph channels, known as canals of Recklinghausen.

[125] Owsei Temkin, "Basic Science, Medicine, and the Romantic Era," in *The Double Face of Janus and Other Essays in the History of Medicine* [Baltimore, MD: Johns Hopkins University Press, 1977], 254. In 1877 in Strassburg, Welch studied gross pathology with von Recklinghausen, normal histology with Waldeyer, and physiological chemistry with Hoppe-Seyler. Page 258. It was von Recklinghausen who pointed out to Welch the significance of bacteria.

enced an awakening.[126] The famous German pathologist, the 63-year-old Professor Friedrich von Recklinghausen, had theorized the pathogenesis of uterine and tubal adenomyomas from embryonic mesonephric rests. Suddenly, Cullen realized the significance of his own work. His microscopic findings differed from those of the great German pathologist. In two cases of uterine adenomyomas, he had demonstrated the endometrial mucosa invaded the underlying uterine muscle. Until that moment, Cullen had had no idea of the significance of his own microscopic analysis. Cullen's awakening by von Recklinghausen is reminiscent of Schwann's dramatic awakening by Schleiden.[127]

Cullen pulled the large microscopic slides of his two cases and restudied them in the light of von Recklinghausen's research. In hindsight, Cullen realized he had demonstrated the mucosal origin of benign diffuse uterine adenomyomas in 1894 and 1895. His mucosal invasion pathogenesis of uterine adenomyomas conflicted directly with von Recklinghausen's mesonephric theory of origin from Wolffian remnants. Confident of his microscopic analysis, he sought consultation.

Armed with his giant microscopic slides, Cullen took his case to Welch. He too had read *Die Adenomyome und Cystadenome der Uterus und Tubenwandung*. Welch defended his old teacher, saying to Cullen: "You're wrong in your interpretation." Cullen recalled his retort to Welch: "I don't care a hoot what von Recklinghausen says...look down the barrel of that microscope." Welch examined the slides without comment.[128] But, Welch's lack of comment to Cullen was not lack of concern or involvement. Welch, affectionately and quietly known among his admirers as "Popsy,"[129] suspected – as Cullen could not – that he knew the basis for the difference of opinion between Cullen and von Recklinghausen.[130]

From Welch's active defense of von Recklinghausen to silence was confirmation enough for Cullen. He determined to write up his findings. Cullen would take issue with von Recklinghausen. Von Recklinghausen had developed a theory to explain the pathogenesis of uterine adenomyomas in the periphery of the uterus and in the proximal fallopian tube: adenomyomas remote from the uterine cavity and its mucosa. Cullen developed no theory. Instead, he demonstrated – by technology unavailable to von Recklinghausen – the

---

126 Cullen, Thomas Stephen. Adeno-myoma of the round ligament. Johns Hopkins Hospital Bulletin. 1896;7:112–114. In a carefully crafted understatement, Cullen recorded his reaction. "Recently our interest in these cases has been awakened by the excellent work of v. Recklinghausen." In the references, see: Cullen: Adeno-myoma uteri diffusum benignum. Johns Hopkins Hospital Reports, Vol. VI (in press). That Volume 7 of the Johns Hopkins Hospital Bulletin was published before Volume 6 was not the first time the Hospital reports were published out of sequence. See: Simon Flexner and James Thomas Flexner, *William Henry Welch and the Heroic Age of American Medicine* [Baltimore, MD: Johns Hopkins University Press, 1993], 243. Volume II written by William Osler was published 7 years before Volume I written by William Welch.

127 Laura Otis, *Müller's Lab* [Oxford: Oxford University Press, 2007], 63. Otis quotes Schwann's dramatic awakening, which illustrates the role of analogy in the formulation of his biological cell theory: "One day when I was having dinner with Schleiden [in October 1837] that illustrious botanist indicated to me the important role that the nucleus plays in the development of plant cells. Suddenly, I remembered having seen a similar structure [*un organe pareil*] in cells of the chorda dorsalis, and at that very instant I grasped the extreme importance the discovery would have if I succeeded in showing that, in the cells of the chorda dorsalis, the nucleus plays the same role that it plays in the development of plant cells...This fact, if solidly established through observation, would imply the negation of a vital force common to animals and would make it necessary to admit the individual life of the elementary parts of other tissues and a common means of formation through cells. This recognition of a principle, later verified by observation, constitutes the discovery I had the good fortune to make...I invited Schleiden to accompany me to the Anatomical Theater, where I showed him the nuclei in the chorda dorsalis cells. He saw [reconnut] a perfect resemblance to the nuclei of plants."

128 Judith Robinson, *Tom Cullen of Baltimore* [London, Toronto, New York: Oxford University Press, 1949], 125.

129 Simon Flexner and James Thomas Flexner, *William Henry Welch and the Heroic Age of American Medicine* [Baltimore, MD: Johns Hopkins University Press, 1993], 170.

130 Donald Fleming, *William H. Welch and the Rise of Modern Medicine* [Boston, MA: Little Brown and Company, 1954], 33–34. From December 1877 to February 1878, Welch had performed a "piece of scientific investigation under von Recklinghausen" in Strassburg. Hence, Welch was familiar with von Recklinghausen's microscopic techniques from that period. Welch also knew that von Recklinghausen was a skilled microscopist as would be expected of an assistant trained by Rudolf Virchow, who was an assistant of Johannes Müller. See also: Simon Flexner and James Thomas Flexner, *William Henry Welch and the Heroic Age of American Medicine* [Baltimore, MD: Johns Hopkins University Press, 1993], 108. Welch might also have remembered the experiment that von Recklinghausen had had him perform nearly 20 years before regarding the origin of pus cells. When it came to interpretation of the experiment, "Welch recognized [von Recklinghausen's] reasoning as fallacious and reserved judgment, assuming there must be some other explanation."

pathogenesis of benign diffuse uterine adenomyoma from the uterine mucosa.[131] Herein lay the crux of the forthcoming debate.

However, Cullen had no dispute with Wilhelm Alexander Freund, the gynecologist who first described the clinical aspects of uterine adenomyoma in an appendix to von Recklinghausen's pathological anatomy.[132] By 1896, the advantages of surgical pathology enabled researchers, like Freund, to correlate the clinical and pathological aspects of chronic diseases hidden in the interior of the living human body. By so doing, Freund elevated the pathological entity adenomyosis to a clinical entity. He demonstrated that a practitioner could diagnose adenomyosis – *Die Adenomyome und Cystadenome der Uterus* – by its signs and symptoms. This empowered him and others to prescribe specific medical or surgical treatment as indicated.[133] Nearly 2 decades earlier in 1878, Freund had published a new method for the removal of the entire uterus, a publication that a century later the medical historian Larry Longo considered among the classic pages in obstetrics and gynecology.[134]

Rokitansky had viewed *Sarcoma adenoids uterinum,* (benign uterine adenomyosis) *Cystosarcoma adenoids uterinum,* (benign cystic uterine adenomyosis), and *Ovarial-Cystosarcoma* (benign ovarian endometriosis) as distinct ontologic disease entities and he gave them descriptive Latin names. In other words, Rokitansky viewed adenomyosis and endometriosis as ontological diseases, distinguishable from healthy bodily tissues and organs.[135] In the ontological view, disease is seen as an independent entity with a history of its own.[136] Pathologists and surgeons tended to adhere to the ontological view of disease; disease was something they excised and separated from the body.[137] By the end of the nineteenth century, the Berlin gynecologist W. A. Freund viewed *Die Adenomyome und Cystadenome der Uterus* of von Recklinghausen, the *Sarcoma adenoids uterinum* of Rokitansky, as a distinct benign clinical entity – an ontological disease with a triad of symptoms and signs that enabled him to diagnose the disease clinically – before surgery.

Louis Pasteur and Robert Koch hastened identification of the role of bacteria as specific external invaders in the causation of specific diseases.[138] The technological inventions of these scientists and their followers strengthened the ancient ontological view that disease was caused by outside factors. The ontological view perceived disease as "essentially *external* in its causation."[139] In the nineteenth century, Claude Bernard in France and Virchow in Germany became exponents of the physiological concept of disease, a concept that expressed doubt about a clear demarcation between health and disease. Claude Bernard's *Introduction to the Study of Experimental Medicine* (1836) "became the classical philosophical exposition of the new concept." Bernard wrote: "The words, life, death, health, disease, have no objective reality."[140] Around the time of the Franco-Prussian War of 1870–1871, the dispute over disease

[131] Cullen cut his tissue sections with a microtome, an instrument that von Recklinghausen did not have.

[132] Anhang. Klinische Notizen zu den voluminosen Adenomyomen des Uterus. Von W. A. Freund. [The complete clinical picture of adenomyomas of the uterus.] Friedrich v. Recklinghausen, *Die Adenomyome und Cystadenome der Uterus- und Tubenwandung ihre Abkunft von Resten des Wolff'schen Korpers. Im Anhang: Von W. A. Freund, Klinische Notizen zu den voluminosen Adenomyomen des Uterus* [Berlin: Verlag von August Hirschwald, 1896.] Robert Meyer, *Autobiography of Dr. Robert Meyer: (1864–1947): A Short Abstract of a Long Life* [New York: Henry Schuman, 1949], 33. Robert Meyer confirmed that W. A. Freund first identified the classical clinical symptoms of uterine adenomyoma/ adenomyosis.

[133] Owsei Temkin, "Basic Science, Medicine, and the Romantic Era," in *The Double Face of Janus and Other Essays in the History of Medicine* [Baltimore, MD: Johns Hopkins University Press, 1977], 427.

[134] Freund, Wilhelm Alexander. Eine neue Methode der Extirpation des ganzen Uterus. Sammlung Klinischer Vortage no. 133, Gynkologie, vol. 41, pp. 911–924, 1878. Longo LD. Classic pages in obstetrics and gynecology. Am J Obstet Gynecol 1977;128:117.

[135] Owsei Temkin, "Health and Disease," in *The Double Face of Janus and Other Essays in the History of Medicine* [Baltimore, MD: Johns Hopkins University Press, 1977], 426. "The ontological view of disease, i.e., thinking of them as real, distinct entities, was nothing new. Even the comparison of a disease with an animal was old-Plato (*Timaeus* 89B) had used it, and Varro (116-27B.C.) had actually spoken of animals, too small to be seen by the eye, 'which by mouth and nose through the air enter the body and cause severe diseases.' (*Rerum rusticarium* 1, 2)."

[136] Robert P. Hudson, *Disease and Its Control: The Shaping of Modern Thought* [Westport, CT: Greenwood Press, 1983], 231.

[137] Robert P. Hudson, 229.

[138] Owsei Temkin, "Health and Disease," in *The Double Face of Janus and Other Essays in the History of Medicine* [Baltimore, MD: Johns Hopkins University Press, 1977], 435.

[139] Roy Porter, *Blood and Guts: A Short History of Medicine* [New York: W. W. Norton & Company, 2002], 82.

[140] Owsei Temkin, "Health and Disease," 434–435.

theory turned nationalistic in character. The German Virchow espoused a physiological or "internal" concept of disease and held that the French Pasteurian bacteriology represented the "external" causation of disease.[141]

Georges Canguilhem offered a nuanced explanation in his doctoral thesis written during World War II.[142] "Medical thought has never stopped alternating between these two representations of disease, between these two kinds of optimism, always finding some good reason for one or the other attitude in a newly explained pathogenesis. Deficiency diseases and all infectious or parasitic diseases favor the ontological theory, while endocrine disturbances and all diseases beginning with *dys-* support the dynamic or functional [physiologic] theory. However, these two conceptions do have one point in common: in disease, or better, in the experience of being sick, both envision a polemical situation: either a battle between the organism and a foreign substance, or an internal struggle between opposing forces. Disease differs from a state of health, the pathological from the normal, as one quality differs from another, either by the presence or absence of a definitive principle or by an alternation of the total organism."[143] Note the nuanced definitions of Canguilhem; physiologic theory means a struggle between opposing forces [internal concept of disease], and ontological theory means a battle between the body and a foreign substance [external concept of disease]; without mention that disease is an independent entity with a history of its own.[144]

Owsei Temkin broadened the concept of ontological disease when he related the concept of an *internal ontological orientation*: "The ontologist thus avoids a difficulty which the radical physiologist must face. The difference in attitude between the two is expressed in the encounter between Michel Peter and Pasteur as told by Rene Dubos. Peter claimed that 'Disease is in us, of us, by us', whereas 'Pasteur emphasized that contagion and disease could be the expression of the living processes of foreign microbial parasites, introduced from the outside, descending from parents identical to themselves, and incapable of being generated *de novo*.' Pasteur made it clear that contagious disease was the expression of a foreign life. But if disease has to be looked for in our own nature it has to be accounted for differently. If we attribute it to genes [or shed endometrium in the case of endometriosis] we still have recourse to ontology, as I indicated previously, an 'internal' ontological orientation in contrast to the external of the bacteriologist. It is probably neither possible nor advisable to renounce ontology completely."[145] Still to be realized for the chronic müllerian (endometriotic) diseases is a classification founded on etiologic causation.[146]

Learning from von Recklinghausen's inclusion of Freund's clinical description of the signs and symptoms of uterine adenomyomas, Cullen integrated clinical picture and pathological anatomy in his response to von Recklinghausen. The medical history of patients and their families reported by Cullen illustrate the background of serious infectious diseases prevalent at the end of the nineteenth century. Such diseases as tuberculosis, diphtheria, influenza, malaria, pneumonia, typhoid fever, and meningitis were endemic. Women with a history of any of these diseases were further weakened by the profuse uterine bleeding and uterine pain and tenderness that accompanied diffuse adenomyosis of the uterus.

Before writing up his scientific report, Cullen carefully reexamined his thinly sliced, microscopic sections mounted in celloidin. They were giant full-thickness *serial sections* that included the diffuse inner muscular thickening of the anterior uterine wall in the first specimen and of the posterior uterine wall in the second specimen. In both specimens, Cullen clearly demonstrated that the adenomyomatous tissue originated from

[141] Roy Porter, *Blood and Guts: A Short History of Medicine* [New York: W. W. Norton & Company, 2002], 82.

[142] Georges Canguilhem, *The Normal and the Pathological.* Trans. Carolyn R. Fawcett in collaboration with Robert S. Cohen [New York: Zone Books, 1991], 29. In the Preface to the Second Edition (1950), Canguilhem wrote: "This second edition of my doctoral thesis in medicine exactly reproduces the text of the first, published in 1943." The text quoted above was originally published in 1966 as *Le normal et le pathologique* and copyrighted by Presses Universitaires de France. It was originally published in English and copyrighted in 1978 by D. Reidel Publishing Company, Dordrecht, Holland.

[143] Georges Canguilhem, *The Normal and the Pathological.* Trans. Carolyn R. Fawcett in collaboration with Robert S. Cohen [New York: Zone Books, 1991], 41.

[144] Robert P. Hudson, *Disease and Its Control: The Shaping of Modern Thought* [Westport, CT: Greenwood Press, 1983], 231.

[145] Owsei Temkin, "The Scientific Approach to Disease: Specific Entity and Individual Sickness," in *The Double Face of Janus and Other Essays in the History of Medicine* [Baltimore, MD: Johns Hopkins University Press, 1977], 450.

[146] Knud Faber, *Nosography in Modern Internal Medicine* [New York: Paul B. Hoeber, Inc., 1923], 98.

direct invasion of the uterine musculature by stroma and glands of the uterine mucosa. Cullen's detailed report of his two cases of mucosal invasion included a third case of "pseudo-invasion." The third case revealed the sophistication of his response. Max Broedel's explicit illustrations of the gross and microscopic pathology proved beyond question the origin in the two cases of uterine adenomyomas from endometrial mucosa.[147] "Adeno-myoma Uteri Diffusum Benignum" by Thomas S. Cullen, MB (Toronto) appeared in the Johns Hopkins Hospital Reports, volume 6, 1896.[148]

Cullen's observations benefited from the application of scientific advances to the processing of tissue, improvements in microscopy, and the emergence of surgical pathology following wider use of aseptic surgery and decreased surgical mortality during the late nineteenth century. He processed his surgical specimens by first hardening them in Müller's solution, a legacy from Johannes Müller via Virchow to von Recklinghausen to Welch to Cullen.[149] "Thereafter, the tissue to be examined had to be immersed for fixed periods in alcohols of varying strength and in celloidin, before it could be blocked, sectioned, stained, and mounted for microscopic examination."[150] Celloidin, a solution of pyroxylin in ether and alcohol, used for embedding histological specimens, was in wide use by 1890 as were the giant histologic sections of an entire organ such as a kidney or a large specimen such as a uterine adenomyoma.[151] Cullen used Weigert's hematoxylin stain for his study of uterine adenomyomas in 1896.[152] Having bought a microscope in Germany in 1893 while studying with Orth, Cullen examined his specimens through an instrument with the latest refinements introduced by the German optical genius Ernst Abbe (1840–1905) between the years 1872 and 1886: the Abbe condenser and apochromatic objectives with compensating eyepieces.[153] And critically, Cullen had access to a microtome to cut thin tissue slices.[154]

However, compared to Virchow's academic stature when he had criticized Rokitansky 50 years earlier, Cullen possessed neither a Ph.D. nor a Habilitation when he challenged von Recklinghausen in 1896. Eschewing his aggressive rhetoric with Welch, Cullen cautiously invited debate with von Recklinghausen by distinguishing adenomyomata "situated in the uterine muscle at some distance from the mucosa" from the *variety* "situated in the inner layers of the uterine wall." Cullen invoked the research of Rokitansky and von Recklinghausen to bolster his argument. To accurately frame the debate, the introduction is presented as Cullen wrote it: "Glandular elements in myomata of the uterus are not at all infrequent, and numerous cases have been reported. There is a difference of opinion as to the source of the glands, some believing that they originate from remains of the Wolffian body, others that they are due to down-growths from the uterine mucosa. In the majority of the reported cases the adeno-myomata have been situated in the uterine muscle at some distance from the mucosa, or have been subperitoneal. From

[147] Judith Robinson, *Tom Cullen of Baltimore* [London, Toronto, New York: Oxford University Press, 1949], 196. Years later, Cullen recalled: "Microscopic examination of large sections of the first two specimens had clearly shown the glandular element in adenomyomata… originated in a flowing outward of the normal uterine mucosa."

[148] Cullen TS. Adeno-myoma uteri diffusum benignum. Johns Hopkins Hospital Reports 1896;6:133–157. Cullen was unaware of two brief notes on the subject that von Recklinghausen had published, the first on May 19, 1893, the second on June 14, 1895. Von Recklinghausen F. Ueber die Adenocysten der Uterustumoren und Ueberreste des Wolff'schen Organs. Deutsche Medicinische Wochenschrift 1893;xix:325–326. Von Recklinghausen F. Ueber die Adenomyome des Uterus und der Tuba. Wiener Klinische Wochenschrift 1895;29:530.

[149] Judith Robinson, *Tom Cullen of Baltimore* [London, Toronto, New York: Oxford University Press, 1949], 120.

[150] Judith Robinson, 120.

[151] Robert Meyer, *Autobiography of Dr. Robert Meyer (1864–1947): A Short Abstract of a Long Life.* With a Memoir of Dr. Meyer by Emil Novak, MD. [New York: Henry Schuman, 1949], 29.

[152] Cullen TS. Adeno-myoma uteri diffusum benignum. Johns Hopkins Hospital Reports 1896;6:133–157:136. Fielding H. Garrison, *An Introduction to the History of Medicine.* 4th edition, reprinted [Philadelphia: W. B. Saunders, 1914], 859. Weigert introduced hematoxylin staining in 1885. Fielding H. Garrison, *An Introduction to the History of Medicine.* 4th edition, reprinted [Philadelphia: W. B. Saunders, 1914], 522. "Virchow did practically all his work with carmine [tissue stain]."

[153] RM Allen, *The Microscope* [New York: D. Van Nostrand Company, 1940], 10–12.

[154] Fielding H. Garrison, *An Introduction to the History of Medicine.* 4th edition, reprinted [Philadelphia: W. B. Saunders, 1914], 522. Purkinje (1787–1869 had a microtome. "The microtome was definitely introduced by Wilhelm His in 1866, but was not perfected until about 1875, after which it became an important labor-saving device." Another source gives a later date. Alexander Hellemans and Bryan Bunch, *The Timetables of Science: A Chronology of the Most Important People and Events in the History of Science*, Touchtone Edition [New York: Simon & Schuster], 362–364. However, some advances such as the microtome to slice thin tissue sections were not invented until

these cases one has only been able to deduce theories as to the origin of the glands, but has not been in a position to make any definitive statement. In this article I propose briefly discussing a variety of adeno-myomata which is diffuse in character, is situated in the inner layers of the uterine wall, and which is dependent on the uterine mucosa for its glandular elements. "Tumours of this nature have been mentioned by Rokitansky,[155] Schatz,[156] and Schroeder,[157] and Diesterweg[158] reports a case which was probably of this character. v. Recklinghausen,[159] in the 'Nachtrag'[160] accompanying his recent work 'Die Adenomyome und Cystadenome der Uterus- und Tubenwandung,' carefully depicts a case belonging to this group."[161]

Mindful that he was a young apprentice in pathology[162] compared to the great German Master, Cullen allowed for their differences of opinion regarding the pathogenesis of uterine adenomyomata by diplomatically, but correctly, stating that most of the lesions previously described had been "situated in the uterine muscle at some distance from the mucosa, or have been subperitoneal." Having established the basis for the difference of opinion, Cullen then cited the case that von Recklinghausen had appended in the Nachtrag, as well as cases by Rokitansky, Schatz, Schroeder, and "probably" Diesterweg that supported his observation that the glands and stroma of uterine adenomyomata originate from the uterine mucosa. Finally, Cullen described minutely the gross and microscopic picture of adenomyoma uteri diffusum benignum (diffuse adenomyosis). In the first case, the uterine wall was "divided into two distinct portions: an outer, 1 cm. thick which resembles normal uterine muscle; the remainder of the wall presents a coarsely striated appearance, the striae running in all directions...the diffuse growth as a whole is much paler ['watered silk appearance' of von Recklinghausen] than the outer covering of uterine muscle." Microscopically, "the diffuse thickening is composed of non-striped muscle bundles which run in all directions. They occur as long bands of fibres, which follow a straight or serpiginous course and do not show much tendency to arrange themselves concentrically as in ordinary myomata.... At numerous points the longitudinal glands are seen penetrating the growth for a distance of 1 cm. or more. These glands present exactly the same appearance as those on the surface of the mucosa, and are accompanied by the characteristic stroma of the mucosa....The glands are most abundant near the uterine mucosa, diminish in number as one passes outward, and in the normal uterine muscle are entirely wanting...The stroma surrounding these glands resembles identically that of the uterine mucosa."[163]

Cullen then carefully described von Recklinghausen's and his own interpretation of the microscopic findings. "v. Recklinghausen was in places able to make out a definite arrangement of the muscle around the glands. He believes that the growth of the glands and of the muscle go hand in hand. I was unable to detect any special relation of the muscle to the glands. In both

1885. The microtome was invented by Charles Darwin, son of Charles Darwin, author of *The Origin of Species.*

[155] Rokitansky. Ueber Uterusdrüsen-Neubildung in Uterus u. s. w. Zeitsch. der k. k. Gesellsch. der Aerzte zu Wien, 1860, S. 577. Also: Rokitansky. (klob.) Gusserow in Billroth u. Luecke, 1886, Bd. II, S. 15.

[156] Schatz. Ein Fall von Fibro-adenome cysticum diffusum et polyposum corporis et colli uteri. Archiv f. Gyn., 1884, XXII, S. 456.

[157] Schroder. Handbuch der Krankheiten der weiblichen Geschlechtsorgane. 7. Auflage, Leipzig, 1886, S. 228.

[158] Diesterweg. Ein Fall von Cystofibroma uteri verum. Zeitschr. F. Geb. u. Gyn., Bd. IX, 1883, S. 191.

[159] von Recklinghausen. Ueber die Adenocysten der Uterustumoren und Ueberreste des Wolff'schen Organs. Deutsche Med. Woch., XIX. 1893, S. 825. Also: Von Recklinghausen. Die Adenomyome und Cystadenome der Uterus und Tubenwandung. Berlin, 1896.

[160] Nachtrag means supplement to the main text.

[161] Cullen TS. Adeno-myoma uteri diffusum benignum. Johns Hopkins Hospital Reports 1896;6:133–157:133.

[162] To more fully appreciate the fruit of Welch's philosophy to allow assistants in his laboratory to learn and discover by plunging into the work of the laboratory, consider the early achievement of Cullen with his demonstration of the pathogenesis of uterine adenomyomas. Cullen's short career in pathology at the time of his discovery is summarized: Judith Robinson, *Tom Cullen of Baltimore* [London, Toronto, New York: Oxford University Press, 1949], 78. Cullen started at Johns Hopkins Hospital in late September, 1891. Ibid: 81. Cullen spent the next months in the "Pathological," the pathology laboratory of William Henry Welch. Ibid: 103. Following a year long internship, Cullen spent several months studying pathology in the laboratory of Johannes Orth at Göttingen, Rudolf Virchows "chosen disciple." Ibid: 113–114. Cullen returned to Johns Hopkins Hospital expecting to start his residency in Gynecology only to find that the more senior William Russell had decided to take the gynecologic residency. Unexpectedly, Cullen would spend October 1893 until October 1896 in Welch's Pathological. He would become a well-trained gynecological pathologist before he started his residency in gynecology.

[163] Cullen TS. Adeno-myoma uteri diffusum benignum. Johns Hopkins Hospital Reports 1896;6:133–157: 149–150.

cases it looked as if the mucosa had penetrated into the spaces between the muscle bundles. I am constrained to believe that the muscular growth commenced in the inner zone just beneath the mucosa, and that the bundles of these fibres have been loosely united with one another and have allowed the uterine glands to penetrate into the depth."[164] Thus, Cullen presented his side of the debate with von Recklinghausen.

In sum, Cullen wrote his article on benign diffuse adenomyoma of the uterus as an immediate response to the totality of von Recklinghausen's monograph. He introduced the term *diffuse* to describe adenomyomas with stroma and glands derived by endometrial invasion of the uterine musculature. Cullen's *diffuse* adenomyomatous lesions were the antithesis of the *organoid* structures described by von Recklinghausen. As adenomyosis originates from the uterine mucosa and invades the myometrium, the lesion is diffuse. However, some lesions become cut off from their site of origin as they invade and appear macroscopically more compact or organoid, though microscopically they appear similar. Cullen's histologic descriptions augmented by Max Broedel's illustrations would give rise to a private debate with von Recklinghausen over the pathogenesis of uterine adenomyomata.

Mindful that Cullen wrote "Adeno-myoma uteri diffusum benignum" [165] as a response to von Recklinghausen's monograph, Welch sent a copy to his old teacher in Strassburg.[166] Von Recklinghausen had seen mucosal invasion but interpreted his findings quite differently than Cullen; von Recklinghausen thought that what appeared as mucosal invasion to Cullen was instead erosion of the mucosa by the expanding organoid adenomyoma, just the opposite of what Cullen demonstrated. Years later, Cullen told his biographer: "I soon heard from von Recklinghausen and I answered him and we had a long and interesting correspondence on our subject. I sent him large sections of my tumors – ones I had described in my paper – and it ended with something as near an admission of error as an old and famous Herr Professor could be expected to make: 'On all material points there is no difference between us.'"[167] From the German professor's perspective, he had demonstrated mucosal invasion in one case as Cullen had in two cases. In other words, Cullen had merely confirmed von Recklinghausen's minor thesis, that of mucosal invasion, which he had reported in the Nachtrag or appendix to his monograph.[168] Hence: "On all material points there is no difference between us."[169] Furthermore, Cullen had not disproved his major theory, the origin from remnants of the Wolffian body. Cullen's dissatisfaction arose from the belief that he *had* disproved the German professor's major theory of origin from remnants of the Wolffian body. Dissatisfied with the outcome, Cullen began to collect more surgical cases to prove his point.

Cullen's "awakening" conformed to the historical germ theory of Herbert Baxter Adams.[170] Adams' theory related American history as an outgrowth of Anglo-Saxon and Germanic antecedents.[171] The Adamsonian "intellectual germ" that awakened Thomas Stephen Cullen in 1896 was a direct outgrowth of Germanic antecedents transmitted and transplanted onto American soil in the form of Friedrich von Recklinghausen's monograph.[172] While reviewing a historical monograph by James

[164] Cullen TS. Adeno-myoma uteri diffusum benignum. Johns Hopkins Hospital Reports 1896;6:133–157:150.

[165] Cullen, TS. Adeno-myoma uteri diffusum benignum. Bulletin Johns Hopkins Hospital 1896;6:133–157.

[166] Judith Robinson, *Tom Cullen of Baltimore* [London, Toronto, New York: Oxford University Press, 1949], 125.

[167] Judith Robinson, 125.

[168] Cullen TS. 1896;6:133–157:133. On the first page of his article, Cullen states "v. Recklinghausen in the 'Nachtrag' accompanying his recent work, 'Die Adenomyome und Cystadenome der Uterus-und Tubenwandung,' carefully depicts a case belong to this group [diffuse adenomyomata]."

[169] Judith Robinson, 125. What Cullen long remembered as v. Recklinghausen's expression of "scientific equivalency" may have been tinged with "chagrin;" the German professor's mental distress caused by humiliation at the hands of an apprentice armed with a microtome.

[170] Adams was Frederick Jackson Turner's dissertation advisor at Johns Hopkins University late in the nineteenth century.

[171] Frederick Jackson Turner, "The Significance of the Frontier in American History," in *The Early Writings of Frederick Jackson Turner*, ed. Frederick Jackson Turner [Madison WI, [1893] 1938], 185–229. The essence of Turner's Frontier Thesis is contained in the last sentence of the first paragraph of his famous 1893 essay: "The existence of an area of free land, its continuous recession, and the advance of American settlement westward explain American development." See also: Harry Ritter, *Dictionary of Concepts in History* [New York: Greenwood Press, 1986], 170–178.

[172] Martzloff, KH. Thomas Stephen Cullen [Presidential Address]. Am J Obstet Gynecol 1960;80:833–843. In 1960, Karl Martzloff gave his presidential address before the American Gynecological Society; a biographical essay entitled "Thomas Stephen Cullen." Martzloff, a former student of Cullen, confirmed that v. Recklinghausen and Cullen enjoyed a long and cordial professional

V. Ricci,[173] Martzloff casually divulged a 50-year-old first-hand-account of von Recklinghausen's reaction on reading Cullen's article Adenomyoma uteri diffusum benignum in 1896.[174] "Chapter 31 discusses the once highly controversial subject of adenomyomatous changes. It would have been interesting to the reader to know that Cullen, in showing that the adenomyomas he studied were of endometrial (Müllerian) origin and not of Wolffian origin, as espoused by Recklinghausen, did so by means of studying serial sections. This he was able to do accurately because he had a microtome! When the great Recklinghausen read Cullen's article he turned somewhat chagrinned to Emil Ries (as told to me by the late E. R.) who was in Recklinghausen's laboratory at that time, and said 'Cullen has proven his point. This merely shows what this young ingenious American (junger künstlicher Amerikaner), (Cullen was born a Canadian) has been able to accomplish with the aid of a mechanical device (Ein mechanisches werkzeug) while we still putter around making sections with razor and amyloid liver.'"[175]

Emil Ries was a young German scientist working in von Recklinghausen's laboratory who witnessed first-hand the Professor's body language and verbal reaction to Cullen's article. Years later, Ries related the story to Karl H. Martzloff who not only recorded it in the Western Journal of Surgery, Obstetrics, and Gynecology but undoubtedly, having studied under Cullen, also related the story to Cullen.[176] Cullen told his biographer his version of the same incident that resulted in von Recklinghausen's comment: "On all material points there is no difference between us:" Cullen explained: "There was a difference, of course, and the real reason for it was that von Recklinghausen had obtained his material from autopsies, after the changes due to death had occurred. I was working on living tissue, or on tissue so lately removed from living patients as to be the next thing. So I knew I was right. It is the difference between trying to find the cause of a fire after the house has burned down, and getting there while it is still burning. The earlier you get to a fire, the better your chance of discovering how it began."[177]

That same year 1896, Cullen identified what he claimed was the first adenomyoma of the round ligament, which he promptly published with illustrations by Max Broedel in the Bulletin of the Johns Hopkins Hospital.[178] Cullen sent a copy of "Adeno-myoma of the round ligament" and microscopic sections to "Professor von Recklinghausen in Strasbourg."[179] In the article, Cullen described the histologic findings: "In many places the glands present a peculiar

---

relationship. "They corresponded for years" contrary to the opinion of some that it was a "long period of ill will."

[173] James V. Ricci. *One Hundred Years of Gynaecology 1800–1900. A Comprehensive Review of the Specialty during it Greatest Century with Summaries and Case Reports of All Diseases Pertaining to Women* [Philadelphia: Blakiston, 1945.] Professor James V. Ricci trained Edward J. Winkler, who was my professor of obstetrics and gynecology during medical school, internship and my first year of residency at the University of Buffalo School of Medicine, 1954–1960.

[174] Martzloff, KH. Views and Reviews. Western J Surgery, Obstetrics, and Gynecology 1946;54 (August):338. The pagination is confusing. On the top of the page, immediately it reads: VIEWS and REVIEWS (Continued from page IX). On the bottom of the page, it reads: 338.

[175] Martzloff ended with "Although Recklinghausen had his forthcoming book in press, he added a footnote, according to Dr. Ries, (not Reis, p. 510), recognizing Cullen's work." This last sentence seems counterfactual. Von Recklinghausen had published his book *before* Cullen published his article. Recall that both Welch and Cullen had read the monograph *before* Cullen walked up to Welch's laboratory with his giant slides from the 1894 and 1895 cases. Recall also that it was von Recklinghausen's monograph, with the appendix containing the one case of mucosal invasion (von Recklinghausen's minor thesis), that "awakened" Cullen to the significance of *his* two cases.

[176] Judith Robinson, *Tom Cullen of Baltimore* [London, Toronto, New York: Oxford University Press, 1949], 125.

[177] Judith Robinson, 125. See also: Martzloff, KH. Thomas Stephen Cullen [Presidential Address]. Am J Obstet Gynecol 1960;80:833–843:833–834. Martzloff offered an insight into Cullen's personality that may tangentially shed some light on Cullen's apparent ambiguity toward von Recklinghausen at this early period. Referring to Cullen, Martzloff said: "These comments are designed to be neither fault-finding nor critical, but only to afford an interesting side light to a distinguished, though not a particularly popular individual. It may seem strange that a man so generous, kind, and thoughtful, who always enjoyed the confidence and loyalty of his staff, should lack popular appeal. Always genuinely appreciative and punctilious in acknowledging a kindness or a favor, he nevertheless gave the impression of being constantly pressed for time and of being self-sufficient to the point of apparent brusqueness." Martzloff, KH. 1960;80:833–843:836. I believe Martzloff's assessment of Cullen may be taken at face value. He described his own relationship with Cullen as follows: "One whom it has been my privilege to know, one who encouraged me in my early years."

[178] Cullen, TS. Adeno-myoma of the round ligament. Bulletin Johns Hopkins Hospital 1896;7:112–114.

[179] Judith Robinson, *Tom Cullen of Baltimore* [London, Toronto, New York: Oxford University Press, 1949], 126.

arrangement and correspond to von Recklinghausen's pseudo-glomeruli." Then, Cullen explained: "These pseudo-glomeruli consist of stroma resembling that of the uterine mucosa...What corresponds to Bowman's capsule consists of a layer of cells resting directly upon the muscle fibres...In other words, the space between the capsule and the so-called glomerulus is nothing more than a dilatation of the gland cavity."[180] In sum, Cullen explained to von Recklinghausen – complete with microscopic slides – how endometrial glands and stroma could appear to be pseudo-glomeruli. This time, Cullen was not dissatisfied with the response. Von Recklinghausen wrote to Cullen thanking him and said that he had used Cullen's slides to illustrate his talk at a medical meeting in Frankfurt, Germany. Cullen considered this reply a "peace offering" from the eminent German Professor, a "peace offering," which he "graciously received."[181] It was after this second communication between the two that "an amicable pathological correspondence passed between Strasburg and Baltimore as matters of interest arose,"[182] a scholarly exchange that continued for more than a decade.[183]

Robert Meyer Disproves von Recklinghausen's Wolffian Theory

> Learning to see was never, is never, will never prove effortless...
> Daston and Galison [184]

The 1890s marked the end of an era in the discipline of human pathology, a paradigm shift from morbid pathological anatomy practiced at the autopsy table to surgical pathology practiced with fresh specimens.[185] Surgical pathology laboratories were often improvised as was Cullen's laboratory at Johns Hopkins Hospital in 1893 and Robert Meyer's "closet" sized laboratory in his Berlin apartment in 1895.[186] Meyer bought a small microtome and so was able to make thin microscopic tissue preparations for Johannes Veit, professor of gynecology at the University of Berlin, as Cullen did for Howard Kelly, professor of gynecology at Johns Hopkins University.[187] Once again, technology played a key role in scientific advancement, a generation earlier it had been the microscope of Rokitansky; now it was the microtome of Cullen and Meyer.[188]

---

180 Cullen, TS. 1896;7:112–114:113.

181 Judith Robinson, *Tom Cullen of Baltimore* [London, Toronto, New York: Oxford University Press, 1949], 126.

182 Judith Robinson, 126.

183 Martzloff, KH. Thomas Stephen Cullen [Presidential Address]. Am J Obstet Gynecol 1960;80:833–843.

184 Lorraine Daston and Peter Galison, *Objectivity* [New York: Zone Books, 2007], 161, 49, 27–28. "Learning to see was never, is never, will never prove effortless...We always return to our central question: how does the right depiction of the working objects of science join scientific sight to the scientific self?... However dominant scientific objectivity may have become in the sciences since *circa* 1860, it never had, and still does not have, the epistemological field to itself. Before objectivity, there was truth-to-nature; after the advent of objectivity came trained judgment...The relationship between epistemic virtues may be one of quiet compatibility, or it may be one of rivalry and conflict. In some cases, it is possible to pursue several simultaneously; in others, scientists must choose between truth and objectivity, or between objectivity and judgment. Contradictions exist."

185 Robert E. Fechner, "The Birth and Evolution of American Surgical Pathology," in *Guiding the Surgeon's Hand: The History of American Surgical Pathology*, ed. Juan Rosai [Washington, DC: Armed Forces Institute of Pathology, 1997], 1.

186 Robert Meyer, *Autobiography of Dr. Robert Meyer (1864–1947): A Short Abstract of a Long Life* [New York: Henry Schuman, 1949], 29. Robert Meyer met Viet, Professor of Gynecology, at his uncle's home in 1895. In response to this meeting with Viet, Meyer began his work as a pathologist in a "closet" sized laboratory in his apartment so he could be close to the hospital.

187 Robert Meyer, *Autobiography,* 29. circa 1895–1896: "I had a microscope, bought a small microtome, and learned in a short time to make sections and diagnoses with the help of Veit and books. Soon I was a virtuoso who could make sections through a whole kidney in celloidin, some of which I still have. I learned to bring the unstained sections from the knife into diluted alcohol onto the slide and to observe them with low power in comparing them with stained sections under high power. That technique I needed in order to look for anomalies in the uterus of many fetuses and adults. I stained and preserved only the positive findings. It required the patience and perseverance of a mule, which I had." Later Meyer trained a technician for this work. Meanwhile, unbeknownst to Meyer, his old professor of pathology von Recklinghausen was still cutting tissue sections by hand using a knife as he had taught Meyer in medical school.

188 Lorraine Daston and Peter Galison, *Objectivity* [New York: Zone Books, 2007], 325. "By the end of the nineteenth century... The perfection of the microscope made it possible to go from the organ pathology of Morgagni and the tissue pathology of Xavier Bichat to the cellular concepts of Rudolf Virchow, and the later introduction of the oil immersion lens greatly aided the development of microbiology. The discovery of anesthesia made vivisection practical, thereby providing the physiologist with his most important tool. The microscope and developments in chemistry made it possible to study the morphological and molecular elements of body fluids. ...a huge growth in the size of the scientific community was facilitated by a remarkable expansion and transformation of scientific pedagogy in Europe and North America during the period roughly between 1880 and 1914, especially in Germany, France, Great Britain, and the United States."

Later, makeshift laboratories were replaced by laboratories in universities and university hospitals equipped with the latest technology. Medical scientists had the choice between medical illustrations "able to capture the meaning and essence of a situation," and photographs "which could serve as a form of 'raw material'."[189]

Daston and Galison described the hazards of negotiating the slippery slope of scientific objectivity. "The persistent visual ambiguities of microscopy demanded photographic illustration, to forestall the observer's tendency 'to insert involuntarily his hypothetical explanation into the depiction.' A photograph was deemed scientifically objective because it countered a specific kind of scientific subjectivity: intervention to aestheticize or theorize the seen.[190] Current usage allows a too easy slide among senses of objectivity that are by turns ontological, epistemological, methodological, and moral. Yet these various senses of the objective cohere neither in precept nor in practice. 'Objective knowledge,' understood as 'a systematized theoretical account of how the world really is,' comes as close to truth as today's timorous metaphysics will permit. But even the most fervent advocate of 'objective methods' in the sciences - be those methods statistical, mechanical, numerical, or otherwise - would hesitate to claim that they guarantee the truth of a finding."[191]

The parallelism between Meyer and Cullen continued. Coincidently in 1896, Robert Meyer was already studying the pathogenesis of a uterine myoma "in which some almond-sized nodules of endometrium were encapsulated…when von Recklinghausen published his work on the mesonephric origin of 'adenomyomata' of the uterus (1896), which were in reality adenomyosis."[192] Like Welch and Cullen, Robert Meyer read von Recklinghausen's monograph. Unlike Welch the conciliator and Cullen the debater, Meyer played the role of a scientific detective. In response to von Recklinghausen's *Die Adenomyome und Cystadenome der Uterus- und Tubenwandung*, he began embryological studies to either corroborate or disprove his old professor's theory. In 1897, Meyer took a practical course in embryology from the Oscar Hertwig, famous for the first microscopic description of fertilization in the sea urchin.[193] That same year, he requested the uteri of fetuses and adults. With these specimens, Meyer began extensive embryological studies to test von Recklinghausen's mesonephric theory.[194] Meyer published six cases of adenomyoma of the cornual–tubal angle of the uterus.[195] Torn between the mucosal theory of Cullen and the mesonephric (Wolffian duct) theory of von Recklinghausen, Meyer assigned the pathogenesis of three cases to each of the theories.[196] In the process, Meyer became an outstanding embryologist comparable to Fischel, Keibel, Felix, and Mall. Emil Novak attributed Robert Meyer's preeminence in pathology to his profound knowledge of embryology.[197] Indicative of a latent interest in embryology, Meyer had squirreled away in his desk "an extremely rare specimen, an osteoid tissue in the uterus of a fetus."[198]

In 1897, R. Kossmann of Berlin vigorously opposed the Wolffian rest theory of von Recklinghausen, arguing for the origin of adenomyomas from accessory müllerian ducts.[199] Cuthbert Lockyer, a contemporaneous

---

[189] Lorraine Daston and Peter Galison, *Objectivity*, 164.

[190] Lorraine Daston and Peter Galison, *Objectivity*, 135.

[191] Lorraine Daston and Peter Galison, *Objectivity*, 51.

[192] Robert Meyer, *Autobiography of Dr. Robert Meyer: (1864–1947): A Short Abstract of a Long Life* [New York: Henry Schuman, 1949], 32.

[193] Robert Meyer, *Autobiography,* 32.

[194] Robert Meyer, *Autobiography,* 32.

[195] Meyer R. Uber Genese der Cystadenome und Adenomyome des Uterus, mit Demonstrationen. Zeitschr Geburtsh und Gyn 1897; 37: 327–337.

[196] Cuthbert Lockyer, *Fibroids and Allied Tumours (Myoma and Adenomyoma): Their Pathology, Clinical Features and Surgical Treatment* [London: Macmillan and Company, 1918], 281–282.

[197] Emil Novak, A memoir of Dr. Meyer in Robert Meyer, *Autobiography of Dr. Robert Meyer: (1864–1947): A Short Abstract of a Long Life* [New York: Henry Schuman, 1949], xii. "In my own judgment the one factor above all others which made possible Meyer's preeminence in the field of pathology was his profound knowledge of embryology. He was really one of the great embryologists of his time, the recognized peer of such men as Fischel, Keibel, Felix, and Mall. It was this great asset which gave him a fundamental approach in the interpretation of problems of pathology which was not possessed by any other pathologist of his day."

[198] Robert Meyer, *Autobiography,* 32. Ibid: 38. Meyer wrote: "I had, on occasion, seen and heard Virchow as the President of the Berliner Medizinische Gesellschaft and was deeply impressed by his clarity. He had accepted from me a short article on osteoid tissue in the cervix of the uterus (Virchows Archiv 167 [1902])."

[199] Kossmann R. Die Abstammung der Drüseneinschlüsse in der Uterus und der Tuben. Archiv für Gynak 1897; Bd. liv. S:359, 381. See Cuthbert Lockyer, *Fibroids and Allied Tumours (Myoma and Adenomyoma): Their Pathology, Clinical Features and Surgical Treatment* [London: Macmillan and Company, 1918], 277.

observer of the events, recorded that Kossmann's "destructive criticism…was instrumental in destroying the enthusiasm" for von Recklinghausen's theory, but not the enthusiasm of Robert Meyer.[200] A great controversy arose as to the origin of the gland elements in adenomyomata, a great "*Streitfrage*" between supporters and detractors of v. Recklinghausen's Wolffian theory. Lockyer commented on the universal respect for the judgment of Robert Meyer: "In this great *Streitfrage* it is particularly interesting to watch the evolution of the important part played by Professor Meyer of Berlin, and his final conclusions carry the great weight from the fact that all through the controversy, he kept an open mind, ready to receive new impressions, and to accord fresh findings their full value; being untrammeled by prejudice, he was candid enough to admit a change of view as occasion required, and he seemed able to do this without loss of dignity or prestige."[201]

Meyer made an informal visit to Alsace in 1898 to see his old professor. Alsace was a Germanic province of the Holy Roman Empire lost to France during the 30-Years War (1618–1648) and recaptured from France during the Franco-Prussian War of 1870–1871. There, in Strasbourg, in 1819, the French founded the first chair of pathological anatomy in Europe.[202] But unfortunately, the French deprived provincial universities "of all local initiative and deliberately subordinated [them] to the Sorbonne and the College de France."[203] After the Franco-Prussian War, the Germans sent Friedrich Daniel von Recklinghausen, the very first assistant of Rudolph Virchow and one of their ablest pathologists, to the chair of pathological anatomy at the German University of Strassburg. The Germans set high standards of scholarship. In that era, standards of *Wissenschaft* were so high that German professors, such as von Recklinghausen, were regarded as virtual academic deities.

As a medical student in Strassburg in the mid-1880s, Robert Meyer studied pathological anatomy under von Recklinghausen.[204] In his autobiography, Meyer wrote: "I learned from him the fundamentals of pathology and the art of dissection and of cutting sections by hand. For staining we used the natural dyestuffs known at the time, cochenille and carmine. Both were excellent and durable, even up to the present."[205] Meyer knew that Friedrich von Recklinghausen was a master morbid pathologist and, as a student of Virchow, a skilled microscopist. But he wanted to find out whether von Recklinghausen was still using the same techniques he had taught him in medical school. Meyer related that von Recklinghausen "was kind enough to demonstrate his sections to me, which he still cut by hand. So it was a matter of chance that he did not find the connection of adenomyosis with the endometrium. Only in later cases did he see it and have to admit in a supplement the possibility of the endometrial histogenesis. That was tragic."[206]

Meyer wondered how it had been possible for von Recklinghausen to have overlooked direct endometrial invasion of the uterine muscle as Cullen had demonstrated so clearly in two cases.[207] Meyer was unaware that von Recklinghausen, expert microscopist that he was, had set out to disprove Chiari's inflammatory theory of the pathogenesis of adenomyomas, a theory that postulated mucosal invasion of the muscular wall of the fallopian tube caused by inflammation.[208] Armed with multiple observations of pseudo-glomeruli, von Recklinghausen appears to have thrown out mucosal invasion with inflammation.[209] With respect to pseudo-

[200] Cuthbert Lockyer, *Fibroids and Allied Tumours (Myoma and Adenomyoma): Their Pathology, Clinical Features and Surgical Treatment* [London: Macmillan and Company, 1918], 278–279.

[201] Cuthbert Lockyer, *Fibroids and Allied Tumours*, 281.

[202] Esmond B. Long, *A History of American Pathology* [Springfield, IL: Charles C. Thomas, 1962], 54.

[203] Donald Fleming, *William H. Welch and the Rise of Modern Medicine* [Boston, MA: Little Brown and Company, 1954], 35.

[204] This was approximately the same time when William Henry Welch worked on a project supervised by v. Recklinghausen.

[205] Robert Meyer, *Autobiography of Dr. Robert Meyer: (1864–1947): A Short Abstract of a Long Life* [New York: Henry Schuman, 1949], 16.

[206] Robert Meyer, *Autobiography of Dr. Robert Meyer: (1864–1947): A Short Abstract of a Long Life* [New York: Henry Schuman, 1949], 33.

[207] Robert Meyer, *Autobiography,* 33. Meyer wrote: "Not that theory is almost forgotten but in retrospect one wonders how von Recklinghausen could in thirty cases have overlooked the connection of the adenomyosis with the endometrium, which is now quite clear…Only in later cases did he see it and have to admit in a supplement the possibility of the endometrial histogenesis."

[208] Rabinovitz M. The pathogenesis of adenomyosalpingitis (salpingitis nodosa): report of ten cases. American Journal of Obstetrics and Diseases of Women and Children 1913; lxviii;711–752.

glomeruli and von Recklinghausen's mesonephric theory, Meyer speculated that it was "perhaps the influence of the times which found it interesting to look for the unusual in 'embryonal' histogenesis."[210] Meyer intimated that von Recklinghausen may have learned embryology from books, which Meyer believed was impossible.[211] He continued: "one can understand von Recklinghausen's misconception when one considers his deficient technique."[212] The hand-cut histologic sections were just too thick. Consequently, as he focused up and down, he saw histologic structures that resembled kidney glomeruli, from which he deduced his theory of mesonephric rests. The renowned German professor had been upstaged in the later years of his career by a young pathologist using a superior piece of technical equipment – a microtome.[213] Though Meyer recognized von Recklinghausen's technical error, he had not proved the error of his theory. That would take 5 more years of persistent research by a prepared mind open to the serendipitous finding of rare embryological anomalies.

Meanwhile in 1898, Iwanoff suggested metaplasia of the uterine serosa to explain the pathogenesis of adenomyomas located under the smooth peritoneal covering of the uterus – distant from the uterine endometrial cavity and its mucosa.[214] Iwanoff's theory later gained the support of Pick, Aschoff, Robert Meyer, Emil Novak, and many others.[215] Thus, by 1898, there were five theories of pathogenesis of uterine adenomyomas; (1) from inflammation, (2) from müllerian rests, (3) from mesonephric rests, (4) from direct mucosal invasion of the myometrium, and (5) from metaplasia of the coelomic epithelium.

In 1899, in the course of his embryological research on human fetuses, Meyer described "various kinds of adenomyoma, adenomyosis of the uterus and islands of endometrium in the uterine wall of a fetus of nine months."[216] What Meyer observed was misplaced embryonic müllerian–endometrial tissue. For the first time ever, Meyer demonstrated – unequivocally – developmentally misplaced endometrium, embryonic adenomyosis. This unusual congenital adenomyosis in the unborn was histologically the same as the common acquired adenomyosis of Rokitansky, von Recklinghausen, and Cullen. Contemporaneously, unaware of Robert Meyer's embryological work, William Wood Russell of Johns Hopkins Hospital postulated developmentally misplaced endometrium in the adult ovary that same year, 1899.[217]

At the Berlin Gynecological Society meeting in 1900, Meyer "remarked that von Franque's work had had the effect of shaking his faith in von Recklinghausen's theory."[218] Heretofore, he had defended the mesonephric theory of von Recklinghausen. Earlier that year, von Franque had demonstrated that the "epithelial features" of adenomyomas resulted from inflammatory changes in "mature mucous membrane" of the fallopian tube.[219] Like the uterine mucosa, the tubal mucosa had no submucosa to limit invasion. One month before the Berlin meeting, Meyer had gone to Carl Ruge with 2 years worth of research and requested additional uteri of fetuses and adults. Ruge was so "enchanted" with

[209] To paraphrase the hackneyed expression: thrown out the baby with the bathwater.

[210] Robert Meyer, *Autobiography,* 64. Meyer quoted the physicist Mack to that effect; "The observation is already influenced by the theory."

[211] Robert Meyer, *Autobiography,* 33.

[212] Robert Meyer, *Autobiography,* 33.

[213] Robert Meyer, *Autobiography,* 33.

[214] Iwanoff NS. Drusiges cystenhaltiges Uterusfibromyom compliciert durch Sarcom und Carcinom. Monatsschr. Geburtsh u. Gynak. 1898;7:295. Cited by Emge LA. The elusive adenomyosis of the uterus: its historical past and its present state of recognition. Am J Obstet Gynecol 1962;83:1541–1563. See also Pick L. Ueber Neubildungen am Genitale bei Zwittern nebst Beitragen zur Lehre von den Adenomen des Hodens und Eierstockes. Arch f Gynaek 1905;lxxvi:251–275. In reference 34, Pick gives the bibliographic reference for Iwanoff's dissertation. Iwanoff, Adeno-myome de l'uterus. Inaug.-Diss. Petersburg. (Russisch.) Vergl. auch Frommel's Jahresberichte für 1897. S. 103 u.

[215] Bailey KV. The etiology, classification, and life history of tumors of the ovary and other female pelvic organs containing aberrant müllerian elements, with suggested nomenclature. J Obstet Gynaecol Brit Emp 1924;xxxi:539–57:540.

[216] Robert Meyer, *Autobiography,* 33.

[217] Russell, William Wood. Aberrant portions of the müllerian duct found in an ovary. Johns Hopkins Hospital Bulletin 1899; 10:8–10.

[218] Cuthbert Lockyer, *Fibroids and Allied Tumours (Myoma and Adenomyoma): Their Pathology, Clinical Features and Surgical Treatment* [London: Macmillan and Company, 1918], 282. See: Franque OV. Salpingitis nodosa isthmica und Adenomyoma tubae. Zeitschr f. Geb 1900; Bd. xlii: S. 42. "Von Franque's conclusions were that a *pre-existing inflammation* explained the origin of most of the 'growths,' but that von Recklinghausen's hypothesis must be held as the elucidation of the few."

[219] Cuthbert Lockyer, *Fibroids and Allied Tumours,* 279. Lockyer cited Franque OV. Salpingitis nodosa isthmica und Adenomyoma tubae. Zeitschr f. Geb 1900; Bd. xlii: S. 41.

Meyer's embryological research that he persuaded Meyer to give a lecture on "The Genesis of the Cystadenomata and Adenomyomata of the Uterus," before the Berlin Gynecological Society.[220] Meyer brought his microscopic slides of "islands of endometrium in the uterine wall of a fetus of nine months" to illustrate his lecture."[221] He used a "brand-new projector, an epidiascope" made by Carl Zeiss of Jena.[222] This was the first time that Meyer was able to project actual microscopic slides, in effect achieving enlargement of the image without sacrifice of detail. Before that he could only project microphotographs.[223] In the epidiascope, Meyer found a new instrument vital for his embryologic and pathologic research.

During the years 1900 and 1901, Robert Meyer published articles on the mucosal origin of uterine adenomyomas.[224] Both Lockyer and Meyer[225] would champion inflammation of mature mucous membranes as the pathogenesis of uterine adenomyomas.[226] Lester King traced the theory of inflammation to ancient authors. Celsus in the first century AD "explicitly" described the characteristic signs of inflammation caused by a foreign body, a cinder in the eye: "*dolor, tumor, rubor,* and *calor* – pain, swelling, redness, and heat." A second cause of inflammation also recognized since antiquity was produced by "bad" food [or drink]; "abdominal pain, fever, and diarrhea…The whole theory of inflammation, constantly expanding like the universe, can be intercalated between terms A and B, between 'the' cause (the cinder [or bad food]) and 'the' effect (the full-blown inflammation)."[227] In the early eighteenth century, Herman Boerhaave (1668–1738) believed that "inflammation resulted principally from a mechanical obstruction of vessels…from a contraction of the vessel, an impaction of…red blood cells, or a thickening…of the blood [which could be relieved by] diminishing the force of the arterial blood by bleeding and purging." William Cullen (1710–1790) succeeded Boerhaave as the leading theorist on inflammation of the eighteenth century. Cullen theorized that inflammation arose from a *functional* obstruction of the blood vessels resulting from spasm, not a *mechanical* obstruction as theorized by Boerhaave. But the treatment was the same.[228] John Hunter (1728–1793) in his classic *Treatise on the Blood, Inflammation, and Gunshot Wounds* described three types of inflammation, "the adhesive, the suppurative, and the ulcerative."[229] In *Traite des membranes* published at the turn of the nineteenth century, Marie-Francois-Xavier Bichat (1771–1802) distinguished simple membranes tissues from pathological membranes. "He considered mucous membrane a protective barrier against foreign bodies, comparable to the skin. A mucous membrane exposed to air, he noted, will have a protective power against inflammation, although a serous membrane, similarly exposed, will not."[230] Thomas Hodgkin (1798–1878) of Guy's Hospital in London who praised the English and French – especially Bichat and Laennec – for the study of tissues, realized that serous and mucous membranes "afford[ed] the best opportunity for observing the varieties in the modes of inflammation, in the products to which they give rise, and in the stages through which they pass." But of paramount importance, Hodgkin linked inflammation and disease: the serous

[220] Robert Meyer, *Autobiography,* 32.

[221] Robert Meyer, *Autobiography,* 33.

[222] *Illustrated Stedman's Medical Dictionary.* 24th ed. [Baltimore, MD: Williams & Wilkins, 1982], 474. The epidiascope is a "projector by which images are reflected by a mirror through a lens, or lenses, onto a screen, using reflected light for opaque objects and transmitted light for translucent or transparent ones." Carl Zeiss was the company for which Ernst Abbe worked.

[223] Robert Meyer, *Autobiography,* 32–33.

[224] Meyer R. Uber Drüsen, Cysten und Adenome in Myometrium bei Erwachsenen. Zietschr f. Geb und Gynak 1900–1901; xlii, xliii, xliv.

[225] Robert Meyer, *Autobiography,* 70–71.

[226] Cuthbert Lockyer, *Fibroids and Allied Tumours (Myoma and Adenomyoma): Their Pathology, Clinical Features and Surgical Treatment* [London: Macmillan and Company, 1918], 279. Lockyer cited Franque OV. Salpingitis nodosa isthmica und Adenomyoma tubae. Zeitschr f. Geb 1900; Bd. xlii: S. 41. Robert Meyer believed that inflammation might initiate basal endometrial invasion characteristic of diffuse adenomyosis, a concept harbored by Chiari for initiation of salpingitis isthmica nodosa (endosalpingiosis). Meyer abandoned the inflammatory theory in favor of the hormonal theory introduced by Lauche in 1923. See Emge LA. The elusive adenomyosis of the uterus: its historical past and its present state of recognition. Am J Obstet Gynecol 1962;83:1541–1563. Emge cited Arnold Lauche. Virchow's Arch Path Anat 1923;243:298.

[227] Lester S. King, *Medical Thinking: A Historical Preface* [Princeton, NJ: Princeton University Press, 1982], 197–198.

[228] Lester S. King, *Medical Thinking: A Historical Preface* [Princeton, NJ: Princeton University Press, 1982], 229–233.

[229] Lester S. King, *The Medical World of the Eighteenth Century* [Huntington, NY: Robert E. Krieger Publishing Co., 1958, Reprint 1971], 284, 287.

[230] Lester S. King, *The Medical World of the Eighteenth Century,* 291–292.

and mucous tissues were subject not only to inflammation but also to an "overwhelming frequency of disease."[231] He accused the followers of Broussaisism, the "so-called physiological doctrine" of Francois-Joseph-Victor Broussais (1772–1838), of seeing nothing but inflammation, "inflammation everywhere."[232] Broussais theorized that disease was the result of inflammation resulting from chemical, mechanical, or emotional stimuli; Laennec opposed the idea.[233] Relating the theory of inflammation to the müllerian diseases; Rokitansky mentioned inflammation several times when he discussed endometriotic lesions in 1860 and Chiari specifically postulated inflammation as the pathogenesis of endosalpingiosis in 1887.

Only von Recklinghausen challenged the inflammatory theory of pathogenesis during the nineteenth century. Lockyer and Robert Meyer held fast to the inflammatory theory. From the historical distance of mid-twentieth century, Robert Meyer reassessed the inflammatory theory as an explanation of the pathogenesis of adenomyosis: "In the Zeitschrift für Gynakologie (1924) in Virchows Archiv (1924), and in Deutsche Pathologische Gesellshaft (1925) I published articles on adenomyosis and endometriosis. As early as 1909 I had observed that it was the stroma of the endometrium which had the ability to destroy other tissue, especially elastic tissues (Virchows Archiv). At that time it was not known that one tissue could dissolve another without being malignant. There was a similarity between inflammation and this dissolving potentiality that induced me to call it adenomyometritis. This was an error and I had to struggle with myself for a long time until I was at length persuaded that it was an adenomyohyperplasia and accepted the expression adenomyosis uteri et tubae (Frankl) and endometriosis from the Americans for the identical ectopic proliferation of the endometrium without musculature. This mostly occurs independently of adenomyosis of the uterus. I found that the histolytic quality is not only responsible for the destruction of the interfascicular connective tissue but also for the musculature which undergoes necrosis to a greater or lesser degree."[234]

Von Franque's theory of the inflammatory pathogenesis of tubal adenomyoma[235] (a theory put forth earlier by Chiari in 1887) and the inflammatory theory of pathogenesis of uterine adenomyoma postulated by "Felix Legueu and Marien of Montreal" had influenced Lockyer.[236] In the years 1901 and 1902, Meyer commented on adenomyomas at the tubal angle of the uterus that von Recklinghausen contended originated from mesonephric (Wolffian) rests. "It is a definitely *post-foetal* phenomenon: all stages are present, from the cutting off of a single cyst in the mucosa (*salpingitis pseudo-follicularis*) and the intrusion of a single short follicles in the muscularis (*salpingitis follicularis*) to an enormous adenomatous branching through all the layers of the tube-wall and into the broad ligament…It was true that the normal tube had no glands, but the pathological tube was different – it could make them."[237] Meyer spoke of the "sprouting-faculty" of the epithelium of the fallopian tube, likening it to "water under a high pressure bursting out in jets to form a fountain; the epithelium of an inflamed tube is under such a pressure, and is ready to make use of the smallest aperture for proliferation and for spreading through countless interstices."[238] Speaking about the pathogenesis of uterine adenomyosis, Meyer continued: "The stroma of the invading mucosa is of great significance: it clothes all the epithelial spaces; it is spindle-celled and thick, but never sarcomatous…The invasion is *post-foetal*; it is a disease of the adult uterus."[239] As with the fallopian tube, absence of a true submucosa favored mucosal invasion of the uterine musculature.

[231] Russell C. Maulitz, *Morbid Appearances: The Anatomy of Pathology in the Early Nineteenth Century* [New York: Cambridge University Press, 1987], 207.

[232] Russell C. Maulitz, *Morbid Appearances,* 205.

[233] Jacalyn Duffin, "Laennec and Broussais: The 'Sympathetic' Duel" in *Constructing Paris Medicine,* ed. Caroline Hannaway and Ann La Berge [Amsterdam, NL: Editions Rodopi B. V., 1998], 251–274: 254, 262.

[234] Robert Meyer, *Autobiography*, 70–71.

[235] Franque OV. Salpingitis nodosa isthmica und Adenomyoma tubae. Zeitschr f. Geb 1900; Bd. xlii: S. 41.

[236] Cuthbert Lockyer, *Fibroids and Allied Tumours (Myoma and Adenomyoma): Their Pathology, Clinical Features and Surgical Treatment* [London: Macmillan and Company, 1918], 279–280. Lockyer cited: Legueu F, Marien. Ann de gyn et d'obstet 1897:134

[237] Cuthbert Lockyer, *Fibroids and Allied Tumours,* 285–286.

[238] Cuthbert Lockyer, *Fibroids and Allied Tumours,* 285–286. Meyer R. Uber Drüsen, Cysten und Adenome in Myometrium bei Erwachsenen. Zietschr f. Geb und Gynak 1900–1901; xlii, xliii, xliv.

[239] Cuthbert Lockyer, *Fibroids and Allied Tumours,* 288. Meyer R. Uber Drüsen, Cysten und Adenome in Myometrium bei Erwachsenen. Zietschr f. Geb und Gynak 1900–1901; xlii, xliii, xliv.

1902 was an eventful year for Robert Meyer's research. That year, Rudolf Virchow accepted an article from Meyer describing an "extremely rare specimen, an osteoid tissue in the uterus of a fetus." It was the specimen he had squirreled away in his desk years before. During the negotiations for publication, Meyer requested and received from Virchow the genitals of a 6-year-old orangutan. On examination, he found "an island of endometrium in the middle of the posterior wall of the fundus" in exactly the same place that he had found a similar lesion in the uterus of the 9 month fetus 3 years previously.[240] Meyer thus had documented developmental adenomyosis in a nonhuman primate and in a human fetus.

Also in 1902, Meyer obtained another unique uterine specimen, this one human. With the Zeiss epidiascope,[241] he studied a "new kind of giant adenofibromyoma proceeding from a horn of the uterus…an organoid structure [that] in no way resemble[d] adenomyosis but strikingly resemble[d] epididymis."[242] Meyer had demonstrated a "real adenomyoma of mesonephric origin imitating the epoophoron or epididymis of the adults."[243] This adenomyoma was not composed of endometrial glands and stroma. Meyer stated that this case was decisive for his renunciation of von Recklinghausen's mesonephric theory of pathogenesis of uterine and tubal adenomyomas.[244] When he published his findings in 1903, he criticized the mesonephric theory "point by point" after which it was "generally and definitely abandoned."[245] Meyer achieved with his embryological expertise what Cullen was unqualified to do; he scientifically refuted von Recklinghausen's mesonephric theory.[246] Meyer could only refute von Recklinghausen by demonstrating an actual Wolffian mesonephric rest in a fetal uterus; he had had to prove that it did not resemble a pseudoglomeruli; in fact, it resembled epididymis. Recall also that Meyer had taken a practical course in embryology from Oscar Hertwig in 1897 and subsequently devoted years to embryological research.[247] Cullen had no such training in embryology; he simply accepted the müllerian theory of pathogenesis of uterine and extrauterine adenomyomas, relying on their histologic identity.

Refuting the theory was one thing, but explaining it to von Recklinghausen was another. Meyer convinced his old professor "of this faulty reasoning" based on misinterpretation of thick, hand-cut histologic sections.[248] While Cullen had demonstrated an alternative pathogenesis by mucosal invasion, he had not disproved von Recklinghausen's theory. It took Robert Meyer's embryological research in fetal uteri and the uteri of children and adults to definitively disprove von Recklinghausen's Wolffian theory of origin of uterine and tubal adenomyomas. The meeting in 1903 between von Recklinghausen and Robert Meyer must have been painful for both men.

---

240 Robert Meyer, *Autobiography,* 38.

241 *Illustrated Stedman's Medical Dictionary,* 24th ed. [Baltimore, MD: Williams & Wilkins, 1982], 474. A projector by which images are reflected by a mirror through a lens, or lenses, onto a screen, using reflected light for opaque objects and transmitted light for translucent or transparent one.

242 Robert Meyer, *Autobiography,* 35. See also: Robert Meyer, Eine unbekannte Art von Adenomyom des Uterus mit einer kritischen Besprechung der Urnierenhypothese v. Recklinghausen's. Zeitschr. f. Geburtsh. Gyn. 1903;49:464–507.

243 Robert Meyer, *Autobiography,* 33.

244 Robert Meyer, *Autobiography,* 35.

245 Robert Meyer, Eine unbekannte Art von Adenomyom des Uterus mit einer kritischen Besprechung der Urnierenhypothese v. Recklinghausen's. Zeitschr. f. Geburtsh. Gyn. 1903;49: 464–507.

246 Emil Novak, "A Memoir of Dr. Meyer," in Robert Meyer, *Autobiography of Dr. Robert Meyer (1864–1947): A Short Abstract of a Long Life* [New York: Henry Schuman, 1949], xii. Novak opined: "In my judgment the one factor above all others which made possible Meyer's preeminence in the field of pathology was his profound knowledge of embryology. He was really one of the great embryologists of his time, the recognized peer of such men as Fischel, Keibel, Felix, and Mall. It was this great asset which gave him a fundamental approach in the interpretation of problems of pathology which was not possessed by any other pathologist of his day."

247 Robert Meyer, *Autobiography,* 32.

248 Emge LA. The elusive adenomyosis of the uterus: its historical past and its present state of recognition. Am J Obstet Gynecol 1962;83:1541–1563:1543.

Cullen's Research at Johns Hopkins Hospital

5

Cullen's Research at Johns Hopkins Hospital 1898–1906

From available evidence, Thomas Cullen remained unaware of the active role Robert Meyer played in resolving Cullen's differences with Professor Friedrich von Recklinghausen. However, Cullen may have relieved von Recklinghausen's embarrassment with his discussion of the origin of the glands in his case of adeno-myoma of the round ligament: "While admitting the probability of the glands in our case being due to remains of the Wolffian body, we cannot, from their striking resemblance to those of the uterine mucosa, and from the fact that their stroma resembles that of the mucosa, refrain from suggesting the possibility that they may be due to an abnormal embryonic deposit of a portion of Müller's duct."[1] Heartened by the "peace offering" he received from Strassburg, von Recklinghausen and Cullen would continue their professional exchange for a decade. Cullen returned to the daily routine of the pathology laboratory of analyzing gynecologic surgical specimens. He focused his attention on completing a study of uterine cancer.[2] Notwithstanding all the work he would do on adenomyomas, Cullen's real interest lay in the pathology and early detection of uterine cancer.

Two years later, in 1898, William W. Russell operated on a postmenopausal patient for cystic adenocarcinoma of the left ovary.[3] The woman had experienced a natural menopause. Russell removed a normal size right ovary "enveloped in adhesions on the posterior surface of the broad ligament, while the tube was free and patent."[4] In the January-February-March 1899 issue of the Johns Hopkins Hospital Bulletin, Russell published the results of his analysis. On microscopic examination of longitudinal serial sections of the ovary, Russell reported: "we were astonished to find areas which were an exact prototype of the uterine glands and interglandular connective tissue."[5] Plate III of Max Broedel's illustrations shows a portion of a wall surrounding a cystic space with what might be interpreted as an organoid structure within the substance of the ovary. "The whole [of the organoid structure] formed an exact reproduction of a portion of the uterine

[1] Cullen, TS. Adeno-myoma of the round ligament. Bulletin Johns Hopkins Hospital 1896;7:112–114:114. See also: Thomas Stephen Cullen, *Adenomyoma of the Uterus* [Philadelphia: WB Saunders, 1908], 253.

[2] Howard A. Kelly and Thomas S. Cullen, *Myomata of the Uterus* [Philadelphia: WB Saunders, 1909], v. "In 1894 we commenced a careful study of uterine myomata and contemplated publishing the results of our findings. A year later, however, the work was temporarily laid aside, as it was deemed wiser to take up the subject of carcinoma of the uterus. After the publication of that work in 1900 we again turned our attention to uterine myomata, and since that time we have been continually gathering data on that subject." Thomas Stephen Cullen, *Cancer of the Uterus: Its Pathology, Symptomatology, Diagnosis, and Treatment. Also the Pathology of Diseases of the Endometrium* [New York: D. Appleton and Company, 1900].

[3] Russell, Cullen's senior at Johns Hopkins, was the same William Wood Russell who reclaimed the residency position promised to Cullen in 1894. He was a resident under Howard Kelly and later became an associate professor of gynecology at Johns Hopkins.

[4] Russell, William Wood. Aberrant portions of the müllerian duct found in an ovary. Johns Hopkins Hospital Bulletin 1899; 10:8–10:8.

[5] Russell, William Wood. 1899; 10:8–10:8. Plates I, II, and III are appended to the article.

R.E. Batt, *A History of Endometriosis*,
DOI 10.1007/978-0-85729-585-9_5,

mucous membrane and muscle. The arrangement of these structures gave the impression that they were a continuous system from the groove on the posterior surface to a cystic space on the anterior face."[6] He stipulated: "accepting the studies of Nagel, that the epithelial elements of the Müllerian duct are derived from the germinal epithelium, as correct, I believe we are able to explain the condition found in this instance as due to an anomalous point of development of portions of the Müllerian duct in the germinal epithelium."[7] Russell then reviewed contemporary explanations "in reference to the origin of the epithelium of the Müllerian duct." Russell drew the conclusion "that the epithelium of the Müllerian duct is exclusively derived from true germinal epithelium." [8] Russell contended that his specimen supplied "direct proof that the germinal epithelium is capable of producing glands analogous to those of the uterine mucosa."[9] In other words, Russell believed the germinal epithelium of the right ovary differentiated into aberrant portions of the Müllerian duct by metaplasia. He did not argue for a pathogenesis from mesonephric rests. Nor did he believe the aberrant endometrial tissue of the right ovary originated from müllerian rests.[10]

Years later, Howard Kelly spoke of this case of W. W. Russell. "Without any doubt, his most important contribution was a carefully made objective study of a case, the first one reported, of endometrial tissue in the ovary, far reaching in its consequences in view of the later studies of Thomas S. Cullen and John A. Sampson."[11] Kelly was unaware of Rokitansky's contribution. More than a century later, Benagiano and Brosens also would credit Russell of Johns Hopkins as the first to describe what is now known as an ovarian endometrioma.[12] However, Russell's case was no ordinary endometrioma as defined by Hughesdon.[13] First, the ovary was normal size. Second, the lesion was strikingly different from the ovarian cystic and solid lesions encountered at Johns Hopkins Hospital at that time. Third, the lesion extended from one surface of the ovary to the other as a solid seam of adenomyomatous tissue with small cystic cavities evidencing some

[6] Russell, William Wood. 1899; 10:8–10.

[7] Russell, William Wood. 1899; 10:8–10:8.

[8] Russell, William Wood, 1899; 10:8–10;9.

[9] Russell, William Wood. 1899; 10:8–10:9–10. "In the specimen which I have described there is a collection of glands in a groove on the surface of the ovary. The epithelium covering them is continuous with a single layer of columnar cells at the margin of the groove and extends a short distance over the surrounding surface. Thus we have direct proof that the germinal epithelium is capable of producing glands analogous to those of the uterine mucosa."

[10] *Wolffian or mesonephric rest*: The mesonephros – the primitive vertebrate kidney – comprises two elongated masses in the early vertebrate embryo. A Wolffian rest represents a group of cells or a portion of the mesonephros (Wolffian body) that has become displaced and lies embedded in tissue of another character that persists as an embryonic remnant in the adult. *Müllerian rest*: The paired müllerian tubes – primitive vertebrate fallopian tubes, uterus, cervix, and upper vagina – comprise two elongated masses in the early vertebrae embryo. A müllerian rest represents a group of cells or a portion of the müllerian that has become displaced and lies embedded in tissue of another character that persists as an embryonic remnant in the adult. *Müllerian duct*, also known as the paramesonephric duct, arises from the urogenital ridge in the fetus to form the fallopian tubes, uterus, cervix and upper vagina. *Germinal epithelium* of the ovary consists of low flat mesothelial cells on the surface of the ovary, similar to those lining the peritoneal cavity. Mesothelial cells are derived from the mesoderm which gives rise to the gastrointestinal and reproductive organs. *Metaplasia* is the abnormal transformation of an adult, fully differentiated tissue of one kind into a differentiated tissue of another kind; metaplasia is an acquired condition in contrast to heteroplasia. *Coelomic metaplasia* is a general term that refers to the abnormal transformation of adult, fully differentiated tissue lining the peritoneal cavity into a differentiated tissue of another kind, such as endometrial tissue. *Serosal metaplasia* is a more restricted term that refers to the abnormal transformation of adult, fully differentiated tissue covering the surface of pelvic and abdominal organs – such as the uterus – into a differentiated tissue of another kind, such as endometrial tissue. *Heteroplasia*, on the other hand, is the development of cytologic and histologic elements that are not normal for the organ or part in question, as the growth of bone in a site where there is normal fibrous connective tissue. *Heterotopia* means cells or tissue displaced to an abnormal location.

[11] Howard Kelly did not credit von Franque whom WW Russell had cited as reference #11. Russell, William Wood. Aberrant portions of the müllerian duct found in an ovary. Johns Hopkins Hospital Bulletin 1899; 10:8–10:10. "...von Franque has published the preliminary report of an ovary which apparently confirms the Wolffian theory. His remarks are so brief that one is not justified in criticism, but it would seem that he has in his case positive evidence that the parovarial tubules can, as we have already suggested, enter the ovary through the hilum and produce these glandular formations." Ref. No. 11: Von Franque. Uber Urnierenreste im Ovarium, etc. Sitzungs-Berichte der physikalich-medicinischen Gesellschaft zu Würzburg, July 7, 1898.

[12] Benagiano G, Brosens I. History of adenomyosis. Best Pract Res Clin Obstet Gynecol 2006;20:449–63:450–1.

[13] Hughesdon PE. The structure of the endometrial cyst of the ovary. J Obstet Gynaecol Brit Emp 1957;44:481–487.

bleeding. "The whole formed an exact reproduction of a portion of the uterine mucous membrane and muscle. The arrangement of these structures gave the impression that they were a continuous system from the groove on the posterior surface to a cystic space in the anterior face."[14] Arguably this lesion may have been Sampson's developmentally misplaced endometrium,[15] a choristoma,[16] and an example of müllerianosis.[17]

An editorial appeared in the September 30, 1899 issue of the Journal of the American Medical Association, without reference to Cullen or Russell. It stated flatly that the work of Leopold Landau of Berlin settled the issue of pathogenesis of adenomyomata of the female sexual apparatus and proved von Recklinghausen's theory of origin from Wolffian canals.[18] At this time in North America, there was only one journal devoted to obstetrics and gynecology, the Journal of Obstetrics and the Diseases of Women and Children. So it was not unusual for a subject of general interest to general practitioners and general surgeons to appear in a general interest medical journal such as the Journal of the American Medical Association. What was unusual, perhaps, was the lack of any reference to Cullen's articles on the subject, articles published by the leading American medical school of the time.

Early in his career Cullen decided to follow the Johns Hopkins idea to write definitive books on a subject[19] rather than medical textbooks that required successive editions.[20] This practice cost Cullen between 50 and 60 thousand dollars for the five books he published. He deliberately took the losses rather than profits from textbooks. Cullen clarified: "With each major book I wrote, I took the same course. Insofar as I could, I assembled all the knowledge on that subject available at that date, presented it in as complete a manner as possible and published. That was definitive and I was through. The next man could take on from there."[21]

By 1900 Cullen had finished his cancer research. He wrote his first monograph, *Cancer of the Uterus,* the equivalent of a PhD dissertation. In the dedication, Cullen acknowledged his teacher-advisors, Howard A. Kelly and William H. Welch.[22] Yale offered him the chairmanship of its department of gynecology with the rank of full professor. Johns Hopkins met this challenge with a counter offer of associate professor and Cullen remained at Johns Hopkins.[23] Reflecting in his later years, Cullen said that *Cancer of the Uterus* "was probably the most important book I ever published."[24] Karl Martzloff, his student and biographer agreed: "Cullen's first book…remained the single great unchallenged monograph on uterine cancer until the voluminous and excellent German monograph of Schottlaender and Kermauner appeared 12 years later."[25] Cullen now had an international reputation based on his work with cancer, not adenomyomas.

In 1901, William Welch was consulted for a second opinion on a case with a presumptive diagnosis of osteo-fibromyoma of the uterus.[26] He was given an unusual specimen to examine and found in it smooth muscle, true bone, and embryonic connective tissue. He agreed with the diagnosis, but with qualifications: "The

[14] Russell, William Wood. Aberrant portions of the müllerian duct found in an ovary. Johns Hopkins Hospital Bulletin 1899; 10:8–10:8.

[15] Sampson JA. Heterotopic or misplaced endometrial tissue. Am J Obstet Gynecol 1925;10:649–664.

[16] Choristoma. In *Stedman's Medical Dictionary*. 28th ed. [Philadelphia: Lippincott Williams & Wilkins, 2006], 371. A choristoma is a mass of histologically normal tissue that is "not normally found in the organ or structure in which it is located." Müllerian choristomas are a subset of non-müllerian choristomas found throughout the body.

[17] Ronald E. Batt, Smith RA, Buck Louis GM, Martin DC, Chapron C, Koninckx PR, Yeh J. Müllerianosis. Histol Histopathol 2007;22:1161–1166.

[18] Editorial. Adenomyomata of the female sexual apparatus. Journal American Medical Association 1899;33:863–4.

[19] Judith Robinson, *Tom Cullen of Baltimore* [London, Toronto, New York: Oxford University Press, 1949], 327. "The Hopkins idea is to publish and to publish adequately; to do so thorough a job when you undertake to deal with a subject that it won't be worth anyone's time to touch it again for twenty or thirty years."

[20] Judith Robinson, *Tom Cullen*, 159.

[21] Judith Robinson, *Tom Cullen*, 159.

[22] Thomas Stephen Cullen, *Cancer of the Uterus: Its Pathology, Symptomatology, Diagnosis, and Treatment. Also the Pathology of Diseases of the Endometrium* [New York: D. Appleton and Company, 1900], 535–536.

[23] Judith Robinson, *Tom Cullen*, 159.

[24] Judith Robinson, *Tom Cullen*, 139.

[25] Martzloff, KH. Thomas Stephen Cullen [Presidential Address]. Am J Obstet Gynecol 1960;80:833–843:837.

[26] Johnston, George B. Osteo-Fibromyoma of the Uterus. Am Gynaec & Obst. J., N.Y., 1901, XVIII, 307–308. William Henry Welch, *Pathology, Preventive Medicine*, vol. 1 of *Papers and Addresses by William Henry Welch* [Baltimore, MD: Johns Hopkins Press, 1920], 432–3.

tumor must, I think, be referred to embryonic remnants, and there is no objection to considering it as a teratoid formation, although not a very complex one. Besides the bone and smooth muscle, there is a great deal of peculiar embryonic connective tissue in the growth, partly mucoid in character, and partly more cellular, and this tissue is quite unlike any found in ordinary myomatous tumors."[27] This was an example of a non-müllerian tissue (bone) in müllerian tissue (uterus); a choristoma, a developmental anomaly. Recall that Robert Meyer had identified endometrial islands in the uterus of a 9 month fetus: developmental adenomyosis. W. W. Russell had identified what may have been a choristoma, i.e., developmentally misplaced endometrial tissue in the ovary. Recall also, that Robert Meyer discovered a giant uterine adenofibromyoma that resembled epididymis, misplaced mesonephric tissue in the uterus, a non-müllerian tissue in müllerian tissue – a choristoma. In sum, by the turn of the twentieth century, developmental uterine adenomyosis, a non-mullerian choristoma of the uterus composed of embryonic bone, and possibly developmentally misplaced endometriosis of the ovary had been identified.

Baldy and Longscope reviewed the pertinent literature on uterine adenomyomas in 1902, before resolution of the debate between Cullen and von Recklinghausen. They strongly supported Cullen's mucosal pathogenesis and thought the mesonephric theory of von Recklinghausen "improbable."[28] Baldy and Longscope made no mention of Iwanoff.[29] However, they seemed better informed than the author of the editorial in the Journal of the American Medical Association of 1899 who settled on von Recklinghausen's theory of origin from the Wolffian body.[30] Six years later, Cullen opined that the review by Baldy and Longscope was "probably the best article written in this country on adenomyoma of the uterus."[31] Undoubtedly, their favorable review of his work encouraged Cullen.

In 1903 Cullen published a supplement in German to the Festschrift for his friend, Professor Johannes Orth of Berlin. On this momentous occasion Cullen reported all the cases of diffuse benign uterine adenomyomata that he had accumulated since 1896.[32] The 22 cases supported his earlier demonstration of the mucosal pathogenesis of diffuse uterine adenomyomas. Because the adenomyomatous process was confined to the uterus in most of his cases, Cullen stated that he could "definitely determine 'in most cases' the origin of the glands from the mucous membrane of the uterine cavity."[33] Cullen must have experienced a sense of pride in his newfound professional stature, contributing to the Festschrift of the successor to Virchow's chair, because he distributed hard cover copies of the Festschrift to his friends.[34]

Cullen received further support from Whitridge Williams, Professor of Obstetrics at Johns Hopkins. In 1904, Williams performed an autopsy on a woman who had tragically died 2 h postpartum. The stroma within diffuse islands of adenomyosis throughout the uterine musculature had been converted to decidua.[35] Arguing by analogy, Cullen used this case as proof that the decidual transformation of islands of mucosa was identical to uterine mucosa, a case that "would certainly tend to convince the most skeptical."[36]

In 1906, while in Germany for the fourth time, Cullen telephoned von Recklinghausen and made an appointment to visit him in Strassburg. After 10 years

[27] Johnston, George B. Osteo-Fibromyoma of the Uterus. Am Gynaec & Obst. J., N.Y., 1901, XVIII, 307–308. William Henry Welch, *Pathology, Preventive Medicine*, vol. 1 of *Papers and Addresses by William Henry Welch* [Baltimore, MD: Johns Hopkins Press, 1920], 432–3.

[28] Baldy JM and Longscope WT. Adenomyomata Uteri. Am J Obstetrics and Diseases of Women and Children 1902;xlv:788–802.

[29] Iwanoff NS. Drusiges cystenhaltiges Uterusfibromyom compliciert durch Sarcom und Carcinom. Monatsschr. Geburtsh u. Gynak. 1898;7:295. See: Cuthbert Lockyer, *Fibroids and Allied Tumours (Myoma and Adenomyoma): Their Pathology, Clinical Features and Surgical Treatment* [London: Macmillan and Company, 1918], 297. Iwanoff postulated that an adenomyoma complicated with carcinoma and sarcoma originated from the uterine serosa. See also: Bailey KV. The etiology, classification and life history of tumours of the ovary and other female pelvic organs containing aberrant müllerian elements, with suggested nomenclature. J Obstet Gynaecol Brit Emp 1924;xxxi:539–57:540. Iwanoff's theory would later gained support of Pick Aschoff, Robert Meyer, Emil Novak, and many others.

[30] Editorial. Adenomyomata of the female sexual apparatus. Journal American Medical Association 1899;33:863–4.

[31] Thomas Stephen Cullen, *Adenomyoma of the Uterus* [Philadelphia: WB Saunders, 1908], 2. Fn. No. 2.

[32] Thomas S. Cullen. Adeno-Myome des Uterus. [Berlin: Verlag von August Hirsch, 1903].

[33] Cuthbert Lockyer, *Fibroids and Allied Tumours*, 289.

[34] The author has a hard bound copy from the Library of Dr. John B. Murphy of Chicago, thanks to Dr. Ronald Cyr.

[35] J. Whitridge Williams. Decidual formation through the uterine muscularis: a contribution to the origin of adenomyoma of the uterus. Transactions of the Southern Surgical Association 1904;17:119.

[36] Thomas Stephen Cullen, *Adenomyoma of the Uterus* [Philadelphia: WB Saunders, 1908], 197.

of correspondence the two finally met face-to-face. Cullen had anticipated that their meeting would provide an opportunity for discussion about their mutual interest, the pathogenesis of adenomyomas. Instead, Cullen witnessed a performance.[37] "Though an old man then, von Recklinghausen was still doing original work in pathology and had just published some results of his recent researches in bone infection that were perfectly fascinating. But do you think I could get him talking about them or showing the work going on in his laboratory? Not a bit of it. What he wanted to talk about and show off was an autopsy table his son had sent him from Pittsburgh. We spent nearly all the time I had with him admiring it; just an ordinary American-made autopsy table."[38] Von Recklinghausen's allegorical performance went right over Cullen's head. Despite a "decade of maturing experience" resulting from his correspondence with the great German pathologist,[39] Cullen simply could not fathom the embarrassment that von Recklinghausen had experienced in 1896, an embarrassment that Robert Meyer had seen as tragic. Nor could Cullen seem to grasp that the performance he was witnessing in 1906 was a reenactment of that earlier embarrassment over an American-made microtome. Ironically, what Meyer had perceived in 1898 as tragedy, Cullen perceived in 1906 as comedy.[40]

One might consider von Recklinghausen's reaction to Cullen's article as a four-act play performed episodically between 1896 and 1908. The young German scientist Emil Ries attended the first act of the performance in von Recklinghausen's laboratory in 1896 where he witnessed the body language and *ironic* verbal reaction of the Professor upon reading Cullen's article.[41] In 1898 the mature German scientist, Robert Meyer, attended the second act of the play in von Recklinghausen's laboratory. Meyer saw his old professor *tragically* performing familiar old techniques of tissue preparation from both of their student days. Thomas Cullen saw in 1896 the *comical* performance of von Recklinghausen in the third act, also set in the latter's laboratory, a performance that might better be called a *tragicomedy*.[42] The fourth act was performed in 1908 on a split stage, the eastern half representing the study of von Recklinghausen, the western half the study of Cullen. Both the older and younger protagonists were writing letters that discussed pathological material for the younger man's forthcoming book, *Adenomyoma of the Uterus*. Perhaps each had observed correctly the performances they attended; the observers were not seeing the same text because each saw a different act.[43]

Of course von Recklinghausen's message appears obvious in historical hindsight: had he had a microtome, his minor thesis of mucosal invasion would have been his major thesis. He would have seen with thinner microscopic preparations just what Cullen had seen. And, he would not have been embarrassed by an apprentice pathologist. Even when Cullen visited von Recklinghausen in his laboratory in Strassburg in 1906, the Herr Professor could not bring himself to discuss adenomyomas. Instead he acted out his lingering humiliation in a performance that Cullen could recall clearly many years later, but never with complete understanding.[44]

---

[37] Ann La Berge and Caroline Hannaway, "Paris Medicine: Perspectives Past and Present," in *Constructing Paris Medicine*, ed. Caroline Hannaway and Ann La Berge [Amsterdam, NL: Editions Rodopi B. V., 1998], 1–69: 17. The theatre metaphor has been used in referring to the Paris surgeon Philippe-Joseph Pelletan. Ibid: 22. "Reviewing Paris Medicine from the vantage point of forty years, Bowditch articulated several themes:…Andral, Chomel, and Louis, and the theatrical nature of Paris Medicine; each leading physician had his theatre in which he regularly performed: Andral at the Faculty of Medicine, Chomel at the Charite hospital, and Louis at the Pitie Hospital."

[38] Judith Robinson, *Tom Cullen,* 127.

[39] Judith Robinson, *Tom Cullen,* 127.

[40] Judith Robinson, *Tom Cullen,* 127. Nearly 30 years later, Cullen recalled this meeting as "one of the most comical experiences of my life."

[41] Martzloff, KH. Views and Reviews. Western J Surgery, Obstetrics, and Gynecology 1946;54 (August):338. The pagination is confusing. On the top of the page immediately it reads: VIEWS and REVIEWS (Continued from page IX). On the bottom of the page it reads: 338.

[42] Roger Chartier, "Texts, Printing, Readings," in *The New Cultural History*, ed. Lynn Hunt [Berkeley, CA: University of California Press, 1989],154–175: 166–67. "The final remarks of Rojas in the prologue of the *Celestina* concern the very genre of the text: 'Others have made quite a to-do about the name of the play, saying it was not a comedy but a tragedy, since it ended so sadly. The first author wished to give it a description that would reflect what happens in the beginning, and so he called it a comedy. I have found myself in a dilemma, and I have cut the Gordian knot by calling the play a tragicomedy.'"

[43] Roger Chartier, "Texts, Printing, Readings," in *The New Cultural History*, ed. Lynn Hunt [Berkeley, CA: University of California Press, 1989], 154–175: 154. The question was not simple because each was reading a different text, seeing a difference act, attending a different performance. Most plays do not enjoy a twelve year run.

[44] Judith Robinson, *Tom Cullen*, 127. Nearly thirty years later, Cullen recalled this meeting as "one of the most comical experiences of my life."

The Mutual Legacy of Friedrich von Recklinghausen and Thomas Cullen

Friedrich von Recklinghausen (1833–1910) retired in 1906 after a long and distinguished career. He is best remembered for his description of lymph channels (canals of Recklinghausen) in connective tissue (1862), of multiple neurofibromatosis (1882), and osteitis fibrosa cystica (1891), but not for adenomyomas.[45] Nonetheless, his monograph *Die Adenomyome und Cystadenome der Uterus- und Tubenwandung* catalyzed the careers of both Robert Meyer and Thomas Cullen. Not without a further touch of irony, Hans Chiari (1851–1916) – assistant to Rokitansky – was called to von Recklinghausen's chair of pathological anatomy at Strassburg in 1906.[46] Chiari honored the memory of von Recklinghausen with a biographical essay.[47]

Cullen honored von Recklinghausen in *Adenomyoma of the Uterus* published in 1908.[48] He credited the "masterly work of von Recklinghausen"[49] for bringing the subject to prominence.[50] Cullen mentioned the "considerable controversy" that followed upon the publication of *Die Adenomyome und Cystadenome der Uterus- und Tubenwandung ihre Abkunft von Resten des Wolff'schen Korpers.*[51] To his everlasting credit, von Recklinghausen graciously accepted the consensus of the scientific community regarding the correctness of Cullen's work on uterine adenomyomas. Similarly, Robert Meyer thought von Recklinghausen's work a pedagogic success because it brought adenomyosis to the attention of the medical profession.[52] Lockyer concurred saying that full interest in the subject of adenomyomas was aroused only in 1896 with the appearance of von Recklinghausen's magnificent work, *Die Adenomyome und Cystadenomyome der Uterus und Tubenwandung*. Lockyer cited other strengths of von Recklinghausen's monograph; he classified uterine adenomyomas morphologically into two classes and four varieties and "the description he gives of his second variety, *i.e. the centrally situated growth* holds good to this day."[53] Retirement notwithstanding, von Recklinghausen continued to review microscopic slides and offer "valuable criticism" as Cullen prepared his definitive monograph, *Adenomyoma of the Uterus*.[54] This was an example of professionalism at its finest. In a footnote, Cullen referenced *Die Adenomyome und Cystadenome der Uterus- und Tubenwandung ihre Abkunft von Resten des Wolff'schen Korpers.* Then he added: "I wish to express my deep sense of obligation to *Professor v. Recklinghausen*[55] for his kindness in examining sections from several of the cases and for his valuable criticism of the same."[56] In short, Rokitansky discovered uterine adenomyosis, von Recklinghausen popularized it, and Cullen wrote the definitive monograph on all the permutations of its pathology, diagnosis, treatment, and malignant transformation.

Cullen used von Recklinghausen's unhyphenated *Adenomyoma* in the title of his 1908 monograph. In prior publications on the subject from 1896 to 1903, Cullen had hyphenated *Adenomyoma*, the descriptive name that von Recklinghausen had first used in 1893.[57] Why had

45 Editorial. Friedrich von Recklinghausen (1833–1910). German Pathologist. JAMA 1968 Aug 26;205(9):640–1.

46 Erna Lesky, *The Vienna Medical School of the 19th Century* [Baltimore, MD: Johns Hopkins University Press, 1976], 115.

47 Chiari H. Friedrich Daniel v. Recklinghausen. Vehr Deutsch Path Ges 1912;15:478–488.

48 Thomas Stephen Cullen, *Adenomyoma of the Uterus* [Philadelphia: WB Saunders, 1908].

49 Friedrich v. Recklinghausen, *Die Adenomyome und Cystadenome der Uterus- und Tubenwandung ihre Abkunft von Resten des Wolff'schen Korpers. Im Anhang: Von W. A. Freund, Klinische Notizen zu den voluminosen Adenomyomen des Uterus* [Berlin: Verlag von August Hirschwald, 1896.]

50 Thomas Stephen Cullen, *Adenomyoma of the Uterus*, 1.

51 Thomas Stephen Cullen, *Adenomyoma of the Uterus*, v–vi.

52 Robert Meyer, *Autobiography*, 33.

53 Cuthbert Lockyer, *Fibroids and Allied Tumours*, 266–271.

54 Thomas Stephen Cullen, *Adenomyoma of the Uterus* [Philadelphia: WB Saunders, 1908], 1–2. On page 2, footnote No. 1, Cullen wrote: "I wish to express my deep sense of obligation to Professor v. Recklinghausen for his kindness in examining sections from several of the cases and for his valuable criticism of the same."

55 The author's italic to emphasize the formal address.

56 Thomas Stephen Cullen, *Adenomyoma of the Uterus*, 2, FN. No. 1. The original quotation was in parentheses: "(I wish to express my deep sense of obligation to *Professor v. Recklinghausen* for his kindness in examining sections from several of the cases and for his valuable criticism of the same.)"

57 Cullen, TS. Adeno-myoma uteri diffusum benignum. Bulletin Johns Hopkins Hospital 1896;6:133–157. Cullen, TS. Adenomyoma of the round ligament. Bulletin Johns Hopkins Hospital 1896;7:112–114. Thomas S. Cullen. Adeno-Myoma des Uterus. [Berlin: Verlag von August Hirsch, 1903].

Cullen preferred Adeno-myoma? Did insertion of the hyphen emphasize his conception of the chronological separation of events in the formation of adenomyomas? Was it to emphasize that glacial endometrial mucosa "flowed" into chinks and crevices in preexisting Laurentian myomas?[58] Or was the hyphen simply a declaration of independence? Finally, what caused Cullen to revert to the original unhyphenated Adenomyoma of von Recklinghausen in the title of his 1908 monograph?

The visit to Strassburg in 1906 changed Cullen's perception of von Recklinghausen. When he saw the 73-year-old professor face-to-face for the first and only time, Cullen observed more than a comical performance. Like Emil Ries a decade earlier, Cullen observed not only the words and body language of von Recklinghausen, the eminent professor of pathology; he also observed his department and his laboratory. Cullen would recall: "Though an old man then, von Recklinghausen was still doing original work in pathology and had just published some results of his recent researches in bone infection that were perfectly fascinating."[59] Cullen departed Strassburg with a new found respect for the old German master who at 73 was still conducting original research. Undoubtedly in Strassburg, Cullen experienced the formidable presence and disciplined formality characteristic of a Germanic Vorstand (University Department Chairman), quite unlike the congeniality he experienced with Professor Orth in Göttingen.[60]

Considering Cullen's personal experience with von Recklinghausen, with whom he had corresponded for more than a decade,[61] and the expression of his "deep sense of obligation to him," one may argue with some justification that von Recklinghausen served on a symbolic level as an academic advisor for Cullen's *Habilitation*, his monograph on *Adenomyomas of the Uterus*.[62] Moreover, in expressing his "deep sense of obligation," Cullen also acknowledged his indebtedness to von Recklinghausen for having awakened him in 1896 to Adeno-myoma uteri diffusum benignum. Due to the professionalism of both men, in 1908 Cullen could accept that "on all material points there was no difference between them."

In *Adenomyoma of the Uterus,* Cullen concentrated on analyzing the surgical material from Johns Hopkins Hospital. He explicitly stated he did not do a search of the literature. This may explain why he did not cite Rokitansky in 1908 when he had done so in the article of 1896 and his monograph on cancer in 1900.[63] However, Cullen did not neglect the work of von Recklinghausen. He restated his position of 1896 that he agreed with von Recklinghausen[64] that uterine adenomyomas are benign "perfectly normal endometrial glands…surrounded by the normal stroma of the mucosa."[65] Cullen also addressed the pathogenesis of tubal adenomyomas so important to von Recklinghausen in 1896. Referring to the work of von Franque,[66] Robert

[58] Thomas Stephen Cullen, *Adenomyoma of the Uterus* [Philadelphia: WB Saunders, 1908], v.

[59] Judith Robinson, *Tom Cullen,* 127. As mention before, there are so many direct quotations from interviews, that *Tom Cullen of Baltimore* is more than a biography; in many places it is autobiographical.

[60] Thomas Stephen Cullen (1868–1953) was 38 years old and an associate professor when he visited von Recklinghausen. Coincidently, the author spent his 38th birthday in Austria in 1971 on a six week mini-sabbatical to study pelvic surgery. He witnessed the austere formality and presence of Professor Hüsslein, Vorstand (chairman) of the Department of Obstetrics and Gynecology, Second Frauenklinik, University of Vienna.

[61] Judith Robinson, *Tom Cullen*, 127. Thirty years later, Cullen would tell his biographer that this decade of correspondence with the famous von Recklinghausen of Strasbourg, "the survivor of the age of giants [had been for him] a decade of maturing experience."

[62] Donald Fleming, *William H. Welch and the Rise of Modern Medicine* [Boston, MA: Little Brown and Company, 1954], 37. "The sense that with advanced students only the lightest kind of supervision could be tolerated went very deep in the greater German scientists and characterized most if not all of the men who succeeded in arousing creativity in others."

[63] Cuthbert Lockyer, *Fibroids and Allied Tumours (Myoma and Adenomyoma): Their Pathology, Clinical Features and Surgical Treatment* [London: Macmillan and Company, 1918]. Lockyer's monograph is an invaluable reference resource for professional and clinician historians. He was an authority of the subject, knew the contemporary principals involved, and analyzed the literature at hand in England during World War I. Ironically, Lockyer did not cite Rokitansky either. It was left to Cullen's English friend and colleague, Cuthbert Lockyer, to publish the first major review of uterine and extrauterine adenomyomas.

[64] Friedrich v. Recklinghausen, *Die Adenomyome und Cystadenome der Uterus- und Tubenwandung ihre Abkunft von Resten des Wolff'schen Korpers. Im Anhang: Von W. A. Freund, Klinische Notizen zu den voluminosen Adenomyomen des Uterus* [Berlin: Verlag von August Hirschwald, 1896.]

[65] Thomas Stephen Cullen, *Adenomyoma of the Uterus* [Philadelphia: WB Saunders, 1908], 187. Cuthbert Lockyer, *Fibroids and Allied Tumours (Myoma and Adenomyoma): Their Pathology, Clinical Features and Surgical Treatment* [London: Macmillan and Company, 1918], 423–4. However, as Lockyer pointed out, three of von Recklinghausen's cases were malignant.

[66] Von Franque O. Salpingitis nodosa isthmica und Adenomyoma Tubae. Centralbl. F. Gynaek., 1900, Bd. xxv, S. 660.

Meyer,[67] Gottschalk,[68] and Lockstaedt,[69] Cullen explained that in salpingitis isthmica nodosa [tubal adenomyosis] the tubal mucosa protrudes into the muscle of the tube creating "gland-like spaces" without underlying stroma because "in the tubal mucosa the characteristic stroma of the uterine mucosa is wanting."[70] Cullen also related his understanding of von Recklinghausen's reasoning with regard to the pathogenesis of uterine adenomyomata. Von Recklinghausen reasoned from the "supposed close analogy between elements of the Wolffian duct and the glandular structures" present in uterine adenomyomata and opined that in the "vast majority" of cases the "glandular elements were derivatives of the Wolffian duct." [71] Cullen did not go into details. Whereas von Recklinghausen developed a morphological classification of uterine adenomyomas, Cullen classified adenomyomas clinically:

1. Adenomyomatous uterus with a relatively[72] normal contour
2. Subperitoneal[73] or intraligamentary adenomyomata[74]
3. Submucous adenomyomata[75]

Interestingly, Cullen continued the tradition started by Rokitansky[76] of using colorful non-medical words as "walnut, hen's egg, hazelnuts, bean, pea, cherry " to describe the size of cysts, tumors, and other lesions.[77] He commented on the two large intraligamentary cystic adenomyomas described by Breus; the cavity of one communicated directly with the endometrial cavity of the uterus[78]; and notably, the other specimen that contained 7 L of thick brownish fluid.[79] Cullen explained the pathophysiology of the latter case.

> It is natural that the cysts in the uterine wall should remain small [miniature uterine cavities], as they are compressed by the muscle, on the other hand, when they have once become subperitoneal [and intraligamentary] they may dilate until they can contain several liters of [chocolate-colored] blood.[80]

Cullen recommended scanning the uterine musculature with a magnifying loupe to "discover small, round, irregular, triangular or oblong areas composed of a waxy, fairly homogeneous tissue, lying between myomatous bundles" in order to differentiate adenomyomas from common myomas (fibroids); sometimes he identified "miniature uterine cavities." [81] Cullen found the need for magnification – as had Rokitansky decades before. It is noteworthy also that in 1908, when he wrote the preface to his book, Cullen still used the metaphorical term flowing: "the uterine mucosa was at many

[67] Meyer R. Ztschr. f. Geburtshülfe und Gynaekologie, Bd. xlii, H. 1.

[68] Gottschalk. Demonstration zur Enstehung der Adenome des Tubenisthmus. Ztschr. F. Geburtshülfe und Gynaekologie, 1900, Bd. xlii, S. 616.

[69] Lockstaedt P. Ueber Vorkommen und Bedeutung von Drusenschlauchen in Myomen des Uterus. Monatsschr. f. Geb. u. Gyn., 1898, Bd. vii, S. 188.

[70] Thomas Stephen Cullen, *Adenomyoma of the Uterus* [Philadelphia: WB Saunders, 1908], 236.

[71] Thomas Stephen Cullen, *Adenomyoma of the Uterus*, 193.

[72] Thomas Stephen Cullen, *Adenomyoma of the Uterus*, 2. Cullen qualified his use of the word relatively: "I use the word 'relatively' because if operative interference be long delayed some of the discrete myomata so frequently found may assume large proportions and almost completely overshadow the adenomyoma, while at the same time greatly altering the contour of the uterus."

[73] Thomas Stephen Cullen, *Adenomyoma of the Uterus*, 125. When the adenomyomatous growth extends from the endometrium to the outer surface of the upper half of the uterus it will tend to form a subperitoneal adenomyoma.

[74] Thomas Stephen Cullen, *Adenomyoma of the Uterus*, 125. When the adenomyomatous growth extends from the endometrium to the outer surface of the lower half of the uterus it will tend to "spread out between the fold of the broad ligament" and form an intraligamentary adenomyoma.

[75] When the adenomyomatous growth extends from the endometrium into the uterine cavity it will form a submucous adenomyoma.

[76] Erna Lesky, *The Vienna Medical School of the 19th Century* [Baltimore, MD: Johns Hopkins University Press, 1976], 106. "Starting with the year…1836, the Medical Yearbooks of the Imperial Royal Austrian State carried 'essays which in their form, tendencies and contents differed strikingly not only from the majority of other articles contained in the same publications, but also from almost all the other usually published in Germany'…They were permeated by a 'particular, logical spirit,' using 'impressive, original language.' They were Treatises by Carl Rokitansky (1804–1878)." Among the treatises was the 1838 publication *Uber* die sogenannten Verdoppelungen des Uterus (On the So-Called Duplications of the Uterus.)

[77] Thomas Stephen Cullen, *Adenomyoma of the Uterus* [Philadelphia: WB Saunders, 1908], 127, 157, 197.

[78] Thomas Stephen Cullen, *Adenomyoma of the Uterus*, 197. Cullen believed "beyond doubt" that the lining of this communicating intraligamentary cystic adenomyoma derived from the uterine mucosa.

[79] Carl Breus, *ueber wahre epithelführende Cystenbildung in Uterusmyomen.* Leipzig und Wien: Franz Deuticke, 1894. See also Thomas Stephen Cullen, *Adenomyoma of the Uterus*, 147–8, 197.

[80] Thomas Stephen Cullen, *Adenomyoma of the Uterus*, 196.

[81] Thomas Stephen Cullen, *Adenomyoma of the Uterus*, 3. See also page 126. Some miniature uterine cavities were filled with "chocolate-colored contents," old menstrual blood.

points *flowing* into the diffuse myomatous tissue."[82] Likely, Cullen was inspired to use this metaphor by recollections of his Canadian vacation experience. Early in his medical career, he vacationed in September in the lovely region of Parry Sound, Ontario, Canada.[83] Parry Sound lies on Georgian Bay which was formed when the glaciers receded over the Canadian Shield, also known as the Laurentian Plateau. The Canadian Shield is a large geographic area in eastern and central Canada composed of bare rock dating to the Precambrian era. Thousands of years ago, during the last ice age, the glaciers ground the hard Canadian Shield smooth and in the process gouged out the Great Lakes of North America and many smaller lakes. When lake water is driven by wind or ship's wake it flows and ebbs in the hard smooth crevices of the rocky shorelines. In this northern landscape, glaciations formed the surface contours of the rock, flowing water from the melting glaciers came after. Cullen envisioned rocky myomas as "pre-existing" pathologic entities into the crevices of which the glacial uterine mucosa "flowed" to cause adenomyomas.[84] In *Myomata of the Uterus,* published in 1909, Cullen described the mechanism by which he envisioned uterine mucosa entering chinks in myomatous tissue. "In cases of adenomyoma of the uterus we usually find a diffuse myomatous thickening of the uterine muscle. This thickening may be confined to the inner layers of the anterior, posterior, or lateral walls, but in other cases the myomatous tissue completely encircles the uterine cavity. This diffuse myomatous tissue contains large or small chinks, and into these the normal uterine mucosa flows. If the chinks are small, there is only room for isolated glands, but where the spaces are goodly in size, large masses of mucosa flow into and fill them. We accordingly have a diffuse myomatous growth with normal mucosa flowing in all directions through it. The mucosa lining the uterine cavity is perfectly normal."[85] Benagiano and Brosens captured the essence of this passage.[86] In Cullen's conception, cancer invaded, but benign endometrial mucosa flowed.

Cullen reported that women were usually between 30 and 60 years of age when they sought medical attention for adenomyomata. They complained of increasingly heavy periods to outright continuous hemorrhaging and menstrual cramps. Occasionally a patient would complain of "grinding pain in the uterus."[87] Cullen always attempted to explain the pathophysiology of disease when he could. He attributed the "grind pain" to "increased tension, since all the islands of mucosa scattered throughout the diffuse myoma naturally swell up at the menstrual period, and thus increase the size of the uterus."[88] What remains unspoken but implied in that reasoning was the "grinding pain" resulted from muscular contractions compressing the islands of mucosa in the adenomyoma. Cullen believed clinicians should easily diagnosis symptomatic uterine adenomyomata because (1) usually bleeding was confined to the menstrual period and (2) usually menstrual pain was midline, "referred to the uterus."[89]

The years between 1896 and 1908 – when Freund first described the clinical symptoms and signs of adenomyosis and Cullen described the Johns Hopkins' clinical experience with patients operated for adenomyosis – are nearly synonymous with the emergence of gynecologic surgical pathology. From Rokitansky through von Recklinghausen, virtually all progress resulted from observations on morbid tissues removed at autopsy. By Cullen's time, aseptic surgery, long experience with general anesthesia, and improved surgical technique resulted in consistent low operative mortality and the necessity for clinico-pathologic correlation to arrive at a correct preoperative diagnosis, tissue diagnosis, and prognosis. Physicians began to record the symptoms and the signs of patient with adenomyosis. During the

[82] Thomas Stephen Cullen, *Adenomyoma of the Uterus*, v.

[83] Judith Robinson, *Tom Cullen,* 169. This is beautiful country for vacationing; the author has fished, canoed, and camped in this region often as it lies within easy driving distance from Buffalo, New York.

[84] Cuthbert Lockyer, *Fibroids and Allied Tumours,* 302.

[85] Howard A. Kelly and Thomas S. Cullen, *Myomata of the Uterus* [Philadelphia: WB Saunders, 1909].

[86] Benagiano G and Brosens I. History of adenomyosis. Best Practice & Research Clinical Obstetrics and Gynaecology 2006;20:449–463:451. "Three points in this description are worthy of mention: first, a clear identification of the epithelial tissue as 'uterine mucosa'; second, an equally clear definition of the mechanism through which the mucosa invades the underlying tissue (through the presence in the myometrium of chinks or fissures); third, the existence of a sort of prerequisite for the formation of what we call adenomyosis, namely a 'myomatous' thickening of the uterine muscle. Also noticeable is the claim that 'sometimes its direct connection with the mucosa of the uterine cavity can be traced'."

[87] Thomas Stephen Cullen, *Adenomyoma of the Uterus* [Philadelphia: WB Saunders, 1908], 261.

[88] Thomas Stephen Cullen, *Adenomyoma of the Uterus*, 261.

[89] Thomas Stephen Cullen, *Adenomyoma of the Uterus*, 261.

long decade between 1896 and 1908, the voice of the patient was heard, interpreted, and recorded by physicians as personal medical history in clinic and hospital charts and in the medical literature.

Between 1894 and 1909 Cullen concentrated on diseases of the uterus: cancer, adenomyomas, and myomas (fibroids). He wrote four books, all profusely and beautifully illustrated: *Cancer of the Uterus* in 1900[90]; *Adenomyoma of the Uterus* in 1908[91]; and *Myomata of the Uterus*[92] and *Cancer of the Uterus* in 1909.[93] They earned for Cullen the admiration of historians of pathology such as Robert H. Young.[94] However, for gynecologists, Cullen's reputation with regard to endometriosis has been overshadowed by John Sampson's theory of retrograde menstruation and implantation. Ivo Brosens declared in 2004 that "It is a cruel trick of history that the great contribution of Cullen to the knowledge of the nosographic entity of endometriosis is usually ignored."[95] A cruel trick of history indeed. Thomas Cullen's monumental *Adenomyomas of the Uterus* with its clinical pathologic correlation firmly established the nosography of adenomyosis.

Cullen's monograph *Adenomyoma of the Uterus,* for which von Recklinghausen may be said to have acted as academic advisor, not only served as the equivalent of a German *Habilitation*, it may be viewed also as the second and revised edition of von Recklinghausen's *Die Adenomyome und Cystadenome der Uterus- und Tubenwandung ihre Abkunft von Resten des Wolff'schen Korpers.* And von Recklinghausen lived to see it published. Whereas the genealogy of ideas on adenomyosis flowed from Rokitansky to Chiari to von Recklinghausen to Cullen, the spirit of *Wissenschaft* emanated from Goethe to Müller to Virchow and through Orth and von Recklinghausen to Cullen.

In conclusion, from Rokitansky's description in 1860 until late in the nineteenth century, all scientific investigation of adenomyomas occurred in Europe. For American gynecologists and surgeons, adenomyoma was an unknown disease until Cullen studied the surgical specimens excised by Howard Kelly at the Johns Hopkins Hospital. Since initially gynecological surgical pathology existed nowhere in North America except Johns Hopkins Hospital, virtually all surgeons and gynecologists had to depend on their own naked eye examination of surgical specimens at the operating table. Consequently, until Cullen began publishing his work on adenomyomas, all that American gynecologists had perceived at abdominal surgery were ovarian cysts, fibroids, massive pelvic and abdominal adhesions from infection, and cancer. Cullen made them aware of the existence of uterine adenomyoma, but still they could not diagnose it accurately until they developed gynecologic pathology in their own departments.

Uterine Cancer to Flexner Report to Cancer Prevention

Thomas Cullen maintained a lifelong interest in uterine cancer and its early diagnosis and treatment. As an aspiring academic in 1898, he published on the early diagnosis of carcinoma of the uterus.[96] In the first line of the preface of his first book, *Cancer of the Uterus: Its Pathology, Symptomatology, Diagnosis, and Treatment* (1900), Cullen revealed the origin of his crusade for early diagnosis and treatment of uterine cancer. "The number of cases of cancer of the genital tract coming too late for operation is so appalling that the surgeon is ever seeking to devise ways and means by which the dread malady may be more generally detected at the earliest possible moment – at a time when complete removal of the malignant tissue is still possible."[97]

[90] Thomas Stephen Cullen, *Cancer of the Uterus: Its Pathology, Symptomatology, Diagnosis, and Treatment, also The Pathology of Diseases of the Endometrium* [New York: Appleton, 1900].

[91] Thomas Stephen Cullen, *Adenomyoma of the Uterus* [Philadelphia: WB Saunders, 1908].

[92] Howard A. Kelly and Thomas S. Cullen, *Myomata of the Uterus* [Philadelphia: WB Saunders, 1909].

[93] Thomas Stephen Cullen, *Cancer of the Uterus: Its Pathology, Symptomatology, Diagnosis, and Treatment, also The Pathology of Diseases of the Endometrium* [Philadelphia: WB Saunders, 1909]. In the 1900 and 1909 editions of *Cancer of the Uterus,* Cullen acknowledged his intellectual debt to von Rokitansky and von Recklinghausen and the other Austrian and German scholars for their contributions to the study of adenomyomas of the uterus.

[94] Young RH. The rich history of gynaecological pathology: brief notes on some of its personalities and their contributions. Pathology 2007;39:6–25. Young RH. Dusting off old books: comments on classic gynecologic pathology books of yesteryear. *Int J Gynecol Pathol* 2000;19:67–84. Young RH. History of gynecological pathology. I. Dr. Thomas S. Cullen. *Int J Gynecol Pathol* 1996;15:181–6.

[95] Brosens I. Endometriosis rediscovered? *Hum Reprod* 2004;19:1679–80. See also: Benagiano G and Brosens I. History of adenomyosis. Best Practice & Research Clinical Obstetrics and Gynaecology 2006;20:449–463.

He also revealed the embryonic state of the specialty of gynecology in 1900 when he addressed his volume to family physicians. "In the present volume it has been my aim to give the family physician a clear idea of the early signs of carcinoma, in order that he may always be on his guard, and may not treat too lightly any suspicious indications which may be present."[98] To put Cullen's statement in context it must be realized that, except in large cities, most gynecologic and obstetric care was in the hands of general practitioners and general surgeons until after World War II. In the first decade of the twentieth century Cullen published additional articles, mostly related to the cause and early diagnosis of cancer.[99] He began duplicate publication in an effort to impress upon the medical profession the need for early diagnosis.[100]

Cullen took an active interest in the etiology of uterine cancer. In 1900, he evaluated both the parasitic theory and the older embryonic inclusion theory of origin of uterine cancer and concluded neither was of value, though he delayed final judgment regarding the parasitic theory for another decade. His evaluation is worth reading as it reveals the depth of his knowledge of the cancer literature.

[Embryonic origin of cancer] "Origin of carcinoma from embryonic inclusion of epithelial elements... This theory, generally attributed to Cohnheim, had previously (as was pointed out by Pianese*) been advanced by Durante in 1874, one year before the appearance of Cohnheim's publication. According to these two authorities, during foetal life portions of the epithelium become nipped off and included in the connective tissue. In after years these isolated colonies of cells are in some manner stimulated to activity, and give rise to carcinomata. This theory had many advocates, but in recent years it has gradually been abandoned."[101]

[Parasitic origin of cancer] "Our work has been essentially along histological lines, the chief aim in view being concerned with the early recognition of carcinoma, in order that the organ involved be may be removed at the earliest possible moment....We have become most interested in the so-called parasitic origin of carcinoma, especially in its relation to cancer of the uterus."[102] [Cullen concludes] "Neither the theory of Cohnheim [embryonic rests] nor that of Ribbert[103] explain its origin; and the weight of evidence is against the parasitic theory."[104]

---

96 Cullen TS. The early diagnosis of carcinoma of the uterus. *Memphis Lancet* 1898; December.

97 Thomas Stephen Cullen, *Cancer of the Uterus: Its Pathology, Symptomatology, Diagnosis, and Treatment* [New York: Appleton, 1900]. Cullen intended this remarkable work with three hundred and ten illustrations to be a definitive treatise on the subject, as he did all his books. He did not want to write textbooks that required periodic updating.

98 Cullen, Thomas Stephen. *Cancer of the Uterus: Its Pathology, Symptomatology, Diagnosis, and Treatment. Also the Pathology of Diseases of the Endometrium.* New York: D. Appleton and Company, 1900:v. Preface.

99 Cullen TS. A rare variety of adeno-carcinoma of the uterus. John Hopkins Hospital Reports 1900 IX:401. Cullen TS. The cause of cancer. American Medicine 1901;1:298. Cullen TS. The early diagnosis of cancer of the uterus: operative technic. International Clinics 1909; 4 (19th series): 193. Cullen TS. The early diagnosis of cancer of the uterus: operative technic. *Pennsylvania Medical Journal* 1909–10; vol. 13:110.

100 Later in the twentieth century, editors frowned on duplicate publication as a tactic of padding the number of publications in curriculum vitae. However, Cullen's motives were honest: to educate physicians to listen to patients who complained of vaginal bleeding and to make every effort to diagnosis cancer of the uterus early when it was curable by surgery.

101 Cullen, Thomas Stephen. *Cancer of the Uterus: Its Pathology, Symptomatology, Diagnosis, and Treatment. Also the Pathology of Diseases of the Endometrium.* New York: D. Appleton and Company, 1900:652. *Pianese C. Beitrag zur Histologie und Aetiologie des Carcinomas. Ziegler's Beitrage (Supplementheft), Jena, 1896.

102 Cullen, Thomas Stephen. *Cancer of the Uterus: Its Pathology, Symptomatology, Diagnosis, and Treatment. Also the Pathology of Diseases of the Endometrium.* New York: D. Appleton and Company, 1900:655.

103 Cullen, Thomas Stephen. *Cancer of the Uterus,* 1900: 653–654. "According to this author [Ribbert], then, the connective-tissue cells increase to such an extent that they invade the epithelial layer and nip off epithelial cells or groups of cells; this isolated epithelium at a later period is capable of producing carcinoma." See also: Lockyer, Cuthbert. Fibroids and Allied Tumours (Myoma and Adenomyoma): Their Pathology, Clinical Features and Surgical Treatment. London: Macmillan and Co., 1918:1. "Cohnheim's theory of embryonic 'rests' has been applied to myoma, and corresponds with the view of Ribbert."

104 Cullen, Thomas Stephen. *Cancer of the Uterus,* 1900:657. Roswell Park had secured a grant from the New York State Legislature to investigate the parasitic theory of endometriosis. Cullen was in personal communication with Harvey Gaylord, who with Pease "have for several years been carrying on extensive investigations as to the origin of cancer, and have brought forward some very suggestive data in support of the parasitic theory." Gaylord became the Director of the Gratwick Clinic in Buffalo, New York, now the Roswell Park Cancer Institute.

Cullen seemed much more concerned with the cause of cancer than the cause of adenomyomas, and rightly so, because cancer killed while adenomyomas only wounded. Cancer theory provides a window to Cullen's mental compartmentalization of adenomyomas and cancer. While Cullen was interested in the infectious parasitic theory of the origin of cancer and early on dismissed the embryonic theory of cancer causation, he never believed in an infectious origin for uterine or extrauterine adenomyoma but readily accepted and championed an embryonic theory of origin for extrauterine adenomyomata. From bitter experience early in his career, he considered cancer a lethal invasive disease, pondered its cause, and campaigned for its early diagnosis and treatment. Contrarily, an adenomyoma was a disease of a lesser order of magnitude. After all, cancer had been known since antiquity, but no one in North America even knew uterine adenomyomas existed until he differentiated adenomyomas from the ubiquitous, benign uterine fibroid. Furthermore, the surgical treatment of uterine adenomyoma was straight-forward and successful, unlike the surgical treatment of advanced uterine corpus cancer and cervical cancer.

Compared to his early and bitter experience with cancer, Cullen had a heady initial experience with uterine adenomyoma that brought him instant recognition at Johns Hopkins, led to an exchange with von Recklinghausen, and found expression in his writings in idyllic metaphors from the wilds of the Canadian Bush. Cullen used metaphors – such as *flowing* and *springing from* – in his scientific writing, the latter suggestive of mushrooms "springing from" the floor of the virgin forest of his youth, the former reminiscent of the "flowing" waters of the Magnetawan River and Lake Ahmic where he vacationed "many happy summers" with Howard Kelly, Max Broedel, and Simon Flexner.[105]

In 1909 Cullen published *Myomata of the Uterus* with Howard A. Kelly as the first author.[106] At the time, Kelly was Professor of Gynecology in the Johns Hopkins University and Gynecologist-in-Chief to the Johns Hopkins Hospital, Cullen an Associate Professor of Gynecology and Associate Gynecologist.[107] *Myomata of the Uterus* consisted entirely of myomatous material from the Johns Hopkins University and Hospital. Because of the large number of original cases he had examined, Cullen reported only the Hopkins experience and made no effort to review the "vast amount of current literature" on the disease.[108] Recall that Kelly had assigned Cullen to study the pathology of uterine myomas in 1893, during the course of which Cullen recognized that uterine adenomyomas differed from myomas.

Cullen changed publishers in 1909 when he released a minimally updated *Cancer of the Uterus*.[109] Despite his disclaimer of 1900, Cullen maintained an active interest in the parasitic theory of cancer.[110] In the 1909 edition, Cullen cited WT Councilman[111] and consulted H. Gaylord regarding the parasitic theory of cancer.[112] Councilman had trained under Welch at Johns Hopkins and later served as Shattuck Professor of Pathological Anatomy at Harvard Medical School.[113] Harvey Gaylord was the director of the Gratwick Clinic in Buffalo, New York, an institute dedicated to the study and treatment of cancer. Founded by Roswell Park, it was later designated the Roswell Park Cancer Institute. As in 1900, Cullen considered the "weight of evidence against the parasitic theory" and concluded the etiology of cancer remained "an unsettled question."[114]

1908 and 1909 were banner years for Cullen. He had published three books and held the rank of associate professor of gynecology at the most prestigious medical school in North America. He felt secure academically.[115] The department chairman, Howard Kelly, was busy and happy in his position at Hopkins, though his close friend and associate Osler had departed for Oxford in 1905. Then a revolution in medical education – an insistence on full-time clinical faculty – intervened to disrupt the enormously productive

[105] Te Linde RW. In Memoriam: Thomas Stephen Cullen, 1868–1953. Transactions American Gynecological Society 1953;76:227–229.

[106] Howard A. Kelly and Thomas S. Cullen, *Myomata of the Uterus* [Philadelphia: WB Saunders Company, 1909].

[107] Howard A. Kelly and Thomas S. Cullen. *Myomata of the Uterus*, 1909:title page.

[108] Kelly, Howard A. and Thomas S. Cullen. *Myomata of the Uterus*, 1909:v. This volume was meant to be definitive.

[109] Thomas Stephen Cullen, *Cancer of the Uterus: Its Pathology, Symptomatology, Diagnosis, and Treatment; also The Pathology of Diseases of the Endometrium* [Philadelphia: W. B. Saunders, 1909].

[110] Cullen, Thomas Stephen. *Cancer of the Uterus*, 1909:657.

[111] Cullen, Thomas Stephen. *Cancer of the Uterus*, 1909:657.

[112] Cullen and Gaylord, personal communication.

[113] Young RH. Dr. Thomas S. Cullen. International Journal Gynecological Pathology 1996;15:181–186:181.

[114] Cullen, Thomas Stephen. *Cancer of the Uterus*, 1909:657.

[115] Kelly, Howard A. and Thomas S. Cullen. *Myomata of the Uterus*. Philadelphia: WB Saunders Company, 1909:title page. In 1909, Howard A. Kelly was the Professor of Gynecology in

rhythm of the department of gynecology and changed the lives of both men. In the end, Cullen assumed increasing administrative responsibilities, sought outside interests, and ultimately ceased significant gynecological research.

In 1910, 6 years after the American Medical Association founded its Council on Medical Education, Abraham Flexner published a report of his survey of 155 medical schools in the USA, of which "50, or a little less than a third, were integral parts of universities."[116] *Medical Education in the United States and Canada*,[117] referred to as the "Flexner report," was officially Bulletin Number Four prepared for the Carnegie Foundation for the Advancement of Teaching.[118]

Frederick T. Gates, of the Rockefeller Institute, invited Flexner to lunch and "asked him what he would do with $1,000.000 to be used for medical education." Flexner replied that "I should give it to Dr. Welch."[119] When Flexner was sent to make a detailed investigation of medical education at Johns Hopkins, Welch took the occasion to invite Flexner to dinner with Franklin Mall and William Halsted. At dinner "Mall argued eloquently that every penny of any new funds that might be obtained should be spent on putting the heads of the clinical departments on full-time [salary]."[120] This proposal for salaried full-time professors in clinical departments, thought radical in America by most physicians, was strongly supported by the German physiologist, Carl Ludwig, as well as other German full-time clinicians. Mall had studied under Ludwig and accepted his ideas on clinical reform.[121] Welch, who also had studied under Ludwig, fully supported Mall's position.[122]

Flexner presented three alternative plans for Johns Hopkins, but favored Plan One: "that the school should be endowed and reduced to 250 students, and the main clinical chairs placed on a university, or full-time, basis."[123] Welch's biographers, Flexner and Flexner, recalled that: "This suggestion, involving as it did full-time, contained dynamite, as everyone saw."[124] They continued: "On June 11, 1911, Welch finally reported to Gates that 'the opinion prevails in our medical faculty and among the trustees of the University' that the proposition involving full-time, 'if it can be carried out upon an adequate financial basis, is the one which meets the most urgent needs and promises the largest benefits not to the Johns Hopkins School alone but to medical education in general.'"[125]

According to Howard Kelly's biographer, Flexner's assessment of the clinical faculty at Johns Hopkins "had been grossly unfair. The report brought about heated argument and discord ensued."[126] Kelly was vehemently opposed to full-time clinical faculty, as was his friend Osler. Osler, then at Oxford, wrote: "Against the sin of prosperity which looms large in Mr. Flexner's report the clinical professor must battle hard. I was

---

the Johns Hopkins University and Gynecologist-in-Chief to the Johns Hopkins Hospital. Thomas S. Cullen was an Associate Professor of Gynecology in Johns Hopkins University and Associate Gynecologist to the Johns Hopkins Hospital. Young RH. Dr. Thomas S. Cullen. International Journal Gynecological Pathology 1996;15:181–186:182. Cullen was advanced from associate in gynecology to associate professor of gynecology in 1900 following the publication of his monograph *Cancer of the Uterus* and the offer from Yale University of the chair of the department of gynecology. See also: Judith Robinson, *Tom Cullen of Baltimore* [London, Toronto, New York: Oxford University Press, 1949], 160.

[116] Simon Flexner and James Thomas Flexner, *William Henry Welch and the Heroic Age of American Medicine* [Baltimore, MD: Johns Hopkins University Press, 1993], 307.

[117] Abraham Flexner, *Medical Education in the United States and Canada* [New York: Carnegie Foundation for the Advancement of Teaching, 1910]. Kenneth M. Ludmerer, *Time to Heal: American Medical Education from the Turn of the Century to the Era of Managed Care* [Oxford: Oxford University Press, 1999], 79. "Abraham Flexner's 1910 report did not even mention internship or other hospital training for medical graduates, reflecting the prevailing orthodoxy that the four years of medical school provided sufficient preparation for general practice."

[118] Judith Robinson, *Tom Cullen*, 229.

[119] Simon Flexner and James Thomas Flexner, *William Henry Welch*, 308.

[120] Simon Flexner and James Thomas Flexner, *William Henry Welch*, 308.

[121] Simon Flexner and James Thomas Flexner, *William Henry Welch and the Heroic Age of American Medicine* [Baltimore, MD: Johns Hopkins University Press, 1993], 300. Judith Robinson, *Tom Cullen of Baltimore* [London, Toronto, New York: Oxford University Press, 1949], 228.

[122] Simon Flexner and James Thomas Flexner, *William Henry Welch*, 141–2.

[123] Simon Flexner and James Thomas Flexner, *William Henry Welch*, 308.

[124] Simon Flexner and James Thomas Flexner, *William Henry Welch*, 309.

[125] Simon Flexner and James Thomas Flexner, *William Henry Welch*, 309.

[126] Audrey W. Davis. *Dr. Kelly of Hopkins: Surgeon, Scientist, Christian* [Baltimore, MD: Johns Hopkins Press, 1959], 99.

myself believed to be addicted to it. ... The truth is there is much misunderstanding in the minds and not a little nonsense on the tongues of the people about the large fortunes made by members of the clinical staff. At any rate, let the University and Hospital always remember with gratitude the work of one 'prosperous' surgeon, whose department is so irritatingly misunderstood by Mr. Flexner. I do not believe the history of medicine presents a parallel to the munificence of our colleague Kelly to his clinic. Equal in bulk, in quality and in far-reaching practical value to the work from any department of the University, small wonder that his clinic became the Mecca for surgeons from all parts of the world, and that his laboratory methods, perfected by Drs. Cullen and Hurdon, have become general models, while through the inspiration of Mr. Max Broedel, a new school of artistic illustration in medical works has developed in the United States. And, shades of Marion Sims, Goodell and Gaillard Thomas! this (sic) is the department which the Angel of Bethesda, in the fullness of his ignorance, suggests should be, if not wiped out, at any rate merged with that of Obstetrics!"[127]

The first rumor of Kelly's impending resignation circulated in 1911.[128] By 1912, in line with his deep interest in cancer and cancer prevention, Cullen diverted some of his energy from research to patient education on a national scale. In response to his inquiry concerning cancer education for the public, he was invited to present a paper at the Fourth Clinical Congress of Surgeons of North America in November 1912. Elected chairman of a newly formed cancer campaign committee, he initiated cancer education of the public and endorsed the first popular article on cancer written by a layman, Samuel Hopkins Adams.[129] Adam's article, entitled "What Can We Do About Cancer" appeared in the May 1913 issue of *The Ladies Home Journal*.[130] Many in the medical profession criticized Cullen for endorsing Adam's article. Nonetheless, he persevered in his crusade because he had seen that many patients at Johns Hopkins were diagnosed too late for surgery to cure their disease.[131] Cullen believed firmly that education of the public would lead to early diagnosis and successful surgical treatment.[132] Cullen launched the crusade for early cancer detection and treatment, a crusade that would catch the imagination of the nation and result in ever expansive private and public funding for cancer research that ultimately resulted in the founding of the American Cancer Society.[133] He related the story of "How cancer education of the public got started" in a letter to Dr. Joseph Bloodgood published many years later in the Bulletin of the American College of Surgeons.[134] The diagnosis and treatment of the benign invasive diseases, adenomyosis and endometriosis, did not share the public spotlight now shining on the malignant invasive disease, cancer.

Cancer education was the first among many extracurricular activities that would distract Cullen from his hitherto total immersion in academic work. In 1913 Johns Hopkins University decided to phase in the full-time plan but left Kelly, Cullen and the Department of Gynecology outside the new arrangement for the time being.[135] Howard A. Kelly, the consummate academic entrepreneur and problem solver, an applied scientist who financed his research and his department with relatively token compensation from Johns Hopkins, was not cut out to be a Flexnerian full-time academic. Another rumor of Kelly's impending resignation surfaced in 1916. He went on indefinite leave early in 1917 and officially tendered his resignation as professor and chairman of the Department of Gynecology at Johns Hopkins on February 12, 1919. Kelly reentered private practice to continue clinical research that he had begun in 1904 into the therapeutic uses of radium for benign and malignant gynecologic diseases.[136] With

[127] Osler quoted in Judith Robinson, *Tom Cullen of Baltimore* [London, Toronto, New York: Oxford University Press, 1949], 232.

[128] Audrey W. Davis. *Dr. Kelly of Hopkins: Surgeon, Scientist, Christian* [Baltimore, MD: Johns Hopkins Press, 1959], 101.

[129] Young RH. Dr. Thomas S. Cullen. International Journal Gynecological Pathology 1996;15:181–186:184.

[130] Judith Robinson, *Tom Cullen of Baltimore* [London, Toronto, New York: Oxford University Press, 1949], 241, 248.

[131] Judith Robinson, *Tom Cullen* 243.

[132] Cullen TS. Report of cancer campaign committee. *Surg Gynecol Obstet* 1913; November.

[133] Cullen, Thomas S. How cancer education of the public got started. *Bull Am Coll Surg* 1963;48:87.

[134] Cullen TS. How cancer education of the public got started. *Bull Am Coll Surg* 1963;48:87.

[135] Audrey W. Davis. *Dr. Kelly of Hopkins: Surgeon, Scientist, Christian* [Baltimore, MD: Johns Hopkins Press, 1959], 100.

[136] Audrey W. Davis. *Dr. Kelly of Hopkins,* 102–103, 127. From the dust jacket, we learn that Audrey Davis was a close friend and editor of his published works for over twenty years. "Before his death, Dr. Kelly asked Miss Davis to write his biography and left her the wealth of material used to write this story." Judith Robinson, *Tom Cullen,* 279.

reluctance, The Board of Trustees accepted Kelly's resignation "to take effect at the end of the present school year."[137] Kelly recommended Cullen as his successor to "head of the Department of Gynecology with the title of Professor of Clinical Gynecology."[138]

Despite all that had transpired, Cullen accepted the full-time position at Johns Hopkins. Long before, in 1896, he had declined the invitation from Vanderbilt University to the chair of pathology and in 1900 he had declined the invitation from Yale to the chair of gynecology with the rank of full professor.[139] As early as 1915, Cullen had adopted Kelly's position that gynecology and abdominal surgery belonged together in one department.[140] When Kelly took an indefinite leave of absence in 1917, Cullen became acting Gynecologist-in-Chief, and declined the invitation to the chair of gynecology at Jefferson Medical College in Philadelphia.[141] With Kelly's formal resignation in 1919, Cullen became head of the division of gynecology within the Department of Surgery.[142] But the tensions from years of controversy regarding full-time clinical faculty and the uncertain fate of the Department of Gynecology combined to take a toll on Cullen. His research output diminished as he took on many outside interests.[143] Before he retired as professor of gynecology in 1939, the Flexnerian reforms had brought forth the modern medical schools and teaching hospitals in the USA, although not all with full-time clinical faculty as at Johns Hopkins.[144] The "[Flexnerian] revolution called for medical schools to be university-based, for faculty to be engaged in original research, and for students to participate in 'active' learning through laboratory study and real clinical work."[145]

Looking back, Cullen the pathologist-surgeon proved a steady and reliable academic colleague for Kelly the quintessential clinician-surgeon.[146] Kelly had a genius for recognizing young physicians with the requisite talents to accomplish the objectives he envisioned. Following Cullen's suggestion, Kelly made pathology a foundational experience of his 5-year residency program of clinical and surgical training and research in gynecology.[147] Ambidextrous, Kelly operated with lightening speed, dexterity, and confidence. Cullen, by his own admission, operated step by step, in a deliberate teaching mode reminiscent of an organ recital in the pathology laboratory. At the completion of each step of the operation, Cullen would ask the resident "Satisfied?"[148] Ever loyal and steadfast, and sharing the humanitarian spirit of Kelly, Cullen was perhaps the ideal associate professor. They complemented each other. Each respected the other's talents. Not without a touch of irony, Kelly may be viewed as a quintessential

[137] Audrey W. Davis. *Dr. Kelly of Hopkins: Surgeon, Scientist, Christian* [Baltimore, MD: Johns Hopkins Press, 1959], 104.

[138] Judith Robinson, *Tom Cullen of Baltimore* [London, Toronto, New York: Oxford University Press, 1949], 295. Thomas S. Cullen. *The Distribution of Adenomyomas Containing Uterine Mucosa.* Chicago, IL: American Medical Association Press, 1920, title page. In 1920, Cullen was officially a "Professor of Clinical Gynecology in the Johns Hopkins University and Visiting Gynecologist to the Johns Hopkins Hospital." Audrey W. Davis. *Dr. Kelly of Hopkins: Surgeon, Scientist, Christian* [Baltimore, MD: Johns Hopkins Press, 1959], 105. However, Cullen assumed direction of gynecology, not as an independent department, but as a division of general surgery under Halsted.

[139] Judith Robinson, *Tom Cullen,* 133, 159.

[140] Judith Robinson, *Tom Cullen,* 262–264.

[141] Judith Robinson, *Tom Cullen*, 279, 281.

[142] Judith Robinson, *Tom Cullen*, 295.

[143] Judith Robinson, *Tom Cullen*, 312. "President of the Medical and Chirurgical Faculty of Maryland; a director of the transportation company that linked the eastern and western shores of Maryland with Chesapeake Bay ferries; trustee, chosen by the Episcopal bishop of Maryland, of the Hannah More Academy for girls; deacon in the Presbyterian church of his own choice; thirty-third degree mason; writer still – four papers by Thomas S. Cullen were published in American medical journals in 1927, two in 1928, two in 1929 – speaker by special invitation at the 1929 meeting of the British Medical Association in Manchester; elected by the House of Delegates of the American Medical Association to be one of its nine trustees…member of the Maryland State Board of Health and vice-president of Baltimore's public library system." Judith Robinson, *Tom Cullen of Baltimore* [London, Toronto, New York: Oxford University Press, 1949], 313. Nonetheless, Cullen continued teaching full time and his due diligence was rewarded in 1932 with the designation Professor of Gynecology, a position he had filled since 1919.

[144] Te Linde RW. In Memoriam: Thomas Stephen Cullen, 1868–1953. Transactions American Gynecological Society 1953;76:227–229. Cullen was promoted from Professor of Clinical Gynecology (1919) to Professor of Gynecology in 1932.

[145] Kenneth M. Ludmerer, *Time to Heal: American Medical Education from the Turn of the Century to the Era of Managed Care* [Oxford: Oxford University Press, 1999], xxii.

[146] Judith Robinson, *Tom Cullen of Baltimore* [London, Toronto, New York: Oxford University Press, 1949], 316. "It was in the laboratory that the men in the gynecological service came to know their chief best."

[147] Judith Robinson, *Tom Cullen,* 315. Cullen designed the five-year residency program for Kelly.

[148] Judith Robinson, *Tom Cullen,* 409.

clinical professor and Cullen an early exemplar of a full-time professor of gynecology. In retrospect, Charles Noble and Hunter Robb, former assistants of Kelly, were too much like Kelly to have filled the niche that Cullen fashioned for himself. The very talents and mind-set that made Osler and Kelly so valuable in founding the clinical departments of medicine and gynecology at Johns Hopkins were the least appreciated by Abraham Flexner, the medical educational reformer. Cullen – not Kelly or Osler – more nearly fitted the new academic model and it was Cullen who stayed on to maintain the teaching and research tradition at Johns Hopkins.

***

The reader will find Chaps. 6 and 7 to be ahistorical in the sense that they represent pure analysis and synthesis of Cullen's scientific thought and medical practice during the last years of his scientifically productive career, though far from the end of his long academic career at Johns Hopkins. Set within an international historical context of emergent surgical pathology and more aggressive surgical treatment of deep pelvic adenomyomas, Chap. 6 presents the tortuous history that led to the recognition, surgical management, serious complications of surgery, and efforts to understand the pathogenesis and natural history of adenomyomas (deeply invasive endometriosis) of the rectovaginal septum by constructing meaningful classifications of the disease.

Cullen addressed the problem of uterine mucosa in the ovary late in his investigative career; 70 years after its discovery by Rokitansky, and nearly 15 years after Ludwig Pick confirmed Rokitansky's discovery. It took the unique case of DeWitt Casler to spark investigation into the differential diagnosis of the myriad causes of chocolate cysts of the ovary, and the recognition by John Sampson that ovarian endometriomas could be distinguished from other chocolate cysts of the ovary, by careful histologic examination of surgical specimens. Casler's unique case, which will be described in full, finally brought Cullen out of his 25-year descriptive pathology mode of analysis of surgical specimens to rethink his classification of extrauterine adenomyomas in terms of misplaced uterine mucosa. This mental readjustment prepared Cullen to accept Sampson's theory of pathogenesis of implantation endometriosis.

Chapter 7 is set in the aftermath of World War I, when Cullen lamented the sad and debilitated state of his German colleagues and the downgrading of the independent status of the Department of Gynecology to a division in the Department of Surgery. It analyzes Cullen's last major synthesis of his research into uterine and extrauterine adenomyomas and his fascination with pathogenesis. It recounts the state-of-the-art surgical management of deeply invasive extrauterine adenomyomas at Johns Hopkins Hospital at the end of the second decade of the twentieth century and Cullen's personal struggle to manage adenomyomas of the bowel. By this time, Cullen's work had stimulated improved patient care and clinical research at several universities and at the Mayo Clinic. No longer would Cullen and Johns Hopkins be the epicenter of endometriosis research; soon the torch would pass to John Sampson and the Albany Medical College.

6 Adenomyomas of Vagina, Rectum, Sigmoid Colon, and Ovary

Extrauterine Adenomyomas

Diagnosis and surgical treatment of adenomyomas of the rectovaginal pouch of Douglas, so-called adenomyomas of the rectovaginal septum, awaited emergence of surgical pathology in the late nineteenth century. The subspecialty of surgical pathology in North America developed in academic departments of surgery at Johns Hopkins (gynecology), Columbia-Presbyterian, and Washington University-Barnes Hospital and in non-university settings at Memorial Hospital, The Mayo Clinic, and the Armed Forces Institute of Pathology.[1]

In 1896 Cullen described his first case of an extrauterine adenomyoma, an adenomyoma of the round ligament of the uterus.[2] Recently awakened by von Recklinghausen to the significance of uterine adenomyomas, Cullen adopted his descriptive term adenomyoma.[3] However, Cullen modified the term. He inserted a hyphen separating adeno from myoma – creating adeno-myoma – to comport with his conviction that the adenomatous tissue flowed into chinks and thereby modified a preexisting myoma.

Even more interesting, Cullen found the pseudo-glomerular structures of von Recklinghausen. Examining thin histologic sections cut with a microtome, Cullen recognized, described and illustrated a microscopic section of a pseudo-glomerulus. "Traversing the nodule in all directions are glands … surrounded by stroma similar to that of the uterine mucosa. It would be impossible to distinguish some of these from uterine glands." Cullen continued: "In many places the glands present a peculiar arrangement and correspond to v. Recklinghausen's pseudo-glomeruli."[4] Cullen postulated the pathogenesis of adeno-myoma of the round ligament from müllerian rests, but not without homage to von Recklinghausen. "The glandular elements in our case correspond very closely to those found by v. Recklinghausen in adeno-myomata of the uterus. In those cases he was able to trace a marked resemblance between the tumor glands and remains of the Wolffian body, and came to the conclusion that the glands were derived from this source. While admitting the probability of the glands in our case being due to remains of the Wolffian body, we cannot, from their striking resemblance to those of the

[1] Juan Rosai, ed., *Guiding the Surgeon's Hand: The History of American Surgical Pathology* [Washington, DC: Armed Forces Institute of Pathology, 1997], 3.

[2] Cullen TS. Adenomyoma of the round-ligament. Johns Hopkins Hospital Bulletin. 1896; VII:112–14.

[3] Von Recklinghausen F. Adenomyomas and cystadenomas of the wall of the uterus and tube: Their origin as remnants of the Wolffian body. Wien klin Wschr 1896;8:530.

[4] Cullen TS. Adenomyoma of the round-ligament. Johns Hopkins Hospital Bulletin. 1896; VII:112–14:113.

R.E. Batt, *A History of Endometriosis*,
DOI 10.1007/978-0-85729-585-9_6,

uterine mucosa, and from the fact that their stroma resembles that of the mucosa, refrain from suggesting the possibility that they may be due to an abnormal embryonic deposit of a portion of Müller's duct."[5]

This conclusion indicates that, while Cullen could not attribute an isolated adenomyoma of the round ligament to direct invasion from the uterine mucosa, he could remain consistent with a müllerian pathogenesis of both the uterine and extrauterine lesions by attributing the latter to embryonic müllerian rests. Cullen argued by analogy. The microscopic appearance of the adenomyoma of the round ligament resembled the microscopic appearance of uterine endometrium; hence he concluded both must be derived from müllerian tissue, not Wolffian tissue. In his extrauterine case, Cullen was not as confident of his argument as he was in asserting the demonstrable pathogenesis of diffuse uterine adenomyomas. In 1898, Cullen published further observations on adenomyomata of the round ligament.[6] Despite the commotion raised by the Flexner report, Cullen continued active research and described umbilical tumors containing uterine mucosa in 1911 and 1912 and abdominal wall tumors that he also attributed to misplaced remnants of Müller's duct.[7] He returned to adenomyomas of the round ligament in 1916.[8] Disorders of the umbilicus so fascinated him that as his last definitive work he wrote a large monograph on the *Embryology, Anatomy, and Diseases of the Umbilicus* in 1916.[9]

Notwithstanding his publications on extrauterine adenomyomas of the upper pelvis and abdominal wall, Cullen and his fellow gynecologic surgeons at Johns Hopkins – including Howard Kelly – apparently remained oblivious to the presence of extrauterine adenomyomas deep in the female pelvis.[10] Given the volume of gynecologic surgery at Johns Hopkins Hospital and the severity of the disease encountered, it seems unlikely that Cullen – with his interest in the disease – had not encountered an adenomyoma of the bowel or pelvic floor during manual exploration of the pelvis and abdomen in all those years. How can one explain Cullen's apparent lack of peripheral vision? One must remember that Cullen first encountered a uterine adenomyoma in the laboratory while examining uterine fibroids for one of Howard Kelly's studies. While fibroids may distort the uterus, they are usually confined to the uterus, or if they extend outward and become intraligamentary, they usually remain attached to the uterus. Completely isolated parasitic fibroids are uncommon. Cullen probably assumed that most adenomyomas – like fibroids – were confined to the uterus or the round ligaments and he did not explore elsewhere. Moreover, Cullen and his colleagues usually performed supracervical hysterectomy in noncancerous cases. Given this surgical approach to benign pelvic conditions, they operated above adenomyomas of the rectovaginal septum.

Cullen awakened to the existence of deep pelvic adenomyomas in January 1913 when DSD Jessup, pathologist at the New York Skin and Cancer Hospital, sent him two specimens removed by William S. Bainbridge.[11] Bainbridge, the first North American surgeon to remove adenomyomas of the rectovaginal septum, gave Jessup and his research fellow Archer Brown permission to publish both of his cases.[12] Jessup sent the surgical specimens to Cullen for his expert opinion and expected Cullen to confirm his diagnosis

[5] Cullen TS. Adeno-myoma of the round-ligament. Johns Hopkins Hospital Bulletin. 1896; VII:112–14.

[6] Cullen TS. Further remarks on adeno-myoma of the round ligament. Johns Hopkins Hospital Bulletin 1898; IX:142.

[7] Cullen TS. Umbilical tumors containing uterine mucosa or remnants of Mueller's duct. Transactions Southern Surgical and Gynecological Association, 1911. Cullen TS. Umbilical tumors containing uterine mucosa or remnants of Mueller's duct. Surg Gynecol Obstet 1912;14:479–491.

[8] Cullen TS. Adenomyoma of the round ligament and incarcerated omentum in an inguinal hernia, together forming one tumor. Surg Gyn and Obstet. 1916;23:258–260.

[9] Thomas S. Cullen. *Embryology, Anatomy, and Diseases of the Umbilicus* [Philadelphia: W. B. Saunders, 1916].

[10] Cuthbert Lockyer, *Fibroids and Allied Tumours (Myoma and Adenomyoma): Their Pathology, Clinical Features and Surgical Treatment* [London: Macmillan and Company, 1918], 301. As Lockyer pointed out, Cullen's experience between 1894 and 1908 when he wrote his "monumental" work *Adenomyomata of the Uterus*, published in 1908, was limited to uterine adenomyomata and adenomyomata of the utero-ovarian and round ligaments. Lockyer stated further: "up to that date this well-know author had met with no case of 'adenomyoma' in the recto-genital space."

[11] Cullen TS. The distribution of adenomyomata containing uterine mucosa. Am J Obstetrics Diseases Women and Children 1919;180:130–138:134. In 1913 Jessup's and Lockyer's "communications set me thinking and I at once felt sure that two of my cases undoubtedly belonged to this category, although the histological examination had given no inkling of such a condition. I had many more sections made and was finally rewarded by finding in each case the typical picture in other portions of the specimen. Since then I have been on the look out for this condition and have had in all 15 cases."

[12] Jessup, DSD. Adenomyoma of the rectovaginal septum. JAMA 1914;LXIII: 383–387.

[13] Jessup, DSD. JAMA 1914;LXIII: 383–387:387.

of adenomyoma of the rectovaginal septum.[13] Cullen, long familiar with the naked-eye and microscopic appearances of extrauterine adenomyomas of the round ligament, replied to Jessup: "There is not a shadow of a doubt but that we are dealing with adenomyoma of the uterus in both cases. From what I can gather the growth is undoubtedly of the uterine type and not of the rectal and the fact that the rectal mucosa is perfectly normal and in no way encroached on also favors the idea of the uterine origin. Furthermore, if we are dealing with an adenomyoma of the rectum then we should expect the glands scattered throughout the tumor to consist of rectal glands and not uterine. Both of these growths are essentially adenomyomas of the uterus and they have undoubtedly involved the rectum secondarily. As you know, a certain number of these adenomyomas are particularly prone to form adhesions. This would naturally be more frequent in the cervical portion because the uterus there lies in close contact with the rectum."[14]

Cullen later reported that "Within forty-eight hours after I had sent my report to Dr. Jessup, the February number of the *Proceedings of the Royal Society of Medicine* reached me, and in it was a similar case reported in full by Cuthbert Lockyer of London."[15] Alerted by Jessup in January and Lockyer in February to the existence of adenomyoma of the rectovaginal septum, at the June 1913 meeting of the Canadian Medical Association, Cullen "incidentally referred to two cases of this character that had recently come under [his] care."[16] On December 16, 1913 Cullen read a paper entitled "Adenomyoma of the rectovaginal septum" before the Southern Surgical and Gynecological Society in Atlanta, Georgia.[17] Before the end of 1913, Cullen published his two cases complete with illustrations along with a review of Lockyer's two cases, in the *Transactions of the Southern Surgical and Gynecological Association.*[18] He evidently adopted the "rectovaginal septum" terminology from Lockyer. Cullen published the same data in the March 14, 1914 issue of the *Journal of the American Medical Association.*[19]

Cullen reported Lockyer's cases in some detail and included an excellent microscopic illustration and a superb illustration of the en-bloc specimen of uterus and rectum.[20] An illustration of Lockyer's case 2, labeled adenomyoma of the rectovaginal septum, actually shows a retrocervical adenomyoma with complete obliteration of the rectovaginal pouch of Douglas forming a false or "pseudo-septum" above the true anatomical rectovaginal septum that Denonvilliers described in 1836.[21] The extent of invasion may be gauged by the fact that Lockyer performed a Wertheim radical panhysterectomy and en-bloc segmental resection of the rectum and permanent colostomy on the assumption that he was dealing with malignancy. In his discussion of Lockyer's case, Cullen recognized the need for an accurate preoperative diagnosis. "Cancer of the rectum starts in the mucous membrane, gradually infiltrates the bowel and then extends to the peritoneum and at a later stage may involve the cervix. Clinically there is a history of hemorrhage from the bowel. In adenomyoma of the rectovaginal septum, on the other hand, the only rectal symptom is painful defecation, or there are obstructive symptoms. On rectal examination the bowel mucosa may be found puckered but still intact. Thus it is seen that the differential diagnosis is relative easy."[22]

Cullen saw his first case of adenomyoma of the rectovaginal septum in consultation on March 17, 1913 and operated the patient on 22 March. A classically

---

[14] Jessup, DSD. JAMA 1914;LXIII: 383–387. Jessup preserved Cullen's first assessment of adenomyoma of the rectovaginal septum.

[15] Cullen TS. Adenomyoma of the rectovaginal septum. Transactions of Southern Surgical & Gynecological Association. 1913;26: 106–118. Lockyer, Cuthbert. Adenomyoma of the rectovaginal septum. Proceedings Royal Society Medicine. February 1913; vi, No. 4.

[16] Cullen TS. Adenomyoma of the rectovaginal septum. Trans Southern Surgical and Gynecological Assoc 1913;26:106–118. Cullen made reference to his "Address in Gynecology" before the Canadian Medical Association in June 1913, published in the Canadian Medical Association Journal, August 1913.

[17] Cullen TS. Adenomyoma of the rectovaginal septum. JAMA 1914;62:835–839. See footnote page 835.

[18] Cullen TS. Adenomyoma of the rectovaginal septum. Trans Southern Surgical and Gynecological Assoc 1913;26:106–118.

[19] Cullen TS. Adenomyoma of the rectovaginal septum. JAMA 1914;LXII: 835–839. The only difference, in the 1913 version large full-page illustrations were clustered in mid-article, in 1914 version the illustrations were smaller and integrated within the text.

[20] Cullen TS. Adenomyoma of the rectovaginal septum. Trans Southern Surgical and Gynecological Assoc 1913;26:106–118.

[21] Cullen TS. Adenomyoma of the rectovaginal septum. Trans Southern Surgical and Gynecological Assoc 1913;26:106–118, Figure 1. Lockyer, Cuthbert. Adenomyoma of the rectovaginal septum. Proceedings Royal Society Medicine. February 1913; vi, No. 4. Denonvilliers, CPD. Bull Soc Anatomy of Paris (Series 3) 1836:20:105.

[22] Cullen TS. Adenomyoma of the rectovaginal septum. Trans Southern Surgical and Gynecological Assoc 1913;26: 106–118:116–7.

beautiful illustration by Broedel, labeled as adenomyoma of the rectovaginal septum, actually shows a large retrocervical adenomyoma occupying the rectovaginal pouch of Douglas from its floor to the level of the internal cervical os of the uterus.[23] The adenomyomatous mass formed not a "septum" but a voluminous mass with "islands of typical uterine mucosa and at another point … a miniature uterine cavity,"[24] the whole *directly above*, but not involving, the true anatomical rectovaginal septum of Denonvilliers.[25] Cullen described the operation. "I did a complete hysterectomy, removing the uterus and appendages, and then shelled out a myoma, 1 cm in diameter, from the left side of the pelvic floor and another, about 4 cm in diameter, with a secondary nodule, 1 cm in diameter, lying on its surface. The combined nodule was situated between the rectum and vagina on the left."[26] Cullen dissected the adenomyomatous lesion from the rectovaginal pouch of Douglas without injury to vagina, rectum, or left ureter. His second case proved more challenging.

Cullen's treatment of patients with adenomyoma of the rectovaginal septum was deeply influenced by the fatal outcome of his second surgical case reported in 1913.[27] Two years previously, in San Francisco, the patient had undergone a high subtotal hysterectomy and removal of both large cystic ovaries along with a small portion of the rectum "on account of dense adhesions." The cervix and lower uterus were not removed. During a stormy postoperative course the patient developed a bowel obstruction. "After leaving the hospital she had a great deal of pain in the lower abdomen and for months had had almost continuous bleeding from the cervix." The patient was admitted to Johns Hopkins Hospital on June 4, 1913 "much weakened from the loss of blood." On examination "the right broad ligament was indurated and board-like" with thickening of the left broad ligament. Cullen and his staff tried to stabilize the patient without improvement and "a few days later felt that it was imperative to explore the abdomen." At surgery Cullen found a 6 centimeter cystic adenomyoma with a 2.5 centimeter irregular cavity filled with "chocolate colored fluid;" the whole attached to the rectum. "We removed a greater part of the growth, but left a portion still attached to the rectum and did not dare explore the right broad ligament."[28] At the start of surgery, the pulse was 45, but by the time the mass was partially removed, "the patient's pulse had become almost imperceptible, the rate being between 180 and 190, although she had lost practically no blood." The patient died postoperatively on June 10, 1913.

This case is reported in some detail because it directly influenced Cullen's surgical judgment and led to his aggressive treatment of adenomyoma of the rectum and rectovaginal septum. Also, given his status as an authority on adenomyotic disease, Cullen was in a position to influence the surgical judgment of others. Even though the patient had continued to menstruate profusely, Cullen assumed that both ovaries had been completely removed by the surgeons in San Francisco. Cullen came to believe that even without the ovaries – that is, even with *no ovarian tissue* remaining – severe adenomyotic disease of the rectovaginal septum would continue to worsen. Unfortunately for the patient, all ovarian tissue was not removed at the first surgery in San Francisco due to the dense adhesions encountered at that surgery. Remnants of ovary must have stimulated the uterus and caused profuse and nearly continuous uterine bleeding. The ovarian remnant syndrome was unknown when

[23] Cullen TS. Adenomyoma of the rectovaginal septum. 1913;26:106–118:116–7, Figure 3.

[24] Cullen TS. Adenomyoma of the rectovaginal septum. 1913;26:106–118. In 1918, Lockyer remarked, "The term 'miniature uterine cavities' for small cystic spaces in adenomyomas has often been employed by Thomas S. Cullen." Cuthbert Lockyer, *Fibroids and Allied Tumours (Myoma and Adenomyoma): Their Pathology, Clinical Features and Surgical Treatment* [London: Macmillan and Company, 1918], 401.

[25] Denonvilliers, CPD. Bull Soc Anatomy of Paris (Series 3) 1836:20:105. See also: Nichols DH, Milley PS. Surgical significance of the rectovaginal septum. Am J Obstet Gynecol 1970;108:215–220. See also: Nichols DH, Milley PS. "Clinical anatomy of the vulva, vagina, lower pelvis, and perineum. In *Gynecology and Obstetrics*, Vol. 1. [Hagerstown, MD: Harper & Row Publishers, Inc., 1977], 15. Figure 1–12. "The rectovaginal septum. Sections showing the partly dissected rectovaginal septum. It extends from the pouch of Douglas to the perineal body and forms the anterior surface of the rectovaginal space. Its adherence to the posterior vaginal wall is illustrated along with its posterolateral curve." (From Nichols DH, Milley PS: Surgical significance of the rectovaginal septum. Am J Obstet Gynecol 108:215, 1970.)"

[26] Cullen TS. Adenomyoma of the rectovaginal septum. Transactions of the Southern Surgical & Gynecological Association. 1913;26:106–118:111–112.

[27] Cullen TS. Adenomyoma of the rectovaginal septum. 1913;26:106–118:112–114.

[28] Cullen TS. Adenomyoma of the rectovaginal septum. 1913;26:106–118:112–114.

Cullen was writing.[29] Notwithstanding, even if the San Francisco surgeons had known of the existence of the ovarian remnant syndrome, it is unlikely that they could have successfully found and removed the ovarian remnants deeply buried in adhesions in the pelvic side wall tissues. In 1913, curare was not available for use by anesthetists as an adjunctive agent to relax abdominal muscles to facilitate such tedious exploratory surgery.

On the other hand, had the surgeons in San Francisco removed all uterine tissue above the cervix, the patient would not have menstruated. Without continuous blood loss, she would have recovered her strength. However, the patient would have continued to suffer deep pelvic pain because ovarian hormones from ovarian remnants would have continued to stimulate the deep pelvic adenomyomas. This was a complicated case. Unfortunately, the surgeons in San Francisco did not remove all functioning uterine tissue so the patient continued to bleed profusely. When admitted 2 years later to Johns Hopkins Hospital she was in desperate circumstances and beyond help.

Cullen never did explain the profuse vaginal bleeding, but he did state clearly his theory of origin of these adenomyomatous lesions. "In my group of adenomyomas of the uterus were several of cervical origin. If these grow posteriorly, owing to their inherent tendency to become attached, they will spread out into the rectovaginal septum, and become adherent to the rectum; or the peritoneal surface of the cervix may grow fast to the peritoneal surface of the rectum. In either case the rectum becomes fixed to the cervix.... The glands in these growths undoubtedly arise from the uterine mucosa or from remnants of Müller's duct."[30]

Cullen would consider neither the Wolffian rest theory of von Recklinghausen, nor the serosal theory of Iwanoff.[31] Until a historic day in 1925, when he heard Sampson speak, Cullen held that the pathogenesis of adenomyomas of the rectovaginal septum arose from the uterine mucosa or from remnants of the müllerian duct, müllerian rests.[32] Cullen republished his first two cases of adenomyoma of the rectovaginal septum in identical form in 1914 in volume 62 of the *Journal of the American Medical Association*.[33] Duplicate publication in this instance should not be judged by twenty-first century standards. Before World War I, except for subscribers to the *Transactions of the Southern Surgical and Gynecological Association*, physicians in private practice would have had to browse the printed *Index Medicus* to find his original article. Likely Cullen believed this subject sufficiently important that he needed to bring it to the attention of a national audience that could be reached through duplicate publication in the *Journal of the American Medical Association*.

Jessup read his paper before the Section on Pathology and Physiology of the Sixty-fifth Annual Meeting of the American Medical Association in Atlantic City, New Jersey in June of 1914. His article appeared in 1914 in volume 63 of the *Journal of the American Medical Association*.[34] It was illustrated with two simple drawings and five microscopic sections. The drawings show the retrocervical location of the adenomyoma in each case and also show precisely where the low- and high-power microscopic sections were taken. Jessup's first case was a 36 year old married woman, Mrs. D, without children who presented with a 2 year

---

[29] Shemwell RE, Weed JC. Ovarian remnant syndrome. Obstet Gynecol 1970;36:299. In the ovarian remnant syndrome fragments of ovarian tissue not removed at surgery survive and function by parasitically deriving their blood supply from other organs or tissues. In 1970, Shemwell and Weed demonstrated the existence of the ovarian remnant syndrome in an experimental model. They fixed fragments of ovarian cortex to the pelvic side wall of cats with sutures [creating artificial adhesions]; the isolated ovarian cortical fragments survived as functioning ovarian cortical tissue by acquiring a parasitic blood supply from vessels in the lateral pelvic wall.

[30] Cullen TS. Adenomyoma of the rectovaginal septum. Transactions of the Southern Surgical & Gynecological Association. 1913;26:106–118.

[31] Cuthbert Lockyer, *Fibroids and Allied Tumours (Myoma and Adenomyoma): Their Pathology, Clinical Features and Surgical Treatment* [London: Macmillan and Company, 1918], 320. Referring to page 252 of Cullen's 1908 publication, *Adenomyoma of the Uterus*, Lockyer pointed out that "Cullen will have nothing to do with the serosal theory." In 1898, N.S. Iwanoff published his theory that glandular cystic spaces in fibromyomas originated by an ingrowth of overlying serosa. Iwanoff NS. Drusiges cystenhaltiges Uterusfibromyom compliciert durch Sarcom und Carinom. Monatsschr fur Geb und Gynak 1898; Bd. vii: S. 295.

[32] Sampson JA. Heterotopic or misplaced endometrial tissue. Am J Obstet Gynecol 1925;10:649–664. Cullen TS. Discussion: Symposium on misplaced endometrial tissue. Am J Obstet Gynecol 1925;10:732–33. "We are great debt to Sampson for the careful, painstaking and brilliant work that he has done toward establishing the modes of origin of peritoneal adenomyomata."

[33] Cullen TS. Adenomyoma of the rectovaginal septum. JAMA 1914;62:835–839.

[34] Jessup, DSD. Adenomyoma of the rectovaginal septum. JAMA 1914;LXIII: 383–387.

history of "excessive menstruation, vaginal discharge and pain in the lower part of the abdomen." On admission to the New York Skin and Cancer Hospital, examination revealed a "mass between the uterus and rectum and attached to each." The preoperative diagnosis was "precancerous" uterus and "probable malignant mass in culdesac." The surgeon Bainbridge performed total abdominal hysterectomy and bilateral salpingo-oophorectomy and "partial excision of the rectal wall." In his pathology laboratory, Jessup observed: "To the portion of the posterior wall of the uterus there is attached by a band of fibrous tissue a section of rectal mucous membrane." Microscopic examination showed glands and stroma that "resemble the uterine mucosa." The second patient, a Mrs. F, was a 40 year old mother of two children, the youngest 13 years of age. "A distinct hard mass was felt in the culdesac of Douglas, beginning to adhere to rectum." Again suspecting malignancy, Bainbridge performed a total abdominal hysterectomy, bilateral salpingo-oophorectomy, and partial excision of the rectal wall. Microscopic examination revealed "as in case 1, the rectal mucosa is normal. Beneath it is a growth of smooth muscle which extends through and is continuous with that of the cervix. Glands appear within 2 mm of the rectal epithelium." Jessup noted the importance of Bainbridge's willingness to operate these cases stating: "in both of our cases other surgeons had previously examined the patients and pronounced their condition inoperable on account of the apparent involvement of the rectum by a malignant growth." Jessup continued: "That they may occur should be recognized by the surgeon, as the diagnosis can be made microscopically by a preliminary [histological] section [of a biopsy taken at surgery]. A simple excision of the mass would then cure the patient and there would be avoided the more serious operation of hysterectomy which would have been indicated if clinical diagnosis alone were relied on."[35]

Jessup's reference to "preliminary section" alluded to Cullen's rapid method of making an immediate intraoperative histologic diagnosis in the laboratory from a biopsy specimen while the patient was still on the operating table. Cullen's technique of frozen section diagnosis from intraoperative biopsy specimens allowed the operating surgeon to proceed by selecting with renewed confidence the appropriate operative procedure based on whether the lesion was malignant or benign.[36]

In the first decades of the twentieth century some surgeons like Lockyer, thinking they were operating for cancer of the rectum, initially performed Wertheim radical abdominal hysterectomy, with or without permanent colostomy, for adenomyomas of the rectovaginal septum.[37] Before the availability of frozen section diagnosis, confirmation of the preoperative diagnosis awaited examination of permanent histological sections of the surgical specimen. As surgical pathologists soon realized, adenomyomas of the rectum originated on the outer serosal surface of the rectum and invaded inwardly toward the rectal mucosa, but did not involve the mucosa. Whereas rectal cancer originated on the inner mucosal lining of the rectum and invaded outwardly through the rectal wall to spread to regional lymph nodes and by metastases to distant organs. In rectal cancer, the involved rectal mucosa was fixed to the cancer and did not move on rectal examination; in adenomyoma of the rectal wall the uninvolved rectal mucosa moved easily over the tumor.[38] Consequently, a careful rectal examination was sufficient to make a presumptive diagnosis of adenomyoma before operation. However, a definitive diagnosis required biopsy before or during surgery.

In 1915, Cullen reported his third case and second surgical fatality in a patient with adenomyoma of the rectovaginal septum. A 30 year-old unmarried woman had consulted him with "almost unbearable" pain that incapacitated her for 2 days before and after her menstrual period. The patient insisted on treatment. The fatality followed a complete hysterectomy and trans-anal low anterior resection of the rectum for adenomyoma of the rectovaginal septum with almost complete obstruction of the rectum. Cullen described the situation at surgery. "The growth, situated between the cervix and the rectum, was intimately blended with both … After

[35] Jessup, DSD. Adenomyoma of the rectovaginal septum. JAMA 1914;LXIII: 383–387.

[36] Cullen, TS. A rapid method of making permanent specimens from frozen sections by the use of formalin . Bull Johns Hopkins Hosp 1895;6:67.

[37] Lockyer, Cuthbert. Adenomyoma of the rectovaginal septum. Proceedings Royal Society Medicine. February 1913;vi, No. 4. Not realizing the benign nature of the disease, Lockyer had performed a Wertheim radical hysterectomy, a permanent colostomy, and resection of the rectum.

[38] Cullen TS. Adenomyoma of the rectovaginal septum. Trans Southern Surgical and Gynecological Assoc 1913;26:106–118:117.

[39] Cullen TS. A further case of adenomyoma of the rectovaginal septum. Surg Gynecol Obstet 1915;20:263–265.

the rectum had been freed for about eight inches the pelvis was packed with gauze and the anal margin all the way around was incised … About eight inches of rectum were then drawn through the anus and removed together with the growth. The rectum was then attached to the skin."[39] When he described the surgical specimen, Cullen pondered a less radical surgical approach.

"The growth is a typical adenomyoma of the rectovaginal septum, evidently starting in or near the cervix and gradually invading the rectum by continuity, but respecting the rectal mucosa at all points. The bowel was so nearly obstructed, however, that we were forced to remove at least 8 inches. The ideal method would have been to excise the area of the growth and then close up the defect."[40]

In 1915, Stickney, in a brief five paragraph note, reported what might be the first case in the American literature of a discrete circumscribed extrauterine adenomyoma adherent to the left ureter, an adenomyoma simulating a ureteral calculus. Following a supravaginal hysterectomy for diffuse uterine adenomyoma of the uterus, Stickney dissected the left ureter free and then dissected the adenomyoma from the anterior surface of the ureter.[41]

In 1916, Cullen reported his fourth and fifth cases of adenomyoma of the rectovaginal septum, with illustrations showing the anatomical localization of the disease. He observed that the "growths occur in women, are noted in the childbearing period, are usually situated directly behind the cervix and as a rule, are firmly adherent to the rectum."[42] He carefully surveyed the literature in *Index Medicus* on adenomyomas of the rectovaginal septum; proposed a tentative classification system; detailed typical symptoms that patients complained of; described five surgical options depending on the severity of the disease; and speculated on pathogenesis. By 1916, Cullen had become aware of reports of adenomyomas of the rectovaginal septum dating back as early as 1910: Stevens, 1910[43]; Nadal, 1911[44]; Lockyer, 1913[45]; Jessup, 1914[46]; and Stevens, 1915.[47] In the discussion that followed Cullen's presentation at the annual meeting of the American Medical Association in Detroit, Dr. Culbertson of Chicago called attention to Stevens' claim that he had reported a case in 1909.[48] Culbertson also remarked on cases of "posterior paravaginitis and parametritis with proliferation of epithelium" that Robert Meyer had described in 1908 and to the more recent case of Aman which that author referred to as "retrocervical fibroadenomatous serositis."[49] Contrary to Robert Meyer's suggestion that his lesion resulted from an inflammatory process, Cullen stated in his concluding remarks to the discussion that "In our cases of adenomyoma of the rectovaginal septum there has been no indication whatever of inflammation."[50]

In Cullen's fourth case, clearly and unequivocally the adenomyoma occupied the rectovaginal pouch of Douglas (RVPD) and not the rectovaginal septum which extends from the base of the RVPD to the perineal body.[51] The adenomyoma invaded deeply "extending out to the right pelvic wall and constricting some of the pelvic nerves … The mass in question was about 3 cm long and densely adherent to the side of the rectum, to the posterior vaginal wall, and also to the lateral wall of the pelvis."[52] On histologic examination, the interface between adenomyoma and normal tissue was "particularly instructive": adipose tissue was gradually replaced by "connective tissue and here and there … muscle and connective tissues are enveloping the nerves" and accounted for the pain in the right side of the pelvis extending down the right leg.[53] Cullen described clearly how the invasive adenomyotic dis-

[40] Cullen TS. A further case of adenomyoma of the rectovaginal septum. 1915;20:263–265.

[41] Stickney GL. A case of diffuse adenomyoma of the uterus, with discrete adenomyoma over the left ureter. Johns Hopkins Hospital Bulletin 1915;xxvi:304.

[42] Cullen TS. Adenomyoma of the rectovaginal septum. JAMA 1916;LXVII:401–406:405.

[43] Stevens TG. Adenomyoma of the rectovaginal septum. Proc Roy. Soc Med., 1910;iii:57.

[44] Nadal, Pierre. Bull. de l'Assn. franc. Pour l'etude du cancer. 1911;iv:338.

[45] Lockyer, Cuthbert. Adenomyoma of the rectovaginal septum. Proceedings Royal Society Medicine. February 1913;vi, No. 4.

[46] Jessup, DSD. Adenomyoma of the rectovaginal septum. JAMA 1914;LXIII: 383–387:385.

[47] Stevens TG. Adenomyoma of the rectovaginal septum. Proc Roy. Soc Med., 1916;ix: Obst. and Gynec. Section, p. 1.

[48] Cullen TS. Adenomyoma of the rectovaginal septum. JAMA 1916;LXVII:401–406:406:406.

[49] Cullen TS. JAMA 1916;LXVII:401–406:406:406.

[50] Cullen TS. JAMA 1916;LXVII:401–406:406:406.

[51] Cullen TS. JAMA 1916;LXVII:401–406:406. See Figure 1 (case 4).

[52] Cullen TS. JAMA 1916;LXVII:401–406:401. Figure 2.

[53] Cullen TS. Adenomyoma of the rectovaginal septum. JAMA 1916;LXVII:401–406:402.

ease *replaced adipose tissue* and encircled nerves. "This was well shown in my Case 4 … Here the young connective tissue cells and the muscle fibers gradually replace the adipose tissue of the broad ligament, and finally engulf it completely. They encircle nerves and gradually compress them."[54] Cullen described this tumor as "an adenomyoma of the type usually found in the rectovaginal septum, and in parts cannot be differentiated from an adenomyoma of the uterine wall."[55]

In Cullen's fifth case, the illustration clearly and unequivocally shows an adenomyoma occupying the retrocervical portion of the rectovaginal pouch of Douglas and not the anatomical rectovaginal septum: "Adenomyoma of the rectovaginal septum. The black area between the cervix and rectum indicates the location and approximate size of the supposed inflammatory thickening …"[56] The patient had previously had a subtotal hysterectomy, with removal of the left tube and ovary and part of the right ovary. On August 7, 1912 the operating surgeon, Cullen's colleague Dr. Richardson, described the pelvic mass as the size of a small hen's egg that "was situated 4 cm from the anus. It had infiltrated the anterior surface of the bowel and extended out laterally."[57] Richardson removed the mass composed of cervical stump, adenomyoma, and rectum. He sutured the rectum to the anus. Unfortunately, the patient died of surgical shock 10 h later. This was the third operative mortality for extrauterine adenomyomas at Johns Hopkins Hospital and the second mortality related to low resection of the rectum; the first such had been reported by Cullen in 1915. Cullen proposed a "tentative classification" of adenomyoma of the rectovaginal septum based on the Johns Hopkins experience and from data gleaned from the literature. He assigned cases to the stage he thought appropriate based on the extent of disease. In effect, Cullen made the first attempt to plot the natural history of this invasive lesion.

1. Small adenomyomas lying relatively free in the rectovaginal septum
2. Adenomyomas adherent to the posterior surface of the cervix and at the same time to the anterior surface of the rectum
3. Adenomyomas gluing the cervix and rectum together and spreading out into one or both broad ligaments
4. Adenomyomas involving the posterior surface of the cervix, the rectum and broad ligaments, and forming a dense pelvic mass that cannot be liberated[58]

Even at this relatively early date, Cullen recognized that the adenomyomata of the rectovaginal septum was a progressive disease and that "a case which today belongs to Group 1 may in a few years belong to Group 2 or to Group 3."[59] As the lesions progressed, patients complained of profuse menstruation, rectal pain, and pain with defecation.[60]

At a meeting in Münster, Germany in 1912, Füth had discussed his experience with adenomyomatous lesions of the rectum and rectovaginal pouch and concluded that "although an excision of the rectum might appear to be indicated, the patients get well without it [i.e. if a portion of infiltrated bowel is left behind.]"[61] This was a sensible conservative approach to surgical treatment of bowel adenomyoma in an era before antibiotics, and combined mechanical and antibacterial cleansing preparations of the bowel to neutralize dangerous bacterial flora of the rectum and large bowel. In 1912, surgeons were treating patients for adenomyoma-associated health and pain problems, not infertility. Either Cullen did not know of Füth's conservative approach or rejected conservatism based on his personal experience. Cullen's treatment of patients with

[54] Cullen TS. JAMA 1916;LXVII:401–406:404. See also Figure 3 (Case 4), page 403. "Muscular and fibrous tissue in an adenomyoma of the broad ligament encircling and compressing nerves. This section is from the right broad ligament. It shows the diffuse myomatous and fibrous tissue surrounding nerves. There were definite symptoms of nerve pressure."

[55] Cullen TS. JAMA 1916;LXVII:401–406:402.

[56] Cullen TS. JAMA 1916;LXVII:401–406:402:404. Figure 4 (Case 5). "A reference to the description of the specimen shows that the mass was a typical adenomyoma."

[57] Cullen TS. JAMA 1916;LXVII: 401–406:402. The rectovaginal pouch of Douglas in women with and without children often extends caudally below the mid-level of the vagina. See also: Cullen, Thomas S. The distribution of adenomyomas containing uterine mucosa. Archives of Surgery. 1920;1:215–283. "Adenomyoma of the rectovaginal septum usually starts just behind the cervix, and on bimanual examination, one can feel in this region a small, somewhat moveable nodule scarcely more than a centimeter in diameter."

[58] Cullen TS. Adenomyoma of the rectovaginal septum. JAMA 1916;LXVII:401–406s:403.

[59] Cullen TS. JAMA 1916;LXVII:401–406:403.

[60] Cullen TS. JAMA 1916;LXVII:401–406:404.

[61] Füth. Zentr f Gynak 1912;xxxvi:1356. Cited by Cuthbert Lockyer, *Fibroids and Allied Tumours (Myoma and Adenomyoma): Their Pathology, Clinical Features and Surgical Treatment* [London: Macmillan and Company, 1918], 333.

adenomyoma of the rectovaginal septum was deeply influenced by the fatal outcome of the second case he operated and reported in 1913.[62]

Cullen never did explain the profuse vaginal bleeding in his surgical fatality of 1913. Instead, 3 years later he expressed his conviction: "Some might argue that simple removal of the appendages [both tubes and ovaries] would cause atrophy of the uterine mucosa contained in the adenomyomas of the rectovaginal septum. My Case 2 is a sufficient answer. Although a supracervical hysterectomy had been performed two years before for a myomatous uterus; the pelvic condition had grown steadily worse."[63]

So saying and without further analysis, Cullen outlined his aggressive surgical management of adenomyoma of the rectovaginal septum. His surgical management, like his tentative classification, plotted the natural history of invasive adenomyomas of the rectovaginal septum: "(1) Where small discrete nodules exist in the posterior vaginal vault, these may be readily removed through a vaginal incision, as was so successfully done by Stevens. (2) Where the growth occupies the posterior surface of the cervix and extends laterally, after the ureters have been dissected out carefully, a complete abdominal hysterectomy should be performed. (3) If the growth be firmly adherent to the rectum, a wedge of the rectum should be removed, together with the uterus. It has been found best, after freeing the uterus on all sides, to open up the vagina anteriorly and laterally. The uterus and the rectum can then be lifted farther out of the pelvis, thus facilitating the removal of the necessary wedge of the anterior rectal wall. The uterus really acts as a handle, and the necessary rectal tissue and the uterus rare removed as one piece. (4) Where the lumen of the bowel is greatly narrowed, a complete segment of the rectum should be removed with the uterus, and an anastomosis should be made. (5) In desperate cases, where everything in the pelvis is glued together, as in my Case 2, an ideal operation is out of the question. The patient will not stand a long operation, and, if she could, a satisfactory result could not be obtained. In such a case it would be better to cut across the sigmoid, invert the lower end, close it, and bring the upper end out through the abdominal wall of the left iliac fossa, making a permanent colostomy. When the patient has to some extent regained her strength, the uterus, the lower portion of the rectum and the broad ligament tissue can be shelled out as one piece."[64] Cullen concluded his aggressive surgical management of adenomyomas of the rectovaginal septum with a statement that confirmed his conviction that adenomyomata of the rectum and rectovaginal septum should be completely excised. "These growths, while histologically not malignant, remind one of glue. Unless they are completely removed, further trouble is liable to occur."[65]

Based on his personal experience and his knowledge of the literature, Cullen forcibly opined: "The glands in the adenomyomas of the rectovaginal septum look like, and act exactly like, those of the mucosa of the body of the uterus, and they undoubtedly arise from uterine glands or from remnants of Müller's duct."[66] Cullen's default position, that adenomyomas of the rectovaginal septum were derived from "remnants of Müller's duct," would resurface in the latter part of the twentieth century as a vigorously defended theory for the pathogenesis of adenomyomas of the rectovaginal septum.[67]

In 1916, Stevens related the English experience. "The origin of these tumours is still far from settled." He listed four possible "sources: (1) the endometrium, (2) Müllerian remnants in the recto-vaginal septum, (3) Wolffian remnants in this situation, and (4) the peritoneal endothelium" [Iwanoff-Meyer theory]. Though he thought the origin from Wolffian remnants was "untenable," he believed the origin from "Müllerian ducts …

[62] Cullen TS. Adenomyoma of the rectovaginal septum. Trans Southern Surgical and Gynecological Association 1913;26:106–118:112–114. Cullen was also influenced deeply by the operative mortality of Richardson.

[63] Cullen TS. Adenomyoma of the rectovaginal septum. JAMA 1916;LXVII:401–406:405.

[64] Cullen TS. Adenomyoma of the rectovaginal septum. JAMA 1916;LXVII:401–406:405–6.

[65] Cullen TS. JAMA 1916;LXVII:401–406:406.

[66] Cullen TS. JAMA 1916;LXVII:401–406:405.

[67] Nisolle M, Donnez J. Peritoneal endometriosis, ovarian endometriosis, and adenomyotic nodules of the rectovaginal septum are three different diseases. Fertility Steril 1997;68:585–96. See also: Michelle Nisolle and Jacques Donnez, *Peritoneal, Ovarian and Recto-vaginal Endometriosis: The identification of three separate diseases* [New York: Parthenon Publishing Group, 1997], and J Donnez, O Donnez, J Squifflet, and M. Nisolle, "The concept of retroperitoneal adenomyotic disease is born." *An Atlas of Operative Laparoscopy and Hysteroscopy*, 2nd ed. Ed. J. Donnez and M. Nisolle [New York: Parthenon Publishing Group, 2001], 113–117.

cannot be disproved."[68] Opining that the origin from peritoneal endothelium appeared "to be an unnecessary theory," Stevens mentioned specifically that Archibald Leitch, among others, was "inclined to favour the endometrium as the source of all adenomyomata, including those which, apparently, are isolated in the recto-vaginal septum." Stevens explained: "The suggestion is that endometrial tubules grow out through the muscular coats of the uterus, accompanied by their own stroma and by a new growth of fibro-muscular tissue. This is obviously the case in the more common instances of diffuse adenomyomata of the endometrium, and the continuity of the tubules with the endometrial glands is easily demonstrated. In the case of growths in the recto-vaginal septum, however, the distance from the endometrium is considerable, and although it has been done, it is difficult to trace the continuity of the growth tubules with the endometrial glands. It is quite possible, too, that the connexion between the two has been completely lost during the process of growth. Once started, however, the tumour continues to grow whether it preserves its connexion with the endometrium or not." [69]

Many investigators reported cases, but few analyzed as thoroughly as Thomas G. Stevens. He referred to a case of adenomyoma of the rectovaginal septum that he had "demonstrated" to the Obstetrical and Gynaecological Section of the Royal Society of Medicine in 1909, "as far as I can ascertain, this was the first case of the kind described in this country."[70] In Stevens' Case I, (the same case he demonstrated in 1909) the adenomyoma was accompanied by a cyst of probable Wolffian origin in the anterior vaginal fornix. He then described five additional cases, all with adenomyomas located in the posterior vaginal fornix.[71] Stevens illustrated each case by a sagittal section drawing and by a drawing of the histology. Illustrations of all six cases show retrocervical lesions. In Case IV, "the true pouch of Douglas was … obliterated." In addition to the adenomyoma in Case IV, Stevens considered it "very significant that in this case there was a large vaginal cyst as well as the adenomyoma. The vaginal cyst, there can be no doubt, is of Gartnerian [Wolffian] origin, as it extended some distance up the lateral wall of the vagina."[72] Stevens deduced that in the presence of one abnormality from Wolffian remnants, that "it seems possible" the adenomyomas "may have arisen also from some remnant … possibly a Müllerian duct abnormality."[73] In Case VI the illustration shows the adenomyoma directly continuous with extensive adenomyosis of the posterior uterine wall.

Following his methodical case reports, in the "remarks" section of the article, Stevens stated "the growths were limited to the posterior fornix, but at the same time were closely adherent to the back of the cervix …" He continued: "the *site*[74] in which these growths are found in all my cases was the recto-vaginal septum." It was then that Stevens corrected himself and made the following insightful comment: "Perhaps it is not quite correct to say the septum, because it was really in the loose connective tissue above the posterior fornix, which is bounded by the back of the cervix in front, the rectum behind, and the peritoneum above."[75] To my knowledge this is the first statement in the medical literature that correctly localizes adenomyomas to the retrocervical portion of the rectovaginal pouch of Douglas.[76] Stevens recognized this retrocervical site was not the anatomical rectovaginal septum; rather it

[68] Stevens TG. Adenomyoma of the rectovaginal septum. Proc Roy. Soc Med., Obstet Gynaecol Section 1916;ix:1–17:16–17.

[69] Stevens TG. Proc Roy. Soc Med., Obstet Gynaecol Section 1916;ix:1–17:16.

[70] Stevens TG. Proc Roy. Soc Med., Obstet Gynaecol Section 1916;ix:1–17:1. In a footnote on page 6, Stevens identified Case I as the same case he had "demonstrated" in 1909 and published in a brief note: Stevens TG. Adenomyoma of the vaginal wall. "Proceedings, 1910, iii, p. 57." The author has a copy of the 1910 publication.

[71] The posterior fornix of the vagina is bounded anteriorly by that portion of the uterine cervix that protrudes into the vagina and posteriorly by the rectovaginal pouch of Douglas. See *Illustrated Stedman's Medical Dictionary*. 24th ed. [Baltimore, MD: Williams & Wilkins, 1982], 555. The vaginal fornix or fornix uteri is "the recess at the vault of the vagina; it is divided into a pars anterior, pars posterior, and pars lateralis with respect to its relation the cervix of the uterus."

[72] Stevens TG. Adenomyoma of the rectovaginal septum. Proc Roy. Soc Med., Obstet Gynaecol Section 1916;ix:1–17:6.

[73] Stevens TG. Proc Roy. Soc Med., Obstet Gynaecol Section 1916;ix:1–17:6.

[74] Stevens italicized the word *site* for emphasis.

[75] Stevens TG. Adenomyoma of the rectovaginal septum. Proc Roy. Soc Med., Obstet. and Gynecol. 1916;ix:1–17. When the rectovaginal pouch of Douglas [RVPD] becomes obliterated by disease, the adenomyomatous lesion is enclosed superiorly by adhesion of the serosal surface of the posterior cervix or posterior uterus to the serosal surface of the rectum. This creates the false impression that the floor of the RVPD is above the lesion. Actually the floor of the RVPD is below the lesion. The adenomyoma (deeply invasive endometriosis) is situated between the true floor of the RVPD below (caudad), and the false floor above created by cervix or uterus adherent to rectum above (cephalad).

[76] Stevens' insight was an important step in the evolution of the pathogenesis of deeply invasive endometriosis involving the

was the wall of tissue that separates the posterior vaginal fornix from the anterior rectovaginal pouch of Douglas. Unfortunately, the strength of his conviction was insufficient to advocate a change in terminology. Neither did Stevens change the title of his article. Perhaps he could not think of a better term.

Cullen was well aware of Stevens' article for he referred to it and cited it in a footnote.[77] Needless to say, we can conclude that Cullen was unimpressed with Stevens' insight.[78] For Cullen, Stevens was just another investigator among many who had reported several cases. Cullen's ear was attuned to Lockyer, a friend and fellow gynecologist and pathologist.[79] It was a classic case of initial conditions setting the terminology. In 1913, when Cullen sent his consultation to Jessup and received Lockyer's article in the mail the following day,[80] the precedent for the nomenclature – adenomyoma of the rectovaginal septum – was already set for him; he did not question it. Stevens' insight was published 3 years later in 1916, and apparently was not convincing. Cullen persisted in using the anatomically incorrect term "rectovaginal septum," and thus – adenomyoma of the rectovaginal septum – became entrenched in the medical literature. Stevens made a second insightful comment regarding the life history of adenomyomas of the rectovaginal septum when he wrote: "nothing is known as to their rate of growth or the age at which they commence."[81] Cullen did not comment on that insight either.

Foster S. Kellogg of Boston[82] was directly informed of the existence of adenomyomas of the rectovaginal septum and their aggressive surgical management by reading Cullen's article in the *Journal of the American Medical Association*.[83] Kellogg seems to have been impressed by Cullen's statement: "These growths, while histologically not malignant, remind one of glue. Unless they are completely removed, further trouble is liable to occur."[84] Kellogg reported a pelvic tumor in his patient that eroded through the posterior vaginal wall "with rather free bleeding."[85] He described the findings at surgery. The tumor "was found to be an integral part of the cervix, the vagina and the rectum. It was determined to dissect it from the rectum and remove it with the uterus and vaginal cuff."[86] Kellogg's description of the rectal involvement is both graphic and typical of the invasive pattern of rectal adenomyomas. "The tumor apparently penetrated all coats of the rectum except the mucous membrane, and it was soon apparent that it would be impossible to dissect it free without opening the rectum; in addition, *the rectum was accordioned onto the tumor, so that perhaps four or five inches was in apposition with the one to one and a half inch tumor* (Italics added). In this way a very small nick, as the rectum was freed up, became a long rent."[87]

Kellogg performed a total hysterectomy, removed the vaginal tumor, the fallopian tubes, but did not remove the ovaries. He dissected the adenomyomatous tissue from the rectal wall and in the process opened and repaired three rents in the rectum. "The patient came off the table in shock, which persisted in considerable degree for 48 hours; she gradually improved … On the 8th day a recto-vaginal fistula developed, but the patient continued to pass gas and feces through the anus … At the end of the 7th week … only gas came through the fistula … at the end of the 8th week the fistula closed." Pathology confirmed an infiltrating "adeno-leiomyoma."[88] The patient lived.

---

vagina, cervix, and rectum. It would be left to Johns A. Sampson's implantation theory to place the site of origin of endometriosis on the peritoneum of the rectovaginal pouch of Douglas.

[77] Cullen TS. Adenomyoma of the rectovaginal septum. JAMA 1916;LXVII:401–406:401. Cullen's footnote 5 on page 401 reads: Stevens, T. G.: Adenomyoma of the Rectovaginal Septum, Proc. Roy. Soc. Med., 1916, ix, Obstet. and Gynecol. Section. p. 1.

[78] Cullen TS. JAMA 1916;LXVII:401–406:401.

[79] Judith Robinson, *Tom Cullen of Baltimore* [London, Toronto, New York: Oxford University Press, 1949], 176. Whenever in London, Cullen visited Lockyer for casual evenings; the two corresponded for years.

[80] Cullen TS. The distribution of adenomyomata containing uterine mucosa. American Journal of Obstetrics and Diseases of Women and Children 1919;180:130–138.

[81] Stevens TG. Adenomyoma of the rectovaginal septum. Proc Roy. Soc Med., Obstet. and Gynecol. 1916;ix:1–17.

[82] Kellogg, FS. Adenomyoma of the recto-vaginal septum. Boston Medical and Surgical Journal 1917;176–177:22–24.

[83] Cullen TS. Adenomyoma of the rectovaginal septum. JAMA 1916;LXVII:401–406:401.

[84] Cullen TS. JAMA 1916;LXVII:401–406:406.

[85] Kellogg, FS. Boston Medical and Surgical Journal 1917;176–177:22–24:23.

[86] Kellogg, FS. Adenomyoma of the recto-vaginal septum. Boston Medical and Surgical Journal 1917;176–177:22–24:24.

[87] Kellogg, FS. Boston Medical and Surgical Journal 1917;176–177:22–24:24.

[88] Kellogg, FS. Boston Medical and Surgical Journal 1917;176–177:22–24:24.

Cullen published four more cases of adenomyoma of the rectovaginal septum in 1917. He began his discussion with a description of the constituent elements of deep pelvic adenomyomas of the rectovaginal septum, the precise anatomical area of their origin and their growth pattern. He retained his tentative classification and his aggressive surgical management outlined the previous year: [Description] "Adenomyoma of the recto-vaginal septum is a diffuse growth consisting of non-striated muscle and fibrous tissue with large or small areas of mucosa identical with the mucosa of the body of the uterus scattered throughout it. This mucosa swells at the menstrual period and, as there is usually no escape for the blood, the gland spaces tend to become cystic and are filled with blood; or there is hemorrhage into the matrix of the tumor."[89] [Origin and Growth Pattern] Vaginal involvement was the crucial localizing feature. "The tumor in the beginning is very small and starts in the vaginal vault just behind the cervix; or it may be recognized as a round or irregular thickening, not over 1 cm in diameter, behind and usually attached to the cervix. The growth gradually spreads in a diffuse and irregular manner, involves the adjacent anterior rectal wall and spreads into one or both broad ligaments, until finally, everything in the pelvis may be firmly glued into one mass."[90]

Cullen's Case 6 was the earliest rectovaginal adenomyoma he had seen to date. He removed the entire uterus, but not the tubes and ovaries. "On vaginal examination a small hard nodule could be felt in the vaginal vault just behind the cervix. On opening the abdomen we found in the mid-line just below and behind the cervix a puckered scar, about 1 cm in diameter."[91] Histologic section of the nodule revealed non-striped muscle and fibrous tissue containing "uterine glands surrounded by the characteristic stroma of the uterine mucosa [and in one area] a miniature uterine cavity."[92]

Max Broedel's illustration of Cullen's Case 7 is the most dramatic and explicit depiction of bilateral ureteral encirclement and compression by retrocervical adenomyomatous tissue – resulting in bilateral ureteral obstruction and bilateral hydroureter – that the author has ever seen.[93] Both ureters were encircled and constricted by the adenomyomatous growth in the broad ligaments, so much so that above the point of involvement the ureters were greatly dilated, each being over 1 cm in diameter.[94] The adenomyomatous growth was so aggressive that it "welled into the posterior vaginal vault, forming polypi, and in some places the growth has literally burst into the vagina, uterine mucosa projecting into and lining the vaginal vault."[95] The patient bled from the endometriotic lesion of the posterior vaginal fornix. A very large sagittal section through the uterus, cervix, and vaginal cuff reveals unequivocally and explicitly the retrocervical location of the adenomyoma labeled "adenomyoma of the recto-vaginal septum with formation of vaginal polypi."[96] Very large histological sections reveal typical adenomyomatous tissue consisting of "non-striated muscle and fibrous tissue … tubular glands lined with one layer of cylindrical epithelium and embedded in a stroma identical with that normally found in the mucosa lining the uterine cavity."[97] At surgery in 1914 the left ovary contained an orange-size cyst filled with old blood. However, in 1916 both ovaries appeared normal judging from Broedel's full pelvic illustration depicting bilateral hydroureters.[98] Cullen performed a total hysterectomy and removed the left tube and ovary and dissected both ureters free. He did not attempt to remove the rectal adenomyoma because the patient's condition deteriorated during surgery. Cullen removed the right tube but did not remove the right ovary. One can only surmise that he preserved

[89] Cullen TS. Adenomyoma of the recto-vaginal septum. Johns Hopkins Hospital Bulletin 1917;28:343–349:343.

[90] Cullen TS. Adenomyoma of the recto-vaginal septum. Johns Hopkins Hospital Bulletin 1917;28:343–349:343.

[91] Cullen TS. Johns Hopkins Hospital Bulletin 1917;28:343–9. Plate LXV, Figure 1.

[92] Cullen TS. Johns Hopkins Hospital Bulletin 1917;28:343–9. Plate LXVI, Figure 2.

[93] Cullen TS. Johns Hopkins Hospital Bulletin 1917;28:343–9. Plate LXVII, Figure 3.

[94] Cullen TS. Johns Hopkins Hospital Bulletin 1917;28:343–49. See Figure 3, Plate LXVII.

[95] Cullen TS. Johns Hopkins Hospital Bulletin 1917;28: 343–49:347.

[96] Cullen TS. Adenomyoma of the recto-vaginal septum. Johns Hopkins Hospital Bulletin 1917;28:343–9. Plate LXVIII, Figure 5.

[97] Cullen TS. Johns Hopkins Hospital Bulletin 1917;28:343–9. Plate LXX, Figure 7. See also other large histologic sections: Plate LXIX, Figure 6; Plate LXXL, Figure 8 showing a "miniature uterine cavity;" Plate LXXII, Figure 9; Plate LXXIII, Figure 10; Plate LXXIV, Figure 11, depicting an adenomyomatous polyps projecting into the posterior vaginal vault; and Plate LXXV, Figure 12.

[98] Cullen TS. Johns Hopkins Hospital Bulletin 1917;28:343–9. Plate LXVII, Inset upper left corner, Figure 3. The orange sized cyst filled with blood that was observed in 1914 possibly represented a hemorrhagic corpus luteum cyst. It is unlikely that an endometrioma of that size would have completely resolved in two years leaving the ovary to appear normal.

the right ovary because of the patient's young age, not wanting to precipitate premature menopause. But given the devastatingly aggressive nature of the disease in this 26-year-old woman, did Cullen fully appreciate the potential consequences of leaving an ovary in the presence of invasive rectal adenomyomatous disease in a patient who had complained of "severe pain in the rectum which radiated down the left thigh"? To judge from Cullen's decision, the pathophysiology of invasive adenomyotic disease was not fully appreciated in the World War I era, even at Johns Hopkins Hospital. In support of that conclusion we have the statement by Lockyer: "My own feeling is one of profound respect for the part played by ovarian tissue in convalescence after hysterectomy in the case of younger women."[99]

Whereas Cullen's seventh case was extraordinarily interesting from both medical and medical-historical perspectives, his Case 8 turned desperate when he became entrapped by more extensive disease than he had anticipated. The patient was a 37-year-old woman who "for the past year at least … had menstruated more frequently through the rectum than from the vagina" despite having undergone a supravaginal hysterectomy, removal of both fallopian tubes, appendix and the left ovary 2 years previously.[100] Examination elsewhere had revealed "a good deal of thickening in the vaginal vault behind the cervix" consistent with adenomyoma.[101] The patient was admitted to Johns Hopkins Hospital and at surgery on May 26, 1917 Cullen "found the cervix firmly glued to the rectum over a wide area."[102] He removed the cervix with a cuff of vagina and the adenomyoma of the rectum *en bloc* planning to repair the surgical defect in the rectal wall.[103] However, Cullen ran into the same problem experienced by Kellogg, the accordion effect whereby the extent of the rectal involvement was greater than he anticipated. He found himself confronted with "only a ribbon of the posterior rectal wall about 1.5 cm broad; consequently we had to do a complete resection, removing about 12 cm of the rectum … with a two layer "end-to-end anastomosis."[104] The patient nearly died on the operating table. To compound the problem, a good amount of liquid fecal matter had spilled during the bowel resection. Consequently the postoperative course was "stormy" for two and a half weeks. On the seventh postoperative day feces escaped into the vagina through a rectovaginal fistula; on the tenth postoperative day urine escaped into the vagina through a vesico-vaginal fistula: in essence a cloaca."[105]

Examination of the surgical specimen showed that the "growth [occupied] the posterior wall of the cervix and … had extended to and involved the outer coats of the anterior and lateral rectal walls, and … also extended to the vaginal mucosa posterior to the cervix."[106] A very large sagittal section through the surgical specimen showed a huge adenomyoma emanating from the posterior aspect of the cervix and involving almost the entire 12 cm length of excised rectum, a remarkable illustration.[107] Another large sagittal section– labeled as adenomyoma of the rectovaginal septum – clearly depicts an adenomyoma invading the posterior cervix and "extending into the rectum."[108] A final large histological section shows the adenomyoma invading the rectal wall and "encroaching on the rectal mucosa."[109]

Case 9 was a 28-year-old woman with tuberculosis of both fallopian tubes. On examination, Cullen palpated "marked induration in the vaginal vault behind the cervix."[110] At surgery Cullen observed that "behind the cervix at the level of the internal os was a hard indurated mass, 2.5 cm in diameter. This involved the posterior wall of the cervix and the anterior wall of the rectum. The bowel wall and the uterine wall at this point were intimately blended together, [in other words]

[99] Cuthbert Lockyer, *Fibroids and Allied Tumours (Myoma and Adenomyoma): Their Pathology, Clinical Features and Surgical Treatment* [London: Macmillan and Company, 1918], 262.

[100] Cullen TS. Adenomyoma of the recto-vaginal septum. Johns Hopkins Hospital Bulletin 1917;28:343–9:347.

[101] Cullen TS. Johns Hopkins Hospital Bulletin 1917;28: 343–9:347.

[102] Cullen TS. Johns Hopkins Hospital Bulletin 1917;28: 343–9:348.

[103] Cullen TS. Johns Hopkins Hospital Bulletin 1917;28:343–49:347, Case 8.

[104] Cullen TS. Johns Hopkins Hospital Bulletin 1917;28:343–49:348.

[105] Cullen TS. Johns Hopkins Hospital Bulletin 1917;28: 343–349:348.

[106] Cullen, Thomas S. Adenomyoma of the recto-vaginal septum. Johns Hopkins Hospital Bulletin 1917;28:343–49.

[107] Cullen TS. Johns Hopkins Hospital Bulletin 1917;28:343–9. Plate LXXVI, Figure 13.

[108] Cullen TS. Johns Hopkins Hospital Bulletin 1917;28:343–9. Plate LXXVII, Figure 14.

[109] Cullen TS. Johns Hopkins Hospital Bulletin 1917;28:343–9. Plate LXXVIII, Figure 15.

[110] Cullen TS. Johns Hopkins Hospital Bulletin 1917;28: 343–9:349.

an adenomyoma of the rectovaginal septum."[111] After removing both tubes and ovaries, the patient's pulse rose, varying between 160 and 170 beats/min. Cullen deferred definitive surgery.

Based on his experience with nine patients with adenomyomas of the rectovaginal septum, Cullen described his treatment plan for future cases. "If the growth be firmly adherent to the rectum, a wedge of the rectum should be removed, together with the uterus. It has been found best, after freeing the uterus on all side, to open up the vagina anteriorly and laterally. The uterus and the rectum can then be lifted farther out of the pelvis, thus facilitating the removal of the necessary wedge of the anterior rectal wall. The uterus can be used as a handle, and the necessary rectal tissue and the uterus removed as one piece."[112] This was the same technique he attempted with Case 8 before becoming entrapped.

Cullen viewed adenomyomas of the rectovaginal septum as invasive disease, albeit benign, that had to be totally excised because any remnants would resume growing and cause more problems. It seems likely that he based his aggressive surgical approach upon radical operations for carcinoma of the cervix reported by Sampson in 1905,[113] and the even more successful 5-year survival results reported by Wertheim in 1907.[114] He defended the aggressive treatment he had recommended in 1916 by writing: "Some might argue that simple removal of the appendages (tubes and ovaries) would cause atrophy of the uterine mucosa contained in the adenomyomas of the rectovaginal septum."[115] Recalling his second case that ended in a fatality, Cullen responded: "My Case 2 is a sufficient answer."[116] In desperate cases, "where everything in the pelvis is glued together, as in my Case 2, an ideal operation is out of the question."[117]

For such desperate cases Cullen recommended a two-stage operation, repeating his advice of 1916 in explicit detail. "In desperate cases … it would be better to cut across the sigmoid, invert the lower end, close it, and bring the upper end out through the abdominal wall of the left iliac fossa, making a permanent colostomy. When the patient has to some extent regained her strength, the uterus, the lower portion of the rectum and the broad ligament tissue can be shelled out as one piece."[118]

This would not be the last time that Cullen would offer this advice. Incomplete knowledge of the pathogenesis and pathophysiology of adenomyomata of the deep pelvis often led to heroic surgery as Cullen and other pioneers attempted by trial and error to work out the safe and appropriate surgical management of extensive extrauterine adenomyotic disease. As noted above, the second stage amounted to a posterior exenteration with total removal of the uterus, tubes and ovaries, all adenomyotic disease and the rectum.[119] In effect, Cullen consciously chose a permanent colo-cutaneous fistula (colostomy) in order to avoid a rectovaginal fistula or vesicovaginal fistula or disastrous double fistulas with feces and urine pooled in a vaginal cloaca. In 1908, Sampson had graphically illustrated and discussed a complication of uterine cancer: "a cloaca into which both the rectum and bladder empty."[120] Henceforth Cullen wanted to avoid this dreaded complication.

Lockyer published a monograph in 1918 summarizing the medical literature on uterine fibroids and uterine adenomyomas up to the early years of World War I (1914–1918).[121] Citing Robert Meyer's article in 1903, Lockyer noted that, lacking a true submucosa, the mucosa of the uterus and fallopian tube has the capacity to invade the surrounding muscle. Meyer had gone to

---

[111] Cullen TS. Johns Hopkins Hospital Bulletin 1917;28:343–9. Plate LXXIX, Figures 16 and 17. At surgery Cullen removed both ovaries and both pus filled tubes caused by tuberculosis. The patient was to return to surgery later for removal of adenomyomatous disease.

[112] Cullen TS. Adenomyoma of the recto-vaginal septum. Johns Hopkins Hospital Bulletin 1917;28:343–49:344.

[113] Sampson JA. The importance of early diagnosis in cancer of the uterus. JAMA 1905;xliv:1586–1593.

[114] Wertheim E. The radical abdominal operation in carcinoma of the cervix uteri. Surg Gynecol Obstet 1907;4:1–10, discussion:101–13. Sampson referred to both of these papers in a review article on uterine cancer entitled: The clinical manifestations of uterine cancer. International Clinics 1908; (Series 18) (2):176–201:199.

[115] Cullen TS. Johns Hopkins Hospital Bulletin 1917;28:343–49:344.

[116] Cullen TS. Johns Hopkins Hospital Bulletin 1917;28: 343–49:344.

[117] Cullen TS. Johns Hopkins Hospital Bulletin 1917;28: 343–49:344.

[118] Cullen TS. Adenomyoma of the recto-vaginal septum. Johns Hopkins Hospital Bulletin 1917;28:343–9:344.

[119] Cullen TS. Johns Hopkins Hospital Bulletin 1917;28: 343–49:344.

[120] Sampson JA. The clinical manifestations of uterine cancer. International Clinics 1908;(Series 18 (2)):176–201:196–197. Figure 22, page 196 is particularly graphic!

[121] Cuthbert Lockyer, *Fibroids and Allied Tumours (Myoma and Adenomyoma): Their Pathology, Clinical Features and Surgical Treatment* [London: Macmillan and Company, 1918], vii.

great lengths to explain that mucosal invasion was not synonymous with malignancy.[122] Nonetheless, Lockyer reported cases of carcinomatous change in uterine adenomyoma with metastases to the liver.[123] Cullen acknowledged that Cuthbert Lockyer had a remarkable command of the foreign literature.[124] Lockyer emphasized contributions to the literature on "*extra*uterine" adenomyomas for the benefit of his British audience.[125]

He collected 47 cases of adenomyoma of the recto-genital space between 1897 and 1915. The first was that of the well-known German gynecologist, Johannes Pfannenstiel in 1897.[126] The second case was reported by von Herff the same year.[127] The third report, from Ludwig Pick in 1899 described a diffuse adenomyoma of the posterior vaginal fornix.[128] "The tumor lay above the posterior fornix; it was the size of a plum, and slightly movable, but the vaginal wall was firmly fixed to it; the mucous surface of the vagina was smooth and intact. Histologically the growth consisted of muscle and branching gland-tissue; it resembled the growths shown by Pfannenstiel and von Herff."[129] Much can be learned by consideration of a few more of these early cases, for they give the reader an idea of the invasiveness of adenomyomas of the pelvic floor. Lockyer described the fourth case, that of Schickele.[130] "Schickele described a small hard growth the size of a nut; it lay in the upper half of the posterior vaginal wall, at the level of the *portio vaginalis*,"[131] and the vaginal mucosa was moveable over it, but the growth was very adherent to the rectum, so that a part of the bowel was removed with the tumour … the uterus was removed on the assumption that it was the seat of the hypothetical primary malignant focus. The case was one of an "adenofibroma, the greater part of which lay in the recto-vaginal *septum*, and the smaller part in the submucosa of the vagina."[132] The last of the early cases was that of Füth.[133] In 1903 he performed a Wertheim radical hysterectomy on a 31-year-old woman who had never borne a child. On examination the "posterior vaginal vault was depressed and there was an *ulcerated surface* the size of half-a-crown on the posterior vaginal wall, extending nearly to the external os. A fixed growth the size of a fist lay behind the cervix and uterus; it extended on the right to the pelvic wall, on the left it projected only slightly beyond the cervix. *The rectal mucosa could be moved over the growth.* [This indicated that the growth was not a rectal cancer.] The rectum was not resected." The mass extending to the right pelvic wall was not resected either. In 1905, 2 years after surgery, the patient was in good health.[134] Lockyer's 31st case of adenomyoma of the recto-genital space was his own case that he had reported in 1913.[135]

Lockyer stressed that the differential diagnosis of adenomyoma of the rectovaginal space must include cancer of the rectum and vagina. He did acknowledge

---

[122] Cuthbert Lockyer, *Fibroids and Allied Tumours (Myoma and Adenomyoma): Their Pathology, Clinical Features and Surgical Treatment* [London: Macmillan and Company, 1918], 419. Lockyer cited Robert Meyer. Uber adenomatose Schleimhautwucherungen in der Uterus- und Tubenwand und ihre pathologisch-anatomische Bedeutung. Virchow's Arch 1903;l172:394–409.

[123] Cuthbert Lockyer, *Fibroids and Allied Tumours*, 422, 427.

[124] Cullen TS. Adenomyoma of the recto-vaginal septum. Johns Hopkins Hospital Bulletin 1917;28:343–9:343. See footnote 4. "For an admirable review of the foreign literature on adenomyomas of the recto-vaginal septum consult Cuthbert Lockyer in Eden & Lockyer's New System of Gynaecology, Vol. II, p. 350. It is brim-full of interest." Cuthbert Lockyer, *Fibroids and Allied Tumours* (*Myoma and Adenomyoma*): *Their Pathology, Clinical Features and Surgical Treatment* [London: Macmillan and Company, 1918]. The author is deeply indebted to Cuthbert Lockyer's scholarly scientific monograph of 1918, an indebtedness also acknowledged by Thomas Cullen and John Sampson. Lockyer presented chronologically and in some detail the pertinent German, French, English, and American literature on adenomyomas to the outbreak of World War I.

[125] Cuthbert Lockyer, *Fibroids and Allied Tumours*, viii.

[126] Pfannenstiel JH: Uber die Adenomyoma, etc. Verhdlg d. Deutschen Ges f Gynak, Leipzig 1897: S. 195. Cited by Cuthbert Lockyer, Fibroids and Allied Tumours (Myoma and Adenomyoma): Their Pathology, Clinical Features and Surgical Treatment [London: Macmillan and Company, 1918], 333.

[127] Von Herff. Uber Cystomyome, etc. Verhdlg d. Deutschen Ges f. Gynak, Leipzig 1897: S. 189.

[128] Pick L. Virchow Archiv 1899; Bd clvi: S. 507. Cited by Cuthbert Lockyer, *Fibroids and Allied Tumours (Myoma and Adenomyoma): Their Pathology, Clinical Features and Surgical Treatment* [London: Macmillan and Company, 1918], 333.

[129] Cuthbert Lockyer, *Fibroids and Allied Tumours*, 334.

[130] Schickele G. Weitere Beitrage zur Lehre von den mesonephritischen Tumoren. Beitr z. Geb. Bd. vi. S. 449.

[131] Cuthbert Lockyer, *Fibroids and Allied Tumours*, 275. Lockyer cites: Schickele, Zentr. F. all. Path. und Anat., 1904;xv. S. 275.

[132] Cuthbert Lockyer, *Fibroids and Allied Tumours*, 334.

[133] Cuthbert Lockyer, *Fibroids and Allied Tumours*, 276. Lockyer cites: Firth, Zur Kasuistik der Adenomyome der Uterus. Zentr. F. Gynak 1903, Bd. xxvi: S. 626.

[134] Cuthbert Lockyer, *Fibroids and Allied Tumours (Myoma and Adenomyoma): Their Pathology, Clinical Features and Surgical Treatment* [London: Macmillan and Company, 1918], 335.

[135] Cuthbert Lockyer, *Fibroids and Allied Tumours*, 335. Lockyer C. Proc Roy Soc Med London (Obst and Gyn Sect.), 1913.

the value of the clinical sign of "freedom of movement" of the rectal mucosa over an adenomyomatous lesion,[136] and that rectal malignancy would fix the mucosa to the tumor. Unlike Cullen, who seemed to put more faith in the accuracy of clinical diagnosis, Lockyer did not recommend relying on clinical examination to differentiate carcinoma from benign invasive adenomyomas of the rectovaginal septum. He believed that biopsy was necessary to rule out malignancy. Also, the presence of uterine fibroids or adnexal masses tended to interfere with diagnosis of adenomyoma of the recto-genital space. In such circumstances Lockyer stated that laparotomy may be required for accurate diagnosis.[137]

Lockyer noted that Cullen was dogmatic in stating that "the glands in these growths undoubtedly arise from the uterine mucosa, or from remnants of Müller's duct."[138] According to Lockyer, Cullen was equally dogmatic about treatment, stating, "When the growth has invaded the rectum to a limited extent, it is *necessary* to remove only a small portion of the anterior wall of the rectum … When the rectal involvement is extensive, as in Lockyer's Case 2, resection of that portion of the bowel will, as a rule, be necessary."[139] This aggressive surgical approach coincided with Cullen's views on prognosis: "If portions be left *these will continue to grow*, and will lead to more pelvic adhesions, and finally produce complications that may result in death or permanent invalidism."[140] Relying on their own clinical experience, authorities on this enigmatic disease sometimes found themselves not only physically separated by the Atlantic Ocean, but nearly as separated in their recommendations for treatment.[141]

Lockyer, like Füth, believed it was not necessary to remove all adenomyomatous disease from the rectum: "For extensive growths in the recto-genital space, it has been shown that total removal or excision of the invaded bowel is, as a rule, unnecessary."[142] However Lockyer believed that operation was indicated for invasive lesions of the bowel to relieve stenosis and chronic intestinal obstruction and for invasive lesions of the posterior vaginal fornix to prevent ulceration and bleeding.

Treatment of bowel endometriosis marked a frontier of medical science in the first two decades of the twentieth century. Two of the leading practitioners, Lockyer and Cullen, had completely different approaches to the problem. Lockyer's approach proved better when both tubes and ovaries were removed. Operating in the 1920s, John Sampson set the standard in North America by successfully following the example of Füth and Lockyer. For extensive endometriosis in the absence of bowel obstruction, Sampson performed a hysterectomy, removed both tubes and ovaries as well as easily accessible endometriotic lesions, but he did not resect the bowel. In short, Sampson did not follow the advice of Cullen. How does one account for Cullen's aggressive approach to bowel endometriosis? Likely based on his adverse experience, Cullen came to the belief that hormone-resistant endometriosis would continue to invade the bowel and cause problems even after hysterectomy and removal of both tubes and ovaries. However, such was not the case, except in rare instances. Such a rare case of hormone-resistant endometriosis following total abdominal hysterectomy and bilateral salpingo-oophorectomy with supporting correlative studies of steroid receptor content and histology was reported in the last decade of the twentieth century.[143]

In 1918, less than two decades after the introduction of radiation therapy, Lockyer reported disappointing results with all types of radiation therapy applied to adenomyomas. "All forms of radio-therapy (Radium, X-Rays, Mesothorium) for adenomyoma are disappointing; only in one case, that of Griffith's, have I ever heard of radium doing good. It is my belief that such treatment is liable to excite the inflammatory process, which is the pathological basis of the disease."[144] The year before, Cullen had expressed similar disappointment with the results of

[136] Cuthbert Lockyer, *Fibroids and Allied Tumours*, 371.

[137] Cuthbert Lockyer, *Fibroids and Allied Tumours*, 371.

[138] Cuthbert Lockyer, *Fibroids and Allied Tumours*, 361.

[139] Cuthbert Lockyer, *Fibroids and Allied Tumours*, 361.

[140] Cuthbert Lockyer, *Fibroids and Allied Tumours*, 361.

[141] Surgeons, then as now, often must rely on their clinical experience and clinical judgment. Controlled clinical trials with medication are much easier to justify and conduct than for surgery. In the twentieth century, prospective controlled surgical trials were first accepted in the study of cancer, only later for the study of benign disease. Even then, due to rampant medical legal litigation, studies were more readily conducted in countries with socialized medicine and limited liability.

[142] Cuthbert Lockyer, *Fibroids and Allied Tumours*, 444.

[143] Metzger DA, Lessey BA, Soper JT, McCarty, Jr. KS, Haney AF. Hormone-resistant endometriosis following total abdominal hysterectomy and bilateral salpingo-oophorectomy: correlation with histology and steroid receptor content. Obstet Gynecol 1991;78:946–950.

[144] Cuthbert Lockyer, *Fibroids and Allied Tumours*, 444.

radium treatment of his adenomyoma of the rectovaginal septum. "In Case 7 the patient was too weak to allow us to resect the bowel and a portion of the growth still remains n the anterior recto-vaginal wall. Radium had been used, but the growth in the rectal wall is becoming thicker and sooner or later, I believe, it will be necessary to remove the portion of the rectum that is involved."[145]

By 1918 Lockyer could state: "The literature on adenomyoma of the recto-genital space is already quite extensive, and the condition is now sufficiently well recognized to prevent the error of treating it as a malignant process – an error which more than one operator excusably made, before the true benign character of the infiltrating adenomyoma was properly understood."[146] Lockyer defined adenomyoma. "The term 'adenomyoma' implies a new formation composed of gland-elements, hyperplastic cellular connective tissue, and smooth muscle."[147] The symptoms or complaints of patients with recto-vaginal adenomyomas are "far more distinctive and definite" compared to adenomyomas confined to the uterus. The chief complaint was *pain* – painful intercourse, pain with bowel movement. Over time, some patients suffered from "blood-stained *vaginal discharge*" if the endometriosis invaded anteriorly through the retrocervical area into the posterior vaginal fornix, and *obstinate constipation* leading in some cases to actual bowel obstruction, if the endometriosis invaded posteriorly and deeply into the bowel wall and constricted the lumen of the rectum or sigmoid colon.[148] None of the cases reported by Lockyer experienced rectal bleeding because endometriosis rarely invades through the submucosa of the bowel.[149] Recall that the uterus and vagina have no submucosa to act as a barrier to invasion, but the rectum, large and small intestine do have a submucosa to limit invasion.

Contrary to Cullen's earlier assertion that: "In our cases of adenomyoma of the rectovaginal septum there has been no indication whatever of inflammation,"[150] Lockyer and other investigators believed inflammation was involved in the pathogenesis of pelvic adenomyomas. Many investigators in this period noted the frequent association of adenomyoma with pelvic peritonitis. Lockyer called attention to tuberculosis, with demonstrable tubercle bacilli frequently contributing to the inflammation associated with tubal adenomyomas in the nineteenth and early twentieth centuries.[151] He summarized: "The intimate relationship with pelvic peritonitis is of great importance for the point of view of prognosis. Therefore, if we summarize the outlook, we must regard an 'adenomyoma' as a hemorrhagic and painful structure which is found in bad company, its intimate associates being adnexal tumours, pelvic peritonitis, parametritis, and infiltrations into bowel, whilst it can claim caseating tubercle, carcinoma, and sarcoma as causal acquaintances."[152]

Lockyer described the clinical signs detected by vaginal and rectal examination, in patients with moderate to advanced disease. Reminiscent of Robert Meyer's 1908 theory of an inflammatory pathogenesis, Lockyer stated in 1918 that: "Broadly speaking, the physical picture is that of a spreading inflammatory induration felt in the posterior fornix of the vagina. The posterior vaginal wall in all marked cases is most intimately adherent to, and is penetrated by, the growth. Puckerings, petechiae, actual haemorrhagic points, ulcerations, polypoid fringes, and teat-like projections are to be found on the free surface of the posterior vaginal fornix" when viewed through a vaginal speculum. He continued: "the posterior wall of the cervix *beneath the peritoneal reflection* is fixed by the invading adenomyomatous process. The mobility of the cervix as a whole is lost. The anterior wall of the rectum *beneath the peritoneum* is fixed to the indurated mass ... between the bowel and the cervix uteri."[153] (Lockyer's italics).

Lockyer's descriptions – *Beneath the peritoneum* and *beneath the peritoneal reflection* – refer *not* to the normal peritoneal floor of the anatomical rectovaginal pouch of Douglas, but to a false floor created *above* the invasive disease by fusion of the visceral peritoneum of the cervix and uterus to the visceral peritoneum of the rectum. Thus a vertical pseudo-rectovaginal septum is formed *above* the true anatomical rectovaginal septum

145 Cullen TS. Adenomyoma of the recto-vaginal septum. Johns Hopkins Hospital Bulletin 1917;28:343–349:344. See also: Cullen TS. 1917;28:343–9. Plate LXVII, Figure 3.

146 Cuthbert Lockyer, *Fibroids and Allied Tumours*, 332–3.

147 Cuthbert Lockyer, Fibroids and Allied Tumours, 265.

148 Cuthbert Lockyer, *Fibroids and Allied Tumours*, 366–7.

149 Cuthbert Lockyer, *Fibroids and Allied Tumours*, 366–7.

150 Cullen TS. Adenomyoma of the rectovaginal septum. JAMA 1916;LXVII:401–406:406.

151 Cuthbert Lockyer, *Fibroids and Allied Tumours*, 433.

152 Cuthbert Lockyer, *Fibroids and Allied Tumours*, 443.

153 Cuthbert Lockyer, *Fibroids and Allied Tumours*, 367–8.

of Denonvilliers by fusion of diseased cervix and uterus to the rectum. This obliterates the rectovaginal pouch of Douglas. The true anatomical rectovaginal septum of Denonvilliers located *below* remains intact and uninvolved with invasive adenomyotic disease.

Lockyer had described a completely frozen pelvis with obliteration of the rectovaginal pouch of Douglas by extensive, invasive endometriotic disease. Pioneer pelvic surgeons in the early decades of the twentieth century had to deal with such extensive disease. The more aggressive the surgical approach, the greater risk for complications. Examination of tissue under the microscope revealed the remarkable resistance of the submucosa of the rectum, a barrier that prevented extrauterine adenomyotic disease from burrowing into the lumen of the bowel. In Lockyer's experience: "The invasion has never been proved histologically to go beyond the submucous [submucosa] into the mucous coat of the bowel."[154] In sharp contrast adenomyotic disease invaded completely through the posterior vaginal wall into upper vagina behind the cervix. Furthermore, in the vagina wall – lacking a submucosa – "the gland-tubules have been shown to have burst through the mucous membrane."[155]

From his description of invasive adenomyomas of the rectovaginal pouch of Douglas one can readily appreciate why more research was needed to achieve early diagnosis, safe treatment, and to understand the pathogenesis and pathophysiology of extrauterine pelvic adenomyomas.

At the end of World War I, the debate over pathogenesis of adenomyoma of the intestinal tract centered on "foetal relics or whether it is a purely inflammatory process accompanied by the phenomenon of epithelial heterotopy" of Meyer.[156] Lockyer, referring to Archibald Leitch's recent concept of 'migratory adenomyoma,' was concerned that it was "liable to convey a wrong impression if it is taken to mean that the uterine mucosa is the *fons et origo* [source and origin] of all adenomyomas."[157] Lockyer added emphatically: "Adenomyoma is *not* confined to the uterus, nor is it always dependent upon changes in the *adult* mucosa. It is a pseudo-neoplasm, the result of an inflammatory lesion in the neighborhood of an epithelial tract."[158] Outside of a single case of adenomyoma invading the floor of the urethra, Lockyer did not identify any adenomyomas of the urinary tract. He confirmed that during pregnancy, characteristic decidual changes occur within uterine and extrauterine adenomyomas and noted Cullen's position that Whitridge Williams' famous case of decidual reaction of pregnancy in diffuse uterine adenomyoma "proved" the origin of the tissue from uterine mucosal invasion.[159] Robert Meyer's research indicated that rare cystic adenomyoma in the midline of the uterus might have a fetal origin from the epithelium of the müllerian ducts before the formation of the glands of the uterine mucosa, or cystic adenomyomas might develop from mature mucous membrane of the uterine corpus.[160] "The central sagittal plane of the uterine body is the situation where Meyer has found epithelial rests in foetal uteri and in uteri up to the age of puberty."[161] Frankl described a cystic adenomyoma in the sagittal plane of the uterine fundus and like Meyer attributed its development from embryonic müllerian tissue.[162]

Writing during World War I (1914–1918), Lockyer stated: "I cannot bring myself to admit that the mature uterine mucosa has ever been *proved* to have provided the gland-tissue in any extrauterine growth, wherever situated. [Alluding to the metaplasia theory of Iwanoff-Meyer, Lockyer opined]: It is much more likely that the peritoneum or vagina is the source of the epithelium in the majority of cases. That Müllerian relics may play a part in the formation of some recto-vaginal 'tumours' is quite probable."[163] Such were the convictions of

[154] Cuthbert Lockyer, *Fibroids and Allied Tumours*, 369.

[155] Cuthbert Lockyer, *Fibroids and Allied Tumours*, 369.

[156] Cuthbert Lockyer, *Fibroids and Allied Tumours*, 371.

[157] Cuthbert Lockyer, *Fibroids and Allied Tumours*, 372.

[158] Cuthbert Lockyer, *Fibroids and Allied Tumours*, 372.

[159] Cuthbert Lockyer, *Fibroids and Allied Tumours*, 380. Williams, JW. Decidual formation throughout the uterine muscularis: a contribution to the origin of adenomyoma of the uterus. Trans Southern Surgical Assoc 1904;17:119–132. "In this paper it is my object to describe a case of unusual decidual formation occurring in a uterus, the seat of a placenta praevia, which to my mind offers conclusive proof of the extension downward into the muscularis of processes from the endometrium, which could readily afford the basis from which a adenomyoma might be derived." Williams reviewed the literature on uterine adenomyomas to 1904.

[160] Cuthbert Lockyer, *Fibroids and Allied Tumours*, 395.

[161] Meyer, Robert. Cited by Cuthbert Lockyer, *Fibroids and Allied Tumours*, 398.

[162] Cuthbert Lockyer, *Fibroids and Allied Tumours*, 397. Cited Frankl, Oskar. Archiv fur Gynak Bd. xciii. Tafel xii.

[163] Cuthbert Lockyer, *Fibroids and Allied Tumours*, 371.

Cuthbert Lockyer, who had conducted the most extensive review of the literature on uterine and extrauterine adenomyomas and had weighed the theories of pathogenesis of the leading academic investigators.

Lockyer gathered all the classifications of adenomyotic disease up to 1916 except Cullen's 1916 classification of extrauterine adenomyomas:

Von Recklinghausen classified uterine adenomyomas by pathogenesis into two classes:[164]

1. Those located at the periphery of the uterus and in the tube – derived from Wolffian tubules
2. Those arising centrally – originated from uterine mucous membrane

Von Recklinghausen classified uterine adenomyomas by morphology into four varieties:[165]

1. Hard – "muscle-tissue in excess of gland-elements."
2. Cystic – cavity visible to naked eye, "possessing gland-tissue and muscle in equal amounts."
3. Soft – gland-tissue predominates and "appears microscopically as islands."
4. Telangiectatic – "soft, very vascular growths, which are almost devoid of cysts."

Cullen classified uterine adenomyomas by location.[166]

1. Intramural within a uterus of normal contour that may be two or three times enlarged.
2. Subperitoneal or intraligamentary
3. Submucous

Lockyer classified extrauterine adenomyomas by organ.[167]

1. Fallopian tube
2. Round ligament
3. Ovarian ligament
4. Broad ligament
5. Recto-genital space
6. Alimentary tract
7. Umbilicus (Cullen)

In 1916 Cullen had "tentatively" classified adenomyomas of the rectovaginal septum by extent of disease.[168]

1. Small adenomyomas lying relatively free in the rectovaginal septum.
2. Adenomyomas adherent to the posterior surface of the cervix and at the same time to the anterior surface of the rectum.
3. Adenomyomas gluing the cervix and rectum together and spreading out into one or both broad ligaments.
4. Adenomyomas involving the posterior surface of the cervix, the rectum and broad ligaments, and forming a dense pelvic mass that cannot be liberated.

Cullen's presentation of the "tentative" classification of adenomyomas of the rectovaginal septum before the Section of Obstetrics, Gynecology and Abdominal Surgery at the American Medical Association meeting in June 1916 amounted to a subtle call for early diagnosis and treatment.

By 1919, he was more forceful. In an address before the New York State Medical Society at Syracuse, Cullen expressed his belief that "in time," untreated endometriosis of the rectovaginal septum would render the woman a "chronic invalid, and in some instances" was a potentially lethal disease. He continued: "The growth sometimes encircles one or both ureters … Occasionally, as the growth progresses, the polypoid condition in the vaginal wall directly behind the cervix becomes very prominent, and in those cases in which the growth breaks through the vaginal mucosa, there may be a menstrual flow from the vaginal vault … Finally, if nothing is done, the pelvis may become so choked with growth that the patient dies from the extreme loss of blood coupled with partial intestinal obstruction."[169] This was not Cullen the pathologist, but Cullen the master physician and humanitarian – the ombudsmen for women – pleading for early diagnosis and treatment.

---

[164] Cuthbert Lockyer, *Fibroids and Allied Tumours (Myoma and Adenomyoma): Their Pathology, Clinical Features and Surgical Treatment* [London: Macmillan and Company, 1918], 270–11. Lockyer opined "The description he (v. Recklinghausen) gives of his second variety (actually his second "class"), i.e. the centrally situated growth hold good to this day."

[165] Cuthbert Lockyer, *Fibroids and Allied Tumours*, 270–11

[166] Cuthbert Lockyer, *Fibroids and Allied Tumours*, 303.

[167] Cuthbert Lockyer, *Fibroids and Allied Tumours*, 306.

[168] Cullen TS. Adenomyoma of the rectovaginal septum. JAMA 1916;LXVII:401–406:403. Lockyer did not include Cullen's 1916 classification; it was published too late for inclusion in his book.

[169] Cullen TS. The distribution of adenomyomata containing uterine mucosa. American Journal of Obstetrics and Diseases of Women and Children. 1919;180:130–138. In 1917, Foster S. Kellogg recognized the importance of Cullen's classification by republishing it verbatim in the Boston Medical and Surgical Journal. Kellogg FS. Adenomyoma of the recto-vaginal septum. Boston Medical and Surgical Journal 1917;CLXXVI:22–24.

Perhaps stimulated by Lockyer's classification of extrauterine adenomyomas, in 1919 Cullen also found time to write a short article entitled "The distribution of adenomyomata containing uterine mucosa." He gave a "bird's eye picture" of adenomyomas, their distribution and briefly described "the clinical picture noted in the various localities in which it occurs."[170] The title, "The distribution of adenomyomata containing uterine mucosa," is particularly revealing; Cullen did not quite know how to classify certain ovarian lesions: the solid and cystic lesion of WW Russell and the cystic lesions (later known as endometriomas) lined with uterine mucosa. They did not fall neatly in place with solid adenomyomas elsewhere, hence the modifier "containing uterine mucosa" in the title. Cullen classified and illustrated with a sagittal drawing the anatomical location of all uterine and extrauterine adenomyomata that he had observed. An obviously unsigned preliminary sketch by Max Broedel demonstrates "the various points at which I [Cullen] have found uterine mucosa."[171] Seven number labels indicated seven locations: "adenomyoma of the body of the uterus," rectovaginal septum, round ligament, anterior surface of the ovary,[172] utero-ovarian ligament, uterosacral ligament, and umbilicus.[173]

Cullen followed closely Lockyer's classification of extrauterine adenomyomas with the following notations: Cullen added lesions of the uterosacral ligament and ovary, used the term rectovaginal septum which Lockyer called recto-genital space, and omitted adenomyomas of the gastrointestinal tract. However, Cullen did discuss adenomyomas of the rectum under the heading of rectovaginal septum. Perhaps he was thinking of Kellogg's experience as well as his own when he expressed his by then time-honored caveat: "Sometimes it will be necessary to remove a wedge of the adherent anterior rectal wall with the uterus. In cases in which the growth is widespread, a preliminary permanent colostomy is imperative. Later the pelvis structures can be removed *en bloc*." [174] Thus Cullen revealed that both his experience and terminology differed from that of his London colleague. Then he expressed a truism attested to by all pelvic surgeons: "The removal of an extensive adenomyoma of the rectovaginal septum is infinitely more difficult than a hysterectomy for carcinoma of the cervix."[175]

In a particularly revealing and characteristically honest comment in his "bird's eye picture" address before the New York State Medical Society annual meeting in May 1919, Cullen acknowledged that he had no personal surgical experience with adenomyomas of the uterosacral ligament until "my colleague, Dr. W. W. Russell removed a pea-sized nodule from the uterosacral ligament."[176] Here again is an example of a phenomenon we have seen before. Despite his expertise in uterine adenomyomas, time and again Cullen needed to be alerted to extrauterine phenotypes of this complex disease. Recall that in 1913 Jessup and Lockyer brought the existence of adenomyomata of the rectovaginal septum to his attention. As a young attending in 1899, Cullen seems to have ignored Russell's report of uterine mucosa in the ovary and for the next 20 years was oblivious to ovarian involvement until awakened by Norris in 1918 and Casler in 1919.[177] Many manifestations of extrauterine adenomyomata as well as the ubiquitous chocolate cysts seem to have remained hidden in plain sight, unobserved by Cullen until he was alerted to their presence.

During 1919, Cullen had been preoccupied with the imminent departure of Kelly and the upcoming administrative duties as professor of clinical gynecology and head of the division of gynecology in the department of surgery under Halsted.[178] According to Cullen's successor

[170] Cullen TS. The distribution of adenomyomata containing uterine mucosa. American Journal of Obstetrics and Diseases of Women and Children. 1919;180:130–138:130.

[171] Cullen TS. The distribution of adenomyomata containing uterine mucosa. 1919;180:130–138:136.

[172] Cullen TS. The distribution of adenomyomata containing uterine mucosa. 1919;180:130–138:137. Referring to uterine mucosa in the ovary, Cullen stated: "In due time a sufficient number of such cases will undoubtedly be reported and then we shall be able to give a composite picture of both the clinical course and of the histological changes that occur in this most unusual group of cases."

[173] Cullen TS. The distribution of adenomyomata containing uterine mucosa. 1919;180:130–138:136.

[174] Cullen TS. The distribution of adenomyomata containing uterine mucosa. American Journal of Obstetrics and Diseases of Women and Children. 1919;180:130–138:135.

[175] Cullen TS. The distribution of adenomyomata containing uterine mucosa. 1919;180:130–138:135.

[176] Cullen TS. The distribution of adenomyomata containing uterine mucosa. 1919;180:130–138:133.

[177] Casler DB. A unique, diffuse uterine tumor, really an adenomyoma, with stroma, but no glands. Menstruation after complete hysterectomy due to uterine mucosa in remaining ovary. Transactions American Gynecological Society 1919;44:69–84.

[178] Te Linde, RW. In Memoriam: Thomas Stephen Cullen, 1868–1953. Trans American Gynecological Society 1953;76:227–229:228.

Richard Te Linde, Howard A. Kelly was not only Cullen's chief but also his "idol."[179] To celebrate that momentous occasion, Cullen wrote an informative biographical essay to celebrate the career of Kelly.[180] He also arranged for Minnie Blogg, librarian of Johns Hopkins Hospital, to publish an invaluable bibliography of Kelly's works from 1882 through his retirement in 1919.[181] The bibliography contains 485 titles that included books, pamphlets, and journal articles.[182]

Adenomyomas of the Ovary

During the second decade of the twentieth century, the subject of menstruation and ovulation still remained a "mysterious mechanism."[183] In 1917 Emil Novak – an instructor in clinical gynecology at Johns Hopkins Medical School who also worked in Cullen's gynecologic pathology laboratory – published a study of hemorrhagic cysts of the ovary.[184] Among 85 surgical specimens of ovarian hematomas varying between 2 and 6 cm in diameter, Novak found none that contained uterine glands and stroma, though he was particularly interested in pathogenesis of the smaller cysts which usually had a more intact lining. Interestingly, Novak may have shed some light upon Cullen's lack of interest in ovarian hematomas associated with adenomyomas of the rectovaginal septum when he commented: "There is no organ of the body which is so frequently the seat of hemorrhages as is the ovary. Indeed, so common are they that no clinical significance is attached to the small hematomata so frequently found in the ovaries removed at operation … By far the largest proportion of hematomata studied, as a matter of fact, were quite small, not exceeding 2 cm in diameter. These smaller lesions afford a much better opportunity than the more extensive ones of solving the important question of pathogenesis."[185]

This study, coming from Cullen's own laboratory, explains why Cullen considered an ovary with a small – 3 cm hematoma – unimportant. Furthermore, Novak found the "surface appearance of an ovary of little importance as an index of its internal structure."[186] Novak's observations may explain not only Cullen's apparent disinterest in ovarian hematomas accompanying extrauterine adenomyomas, but also the disinterest of most gynecologists at the time.

In 1918, Lockyer addressed the topic of adenomyomatous tissue in the ovary under the heading of adenomyoma of the ovarian ligament.[187] He began the discussion with an unexpected verbal thrust at Cullen. "Adenomatous elements within the substance of the ovary have been described by Cullen. I suppose he would refer these to the paroophoron."[188] By this Lockyer undoubtedly meant that Cullen considered such adenomyomatous elements to be embryonic remnants, but ironically remnants of the Wolffian duct, not the müllerian duct.[189] Lockyer illustrated a case of Semmelink and de Joselin de Jong[190] in which the adenomyomatous tissue invaded a cystic ovary.[191] A "blood-cyst lined by cytogenous tissue and gland-tissue (Adenomyoma) occupied a central portion of

[179] Te Linde, RW. In Memoriam: Trans American Gynecological Society 1953;76:227–229:228.

[180] Cullen TS. Dr. Howard A. Kelly: Professor of Gynecology in the Johns Hopkins University and Gynecologist-in Chief to the Johns Hopkins Hospital. Bull Johns Hopkins Hospital 1919;xxx:287–293.

[181] Blogg, MW. Bibliography of Howard A. Kelly, M. D., LL.D., Hon. F.R.C.S. Johns Hopkins Hospital Bulletin 1919;xxx:293–302.

[182] Blogg, MW. Bibliography of Howard A. Kelly, 1919;xxx:293–302.

[183] Novak E. Hematoma of the ovary, including corpus luteum cysts. Bulletin Johns Hopkins Hospital 1917;28:349–354:350. Novak actively investigated the interrelationship of the corpus luteum and menstruation. See: Novak E. The corpus luteum –Its life cycle and its role in menstrual disorders. JAMA 1916;lxvii:1285.

[184] Novak E. Hematoma of the ovary, including corpus luteum cysts. Bulletin Johns Hopkins Hospital 1917;28:349–354.

[185] Novak E. Hematoma of the ovary, including corpus luteum cysts. Bulletin Johns Hopkins Hospital 1917;28:349–354: 349–50.

[186] Novak E. Hematoma of the ovary, including corpus luteum cysts. 1917;28:349–354:350.

[187] Cuthbert Lockyer, *Fibroids and Allied Tumours (Myoma and Adenomyoma): Their Pathology, Clinical Features and Surgical Treatment* [London: Macmillan and Company, 1918], 321–329.

[188] Cuthbert Lockyer, *Fibroids and Allied Tumours*, 327.

[189] Illustrated Stedman's Medical Dictionary. 24th ed. [Baltimore, MD: Williams & Wilkins, 1982], 1033. "Paroophoron: Corpus pampiniforme; parovarium; a few scattered rudimentary tubules in the broad ligament between the epoophoron and the uterus; remnants of the tubules and glomeruli of the lower part of the Wolffian body."

[190] Semmelink and de Joselin de Jong. Monatsschr für Beb u Gyun Bd. xxii:244, Figure 7.

[191] Cuthbert Lockyer, *Fibroids and Allied Tumours (Myoma and Adenomyoma): Their Pathology, Clinical Features and Surgical Treatment* [London: Macmillan and Company, 1918], 328. Figure 198.

the ovary." A large amount of adenomyomatous tissue in that specimen was situated in the hilum of the ovary.[192] Lockyer concluded his short discussion with mention of a cherry-sized adenomyoma in the hilum of an ovary reported by Ludwig Pick in 1900.[193]

Casler's Menstruating Ovarian-Uterus

By invitation of the American Gynecological Society in 1919, De Witt Casler of Johns Hopkins Hospital presented one of the more remarkable case reports in the annals of gynecology.[194] In all probability the invitation was arranged by Cullen. The patient was a single 39 year old nurse who first consulted Casler in January 1913 with the complaint of painless excessive menstruation of 2 years duration. Examination revealed an irregular myomatous uterus that filled the pelvis and extended two finger's breaths above the pubic bone. On January 13, 1913 Casler performed a panhysterectomy and removed the right tube and ovary, the left tube, and the appendix. Preoperatively the patient, a nurse, insisted the Casler not remove all ovarian tissue because she dreaded an artificial menopause.[195] Finding the left ovary normal, the surgeon complied with his patient's request. Casler placed a small cigarette drain into the vagina, a surgical decision that would in time contribute to a unique experiment of nature.

Before closing the abdominal incision, Casler opened the uterus as was customary on the Johns Hopkins' gynecologic service. "The uterine cavity was found to contain one large and several smaller liver-colored polypi ... From the mucosa to the peritoneal surface the walls were everywhere converted into a coarse meshwork by tough bands of muscle or fibrous tissue running in all directions, and in the interstices of the meshwork and standing out prominently above the cut surface were small comedo-like areas of an appearance we had never seen before ... They were elevated above the surface, while in a diffuse adenomyoma we would have numerous depressions, with characteristic chocolate-colored fluid."[196] Microscopic examination was equally unusual. The mucosa was composed only of endometrial stroma without glands. The stromal masses consisted of: "an embryonic tissue made up of oval and spindle-shaped nuclei closely packed together ... The pathological process beginning in the polyp is really an orderly overgrowth of the stroma, which has gradually exterminated the uterine glands by strangulation, and then in the same manner has attacked the uterine musculature."[197]

In his autobiography, Robert Meyer recalled "As early as 1909 I had observed that it was the stroma of the endometrium which had the ability to destroy other tissue, especially elastic tissues (Virchows Archiv). At that time it was not known that one tissue could dissolve another without being malignant ... I found that the histolytic quality is not only responsible for the destruction of the interfascicular connective tissue but also for the musculature which undergoes necrosis to a greater or lesser degree."[198] Emge called this lesion "endometrial stromatosis," an aglandular form of internal endometriosis that, unlike adenomyosis, tends to dedifferentiate into sarcoma.[199]

---

[192] Semmelink and de Joselin de Jong. Monatsschr für Beb u Gyn Bd. xxii:244, Figure 7. Cuthbert Lockyer, *Fibroids and Allied Tumours (Myoma and Adenomyoma): Their Pathology, Clinical Features and Surgical Treatment* [London: Macmillan and Company, 1918], 328. Figure 198.

[193] Pick L. Ist das Vorhandensein der Adenomyome des Epoophoron erwiesen? Centr f. Gynak 1900, No. 15, S. 389.

[194] Casler DB. A unique, diffuse uterine tumor, really an adenomyoma, with stroma, but no glands. Menstruation after complete hysterectomy due to uterine mucosa in remaining ovary. Transactions of the American Gynecological Society. 1919;44:69–84.

[195] Casler DB. A unique, diffuse uterine tumor, really an adenomyoma, with stroma, but no glands. Menstruation after complete hysterectomy due to uterine mucosa in remaining ovary. Transactions of the American Gynecological Society. 1919;44:69–84:70–71. A panhysterectomy means removal of the entire uterus including the cervix. A supracervical or partial hysterectomy means removal of the body of the uterus but not the cervix.

[196] Casler DB. Transactions of the American Gynecological Society. 1919;44:69–84:72.

[197] Casler DB. Transactions of the American Gynecological Society. 1919;44:69–84:74.

[198] Robert Meyer, *Autobiography of Dr. Robert Meyer (1864–1947): A Short Abstract of a Long Life* [New York: Henry Schuman, 1949], 70–71.

[199] Emge LA. The elusive adenomyosis of the uterus. Am J Obstet Gynecol 1962;83:1541–1563:1554. Emge added that stromatosis was first described in 1864 by Virchow. Robert Meyer, *Autobiography of Dr. Robert Meyer (1864–1947): A Short Abstract of a Long Life* [New York: Henry Schuman, 1949], 63. "In 1919 I published a case of adenomyosis sarcomatosa, unknown before that. In definite adenomyosis of the uterus, its stroma grows deeper and through the whole uterine wall inside the lymphatics (*Zentralbl. F. Gyn. 1919, 43*). The same sarcoma of the stroma endometrii is described under a different name in the United States."

Casler examined his patient at 3–4 month intervals for 4 years and at each examination the left ovary was "normal in size and not enlarged or tender."[200] "During this period of 4 years, the patient consistently maintained that at regular monthly intervals she menstruated for a part of 1 day each month. Just as constantly I assured her she must be mistaken, for a panhysterectomy had been done and menstruation was out of the question."[201]

Then on January 1, 1917, exactly 4 years after the hysterectomy, the patient returned complaining of "obstinate constipation, with rather flattened stools" followed by diarrhea since November and of severe crampy pains of 2 weeks duration that the patient thought might be a partial bowel obstruction. Casler found "on vaginal examination the old drainage tract in the upper vaginal vault had opened slightly, and through this tract could be felt an irregular, nodular but cystic mass in the region of the left ovary. This was slightly moveable and was evidently the cause of the partial obstruction of the bowel."[202] Recall that at the initial operation on January 13, 1913, before closing the abdomen Casler had inserted a "cigarette drain" through the vaginal cuff.[203] In all probably the drain prevented healing by primary intention and by its presence created a fistulous channel between the vagina and the right ovary, a channel through which the patient menstruated.

At surgery on January 3, 1917 Casler found a grapefruit-sized semicystic ovarian tumor in the left lower pelvis densely adherent to the upper rectum and sigmoid colon with almost complete bowel obstruction.[204] He removed "about 20 cm of the sigmoid and upper part of the rectum with the ovarian tumor," and performed an end-to-end anastomosis. The ovarian tumor ruptured during removal and spilled "several ounces of dirty, chocolate-colored fluid and several reddish, liver-colored polypi escaped."[205] The postoperative course was essentially uneventful until the tenth day when the patient "was seized with a severe attack of abdominal pain, nausea and vomiting, and died from what was apparently a mesenteric thrombosis."[206] While no autopsy was permitted, Casler did have the opportunity to study the surgical specimens. "On opening the ovarian growth … we find a cystic tumor with walls of varying thickness. In the region near the attached sigmoid the walls are quite thick and cartilaginous, measuring 4 cm, while in other portions they are much thinned out and are 2–3 mm in thickness. The walls present an unusual appearance. In that portion adjacent to the sigmoid which forms the thickest portion of the tumor we find a tough and cartilaginous tissue."[207] "Microscopic examination reveals an ovarian cyst made up almost entirely of uterine tissue, the interior of the cyst corresponding to the uterine cavity and filled with blood while the walls contain may normal glands and others which show glandular dilatation. A pathological change has also occurred and we have an overgrowth of the interglandular stroma much resembling that seen 4 years previously in the uterus … The entire cyst, or uterine cavity, as it really is, is lined throughout by a single layer of tall columnar epithelium of the uterine type and in places cilia can be made out."[208]

Casler gave three somewhat ambiguous descriptions of the sigmoid colon, one at operation and two of the pathological specimen, but no microscopic examination. "At operation a semicystic tumor, about the size of a grapefruit was found occupying the left lower portion of the pelvis. Over the top of this cystic mass, and firmly attached to it, and almost completely obstructed by it, coiled the sigmoid flexure and the upper portion of the rectum, displaced by the growth toward the right. The ovarian mass was densely adherent to the lateral wall of the pelvis, was extremely vascular, and there was a marked infiltration of the bowel wall."[209] [The gross specimen.] "The sigmoid

---

[200] Casler DB. A unique, diffuse uterine tumor, really an adenomyoma, with stroma, but no glands. Menstruation after complete hysterectomy due to uterine mucosa in remaining ovary. Transactions of the American Gynecological Society. 1919;44:69–84:75.

[201] Casler DB. Transactions of the American Gynecological Society. 1919;44:69–84:76.

[202] Casler DB. Transactions of the American Gynecological Society. 1919;44:69–84:76.

[203] A cigarette drain is a made from a long tubular piece of thin rubber filled with gauze sponges.

[204] Casler DB. Transactions of the American Gynecological Society. 1919;44:69–84:76–77. See Fig. 6. "Drawing of ovarian tumor and adherent sigmoid, showing almost complete obstruction of the sigmoid, due to growth."

[205] Casler DB. Transactions of the American Gynecological Society. 1919;44:69–84:77. See Figure 6,

[206] Casler DB. Transactions of the American Gynecological Society. 1919;44:69–84:77.

[207] Casler DB. Transactions of the American Gynecological Society. 1919;44:69–84:77–78.

[208] Casler DB. Transactions of the American Gynecological Society. 1919;44:69–84:78–79. Figure 10.

[209] Casler DB. A unique, diffuse uterine tumor, really an adenomyoma, with stroma, but no glands. Menstruation after complete hysterectomy due to uterine mucosa in remaining ovary.

is closely attached to the growth and the lumen of the bowel is almost shut off at its middle portion by the encircling tumor. The mucosa of the bowel is normal while the muscular walls above the obstruction are somewhat hypertrophied."[210] [The gross specimen.] "The mucous membrane of the intestine is normal and the *muscular coats of the bowel have not been invaded*, but this infiltration of the tissue has gone around the sigmoid, so that for fully one-half of its circumference it is surrounded and compressed by this [ovarian] growth, thus causing the almost complete obstruction."[211]

The operative and laboratory descriptions suggest that the ovarian tumor not only bled through the fistulous tract on a monthly basis, but also ruptured into the left pelvis and invaded the wall of the sigmoid colon producing a near "napkin-ringlike constriction" of the bowel wall.[212] Casler opined this unique ovarian tumor originated from remnants of the müllerian duct.[213] From the advantage of historical perspective, the pathogenesis more likely is attributable to transmural spread of aggressive uterine stromal endometriosis through veins and lymphatics to the ovary. In 1920 Casler republished his presentation in *Surgery, Gynecology and Obstetrics*.[214]

Transactions of the American Gynecological Society. 1919;44:69–84:76–77.

210 Casler DB. Transactions of the American Gynecological Society. 1919;44:69–84:77.

211 Casler DB. Transactions of the American Gynecological Society. 1919;44:69–84:77, 80.

212 Ancel Blaustein, "Pelvic endometriosis," in *Pathology of the Female Genital Tract,* ed. Ancel Blaustein [New York: Springer-Verlag, 1977], 404–419. See figure 22.29, page 416. "Napkin-ringlike constriction of the [bowel] wall, intramural endometriosis present."

213 Casler DB. Transactions of the American Gynecological Society. 1919;44:69–84:82.

214 Casler DB. A unique diffuse uterine tumor, really an adenomyoma with stroma but no glands; menstruation after complete hysterectomy due to uterine mucosa in remaining ovary. Surg Gynecol Obstet 1920;31:150.

Distribution of Pelvic and Abdominal Adenomyomas

7

The Distribution of Adenomyomas Containing Uterine Mucosa

By 1920, Cullen accepted three models for the pathogenesis of extrauterine adenomyomas: (1) from embryonic müllerian rests, (2) "springing from" the posterior wall of the cervix or body of the uterus and invading the rectum, and (3) from overflow of uterine mucosa – shed from an adenomyoma of the rectovaginal septum onto tube and ovary – the same flowing metaphor that he used to explain the pathogenesis of diffuse uterine adenomyomas. Cullen came tantalizingly close to – and yet so far from – Sampson's later observations when he wrote: "One gathers the impression that the uterine mucosa from the diffuse adenomyoma on the posterior surface of the cervix and uterus has overflowed upon the adherent tube [and ovary]."[1] Cullen had the implantation pathogenesis in reverse.

In 1920, Cullen published a major review of uterine and extrauterine adenomyomas containing misplaced uterine mucosa.[2] This 69 page scientific article represented the apotheosis of Cullen's research on all phenotypes of adenomyomata. In a comprehensive review of his experience with extrauterine adenomyomata, Cullen emphasized adenomyoma of the rectovaginal septum and included a cursory summary of adenomyomas of the uterus.[3] The article contains the definitive illustration by Max Broedel of a sagittal section of abdomen and pelvis, showing all ten anatomic locations where Cullen had personally observed misplaced uterine mucosa.[4] Whereas in 1919 Cullen had enumerated seven sites,[5] only 1 year later he listed ten locations in which he had "found uterine mucosa" within the pelvis and abdomen.[6] Cullen's classification appears to be an expansion of Lockyer's 1918 classification by organ.[7]

[1] Cullen, TS. The distribution of adenomyomas containing uterine mucosa. Archives of Surgery. 1920;1:215–283: 244.

[2] Cullen TS. Archives of Surgery 1920;1:215–283.

[3] Scholars with a deep interest in this subject may wish to read this chapter with a copy of Cullen's 1920 article in hand so they can compare the illustrations in the article with the text of this chapter.

[4] Cullen TS. Archives of Surgery 1920;1:215–283;217. Fig. 1.

[5] Cullen TS. The distribution of adenomyomata containing uterine mucosa. American Journal of Obstetrics and Diseases of Women and Children. 1919;180:130–138:136. "Figure 1. The abnormal distribution of uterine mucosa. 1. In the wall of the uterus and at the uterine horn. 2. I the rectovaginal septum. 3. In the round ligament. 4. In the ovary. 5. In the utero-ovarian ligament. 6. In the uterosacral ligament. 7. At the umbilicus."

[6] Cullen, Thomas S. The distribution of adenomyomas containing uterine mucosa. Archives of Surgery. 1920;1:215–283.

[7] Cuthbert Lockyer, *Fibroids and Allied Tumours (Myoma and Adenomyoma): Their Pathology, Clinical Features and Surgical Treatment* [London: Macmillan and Company, 1918].

R.E. Batt, *A History of Endometriosis*,
DOI 10.1007/978-0-85729-585-9_7, © Springer-Verlag London Limited 2011

Figure 1 – The various points at which I have found uterine mucosa:[8]

1. Adenomyoma of the body of the uterus[9]
2. Adenomyoma of the rectovaginal septum[10]
3. Adenomyoma of the uterine horn, or of the fallopian tube[11]
4. Adenomyoma of the round ligament
5. Uterine mucosa in [the hilum of] the ovary[12]
6. Adenomyoma of the utero-ovarian ligament
7. Adenomyoma of the uterosacral ligament
8. Adenomyoma of the sigmoid flexure
9. Adenomyoma of the rectus muscle
10. Adenomyoma of the umbilicus[13]

By labeling Figure 1 as various sites where he had observed "uterine mucosa," instead of various sites where he had observed adenomyomata, Cullen gave inordinate emphasis to the ovary, the one location where cystic lesions did not fit neatly into his categorization of solid uterine and extrauterine adenomyomas.[14] Furthermore by so labeling, Cullen identified an outlier – uterine mucosa – as the defining characteristic of both uterine and extrauterine disease. To grasp Cullen's thinking, one may consider the game of billiards. Cullen racked his solid and striped adenomyomas only to find the odd ovarian ball did not fit, so he devised a larger more inclusive rack, relabeled the billiard balls and found that all ten uterine mucosa balls fitted neatly into the new rack. This proved to be the first tentative break from von Recklinghausen's "adenomyoma" terminology.

In Cullen's review of *the distribution of adenomyomas containing uterine mucosa*, Broedel captured Cullen's classification in a famous sagittal view of the female pelvis and abdomen that showed all ten anatomical sites where Cullen had personally observed uterine mucosa.[15] Broedel's illustration, which included a depiction of a large intraluminal adenomyoma of the sigmoid colon, was last reproduced in textbooks in 1958.[16] Uterine mucosa in the hilum of the ovary, in the rectus muscle, and the sigmoid colon was illustrated for the first time.[17,18]

---

[8] Cullen, TS. The distribution of adenomyomas containing uterine mucosa. Archives of Surgery. 1920;1:215–283:217.

[9] Cullen, Thomas S. The distribution of adenomyomas containing uterine mucosa. Archives of Surgery. 1920;1:215–283: 217, Fig. 1. The illustration shows extensive "diffuse adenomyoma" or adenomyosis of the uterus involving not only the anterior and posterior walls but also the fundus of the uterus. Young, RH. Dusting of old books: Comments on classic gynecologic pathology books of yesteryear. International Journal of Gynecological Pathology. 2000;19:67–84. As Robert H. Young pointed out, Cullen used the term adenomyoma of the uterus to include both "diffuse adenomyoma" (adenomyosis) and "discrete adenomyoma" (adenomyoma). This lesion was treated exhaustively in a separate monograph. Thomas Stephen Cullen, *Adenomyoma of the Uterus* [Philadelphia: WB Saunders, 1908].

[10] Cullen, Thomas S. Archives of Surgery. 1920;1:215–283: 217, Fig. 1. Note the discrepancy between terminology and illustration: the lesion labeled adenomyoma of the rectovaginal septum is shown in a retrocervical location involving the tissue between the posterior vaginal fornix and anterior portion of the rectovaginal pouch of Douglas.

[11] Cullen, Thomas S. Archives of Surgery. 1920;1:215–283: 222 Cullen noted: "We have in this tube an adenomyoma of the uterine type, and I am totally at a loss to explain its mode of origin."

[12] Cullen, Thomas S. Archives of Surgery. 1920;1:215–283: 243, Fig. 21. The legend reads: "Uterine mucosa on the surface of the ovary in a case of adenomyoma of the rectovaginal septum…The miniature uterine cavity on the surface of e the right ovary is represented by a. The lining mucosa resembles in every particular that of the body of the uterus. Some of the glands show hypertrophy. The mucosa of the adenomyoma of the rectovaginal septum seems to have overflowed to the surface of the adherent ovary. The same condition was noted on the surface of the corresponding tube." This is an important addition to his classification and the first evidence of his attention directed to the ovary, other than a prior acknowledgement of the case of WW Russell published in 1899.

[13] This lesion was treated exhaustively in a separate monograph. Thomas S. Cullen. *Embryology, Anatomy, and Diseases of the Umbilicus* [Philadelphia: W. B. Saunders, 1916].

[14] Cullen TS. The distribution of adenomyomas containing uterine mucosa. Archives Surgery 1920;1:215–283. In Figure 1, Cullen labeled the various sites at which he had found uterine mucosa, (1) was the body of the uterus; (2) rectovaginal septum, (3) uterine horn or fallopian tube, (4) round ligament, (5) hilum of the ovary, (6) utero-ovarian ligament, (7) uterosacral ligament, (8) sigmoid colon, (9) rectus muscle, and (10) umbilicus.

[15] Cullen TS. Archives of Surgery 1920;1:215–283;217. Figure. 1. As evidence that Cullen valued this contribution, he had it published as a hard cover sixty-nine page monograph in 1920. Thomas S. Cullen. *The Distribution of Adenomyomas Containing Uterine Mucosa.* Chicago, IL: American Medical Association Press, 1920. The author has a copy in his library, thanks to Dr. Ronald Cyr.

[16] E. Stewart Taylor, *Essentials of Gynecology* [Philadelphia: Lea & Febiger, 1958], 256. Figure 194. "The usual locations for endometriosis. (Cullen, courtesy of Arch. Surg.)"

[17] Cullen TS. The distribution of adenomyomas containing uterine mucosa. Archives Surgery 1920;1:215–283:269. Figure 42 (Case 16, rectovaginal septum Case 19). See also Figure 1, page 217; sagittal view of the female pelvis and abdomen.

[18] Cullen TS. Archives Surgery 1920;1:215–283:271, Figure 43 (Case 16, rectovaginal septum Case 19).

Analysis reveals a glaring discontinuity between Broedel's illustrations and Cullen's operative findings and histology recorded in the captions. In the exquisite composite illustration drawn in 1918, Broedel depicted a large spherical polyp with a broad base – originating in the *musculature* of the wall of the sigmoid colon.[19] Broedel's broad based spherical polyp projects far into the lumen of the sigmoid colon causing a blockage analogous to a tennis ball obstructing the downspout on a gutter.[20] First of all, adenomyomas of the bowel – be they of the sigmoid colon, rectum, ileum, or appendix – originate on the *serosa*, not from within the musculature of the bowel wall. Second, as adenomyomatous tissue invades from outside inward it puckers and gathers the serosa, distorting and kinking the bowel and causing partial to complete obstruction. This kinking and distortion of the bowel, the "accordion effect," was observed by Kellogg[21] and subsequently by all pelvic surgeons treating obstructive endometriotic bowel lesions. In Broedel's illustration, there is no evidence of Kellogg's accordion effect, no puckering and gathering of the serosa.[22] In Broedel's illustration, the serosa of the sigmoid colon – in the area where the broad based polyp originates – is completely normal! For emphasis, there is no sign of puckering of the serosa, no accordion effect so well described by Kellogg. In other words, Broedel's large spherical polyp with a broad base, originating in the *musculature* of the wall of the sigmoid colon, was not an adenomyoma. If not an adenomyoma, what was it? More than likely the large spherical polyp was a gastrointestinal stromal tumor such as a myoma, leiomyoma, or neurofibroma of the wall of the sigmoid colon.[23]

Whereas Broedel illustrated an obstructive intraluminal spherical polyp of the sigmoid colon with normal bowel serosa, at surgery Cullen described a "puckered area [serosa of sigmoid colon] at the pelvic brim."[24] Furthermore, "a photomicrograph of a [histologic] section taken from the sigmoid growth" shows no evidence of the large spherical intraluminal tumor depicted by Broedel. On the contrary, the histology shows a normal rectal (sic) mucosa with great thickening of the underlying muscular wall.[25] "Scattered throughout the muscular tissue were uterine glands surrounded by the characteristic stroma."[26] In other

[19] Cullen TS. Archives Surgery 1920;1:215–283:269. Figure 42 (Case 16, rectovaginal septum case 19) inset showing "independent adenomyoma of the sigmoid almost completely blocking the lumen of the bowel." This beautiful illustration depicts deeply invasive endometriosis (adenomyoma) of the rectovaginal pouch of Douglas that has penetrated the posterior fornix of the vagina. It also purports to show an adenomyoma partially obstructing the sigmoid colon.

[20] In the illustration the mucosa – though distended over the intraluminal spherical polyp – is normal.

[21] Kellogg FS. Adenomyoma of the recto-vaginal septum. Boston Medical and Surgical Journal 1917; 176 or 177: 22–24:24. Puckering and gathering of bowel serosa is a universally recognized phenotypic feature of advanced bowel adenomyomas that surgeons routinely observe with adenomyomas of the rectum, sigmoid colon, descending colon, ascending colon, and ileum. On numerous occasions of partial to complete obstruction of the sigmoid colon or the ileum, the author has observed an "Omega deformation of the bowel segment" where the adenomyoma (endometriosis) has invaded.

[22] Cullen TS Archives Surgery 1920;1:215–283:269. Figure 42 (Case 16) inset showing "independent adenomyoma of the sigmoid almost completely blocking the lumen of the bowel." This illustration depicts deeply invasive adenomyoma (endometriosis) that has penetrated through the anterior rectovaginal pouch of Douglas into the posterior fornix of the vagina. It also purports to show an adenomyoma obstructing the sigmoid colon.

[23] Stacey E. Mills, ed., *Sternberg's Diagnostic Surgical Pathology*, 4th ed., vol. 2. [Philadelphia: Lippincott Williams & Wilkins, 2004], 1589–1591. Juan Rosai, ed., *Ackerman's Surgical Pathology*, 8th ed., vol. 1. [St. Louis: Mosby, 1996], 645–647:645. "Gastrointestinal stromal tumors, (GISTs) constitute the largest category of primary nonepithelial neoplasms of the stomach and small intestine." Dr. Salvador Udagawa, my colo-rectal surgical colleague with whom I have worked closely for 25 years has removed gastrointestinal stromal tumors from the large intestine including the sigmoid colon; the largest GIST he removed was obstructing the distal transverse colon. See also Ancel Blaustein, "Pelvic endometriosis," in *Pathology of the Female Genital Tract*, ed. Ancel Blaustein [New York: Springer-Verlag, 1977], 404–419. See figure 22.29, page 416. "Napkin-ringlike constriction of the [bowel] wall, intramural endometriosis present." See figure 22.30, page 417. "Sigmoid colon. Endometrial implants in the smooth muscle layer. There is a hypertrophy of muscle about the implants." See Figure 22.31 "Sigmoid colon. Lesions of endometriosis that on gross inspection have a high index of suspicion for carcinoma. There is a raised submucosal lesion and puckering on the serosal surface."

[24] Cullen TS. The distribution of adenomyomas containing uterine mucosa. Archives Surgery 1920;1:215–283:269–270. See caption under Figure 42 (Case 16, rectovaginal septum Case 19), page 269 that is titled "Adenomyoma of the rectovaginal septum, independent adenomyoma of the sigmoid almost completely blocking the lumen of the bowel."

[25] Cullen labeled the specimen rectal mucosa instead of mucosa of sigmoid colon.

[26] Cullen TS. The distribution of adenomyomas containing uterine mucosa. Archives Surgery 1920;1:215–283:271. See caption under Figure 43 (Case 16, rectovaginal septum Case 19) labeled "Adenomyoma of the sigmoid flexure totally independent of a coexisting adenomyoma of the rectovaginal septum."

words, the operative description and the histologic findings indicated typical adenomyoma that had invaded through the serosa into the muscularis of the sigmoid colon.

For years these two illustrations have been accepted as representing an adenomyoma of the sigmoid colon; accepted without question on the authority of Cullen and his premier medical illustrator, Broedel. One can only speculate how this error happened. The explanation may lie in the stressful circumstances at Johns Hopkins Hospital and Medical School in 1918 when Broedel drew this illustration. First of all, following the effective date of Howard Kelly's resignation as chairman of the Department of Gynecology, Cullen's status was diminished twice: from the unqualified rank of associate professor to the higher but qualified rank of professor of clinical gynecology, and, when his responsibilities were formalized Cullen was appointed head of the new division of gynecology in Halsted's Department of Surgery, not chairman of Kelly's Department of Gynecology. Secondly, Cullen was distracted by extramural obligations such as preparation of a paper on "Cullen sign" for inclusion in a gift volume to celebrate Osler's 70th birthday.[27] Cullen also endured "deepening loneliness" due to the absence of "Popsy" Welch and Cullen's brother Ernst in military service in World War I and the suffering and death of his wife Emma Beckwith Cullen from a brain tumor in 1918.[28] Finally, he found himself unable to comfort his dear friend Broedel, who was "bereft of the Germany he loved."[29] All of these difficulties were compounded by the outbreak of the influenza pandemic of 1918. "All Baltimore, all of the East Coast, was erupting in flames. The virus struck the Hopkins itself so hard that the university closed its hospital to all but its own staff and students. Three Hopkins medical students, three Hopkins nurses, and three Hopkins doctors would die."[30] In short, under such stress Cullen had little time to devote to details of medical illustration, which he left to Broedel.[31] The normal two-way flow of communications between collaborators was disrupted by events beyond their control. The disconnect between illustration and caption went into print without being detected. Thus the error entered the medical literature in 1920[32] and proceeded from there into gynecologic textbooks.[33]

Uterus

Though he devoted less than two pages of text to adenomyomas of the body of the uterus, several points are clinically relevant. "The line of demarcation between the normal outer uterine muscle wall and the diffuse myomatous growth just beneath the mucosa is invariably sharply defined, but the two are nevertheless so closely blended that it would be absolutely impossible to separate them."[34] Gynecologic surgeons experienced in performing conservative uterine and pelvic surgery will immediately recognize why they must "cut out" adenomyomas which do not have a capsule while they can "shell out" fibroids because they do have a capsule. Cullen went on to say that "the histologic picture in a typical case [of diffuse uterine adenomyoma –

[27] Judith Robinson, *Tom Cullen of Baltimore* [London, Toronto, New York: Oxford University Press, 1949], 330.

[28] Judith Robinson, *Tom Cullen*, 280, 282.

[29] Judith Robinson, *Tom Cullen*, 279–80.

[30] John M. Barry, The Great Influenza: The Epic Story of the Deadliest Plague in History. [New York: Penguin Books, 2005], 258.

[31] Martzloff KA. Thomas Stephen Cullen. *Am J Obstet Gynecol* 1960;80:833–843:837. "The artistry of Max Broedel was a priceless adjunct to the books written by Kelly and by Cullen; Broedel was, in fact, an indispensable collaborator. While it was his judgment that frequently decided the type and form of illustration to be used in a given situation, of equal importance were some of his dissections and microscopic studies."

[32] Cullen TS. The distribution of adenomyomas containing uterine mucosa. Archives Surgery 1920;1:215–283:269. Figure 42 (Case 16, rectovaginal case 19).

[33] Ancel Blaustein, "Pelvic endometriosis," in *Pathology of the Female Genital Tract,* ed. Ancel Blaustein [New York: Springer-Verlag, 1977], 404–419. See Blaustein illustration 22.2, on page 405, labeled "Pelvic and abdominal sites of endometriosis." It is a reproduction of Broedel's sagittal illustration of abdomen and pelvis, showing all ten anatomic locations where Cullen had personally observed misplaced uterine mucosa: Cullen TS. The distribution of adenomyomata containing uterine mucosa. Archives of Surgery 1920;1:215–283;217. However, it was not attributed to Cullen. Instead it was reprinted in Blaustein by permission from C. Javert, Pathogenesis of endometriosis, Cancer 1949;2:399. In other words, Broedel's sagittal illustration of abdomen and pelvis showing the sites of misplaced uterine mucosa had taken on a life of its own; the original reference to Cullen was not mentioned, another "disconnect" helped to perpetuate the error.

[34] Cullen TS. The distribution of adenomyomas containing uterine mucosa. Archives of Surgery 1920;1:215–283:216.

adenomyosis] is very characteristic: the uterine mucosa is often of normal thickness and looks perfectly natural, but as we approach the underlying diffuse myomatous tissue, the mucosa is seen to penetrate it in all directions."[35] And perhaps with a final unreferenced nod to Rokitansky, Cullen wrote: "In the course of time, portions of the diffuse adenomyoma may project into the uterine cavity and be expelled through the cervix as submucous adenomyomas."[36] He also expressed his opinion of the pathophysiology of uterine hemorrhage and uterine crampy pain associated with diffuse uterine adenomyomata. With onset of menstruation, "the patient will not only lose her normal quota of blood, but this will be greatly increased by the flow coming from the large areas of mucosa which are scattered throughout the diffuse myomatous growth....There will, as a rule, be a great deal of pain in the uterus at the period due primarily to the swelling of the mucosa which is scattered throughout the uterine walls."[37]

The most "widespread" and extensive adenomyoma of the uterus that Cullen ever saw was located in the right horn of a bicornuate uterus, an anomalous uterus.[38] "Islands of normal-appearing uterine mucosa are seen scattered everywhere throughout the diffusely thickened uterine walls, and the glands extend right up to the peritoneal surface."[39] In the same anomalous specimen, Cullen described a 1 cm adenomyoma of the left tube located 2 cm "beyond the [left] uterine horn," an "adenomyoma of the uterine type."[40] This particular lesion was unique in his experience and is worth describing in some detail. "Even with low power it is noted that it is almost solid... Its center is occupied by diffuse myomatous tissue, and scattered everywhere throughout this are glands which resemble in every particular uterine glands. The majority of these lie in direct contact with the muscle, but here and there are several glands embedded in the characteristic stroma of the uterine mucosa. Some of the glands are dilated and at one or two points we can see miniature uterine cavities. We have in this tube an adenomyoma of the uterine type, and I am totally at a loss to explain its mode of origin."[41]

Nonetheless, Cullen may have given a clue to its origin. "In this case, we have a most unusual combination; a bicornuate uterus, the right horn of which presents a most beautiful example of diffuse adenomyoma; a right tubal ectopic pregnancy; adenomyoma of the inner end of the left tube and a hydrosalpinx of its outer end."[42] Could the "adenomyoma of the inner end of the left tube" represent "salpingitis nodosum isthmica" of Chiari[43] that had undergone metaplasia under the hormonal stimulus associated with the tubal pregnancy? Another clue to the original tubal morphology is that the majority of the glands had no stroma and lay in direct contact with the muscle, a characteristic of tubular epithelium.

Rectovaginal Septum

The substance of this article rests in the long section on adenomyoma of the rectovaginal septum. Cullen wished to lay "unusual emphasis" on these lesions because of their "unusual importance," describing in some detail pervasive invasiveness with the risk of chronic invalidism or even death if not diagnosed and treated in time.[44] Death was no stranger to Cullen, as we shall see when we come to discussion of adenomyomas of the sigmoid colon. This socially conscious physician wanted to caution his audience that they might avoid his terrible experience. He retold the 1913 story of Dr. Jessup sending him specimens of two adenomyomas of the rectovaginal septum and of receiving the "*Proceedings of the Royal Medical and Chirurgical Society of London,* containing Cuthbert Lockyer's article on 'Adenomyoma of the Rectovaginal

[35] Cullen TS. Archives of Surgery 1920;1:215–283:216.

[36] Cullen TS. Archives of Surgery 1920;1:215–283:216.

[37] Cullen TS. Archives of Surgery 1920;1:215–283:216–17.

[38] Cullen TS. Archives of Surgery 1920;1:215–283:221. Figure 4 (Case 1). Adenomyoma of the right uterine horn.

[39] Cullen TS. The distribution of adenomyomas containing uterine mucosa. Archives of Surgery 1920;1:215–283:221.

[40] Cullen TS. Archives of Surgery 1920;1:215–283:222.

[41] Cullen TS. Archives of Surgery 1920;1:215–283:224. See Figure 6, Case I. Adenomyoma of the left fallopian tube.

[42] Cullen TS. Archives of Surgery 1920;1:215–283:222.

[43] Chiari H. Zur pathologischen Anatomie des Eileiter-Catarrhs. Pager Ztschr. Heilkunde 1887;8:457–473. That same year, Martin reported cases similar to Chiari. Martin. Uber Tubenkrankung. Zeitschr für Geb und Gynak 1887;13. S. 299. Martin cited by: Cuthbert Lockyer, *Fibroids and Allied Tumours (Myoma and Adenomyoma): Their Pathology, Clinical Features and Surgical Treatment* [London: Macmillan and Company, 1918], 284.

[44] Cullen TS. The distribution of adenomyomas containing uterine mucosa. Archives of Surgery 1920;1:215–283:223–224.

Septum.'"[45] Compared to his first awakening and "gotcha" experience in 1896,[46] the second awakening must have deeply impressed Cullen, for he had told the story several times before: in 1914,[47] 1916,[48] and again in Syracuse in 1919.[49]

Returning to the seriousness of "widespread" adenomyomas of the rectovaginal septum, Cullen exhorted surgeons to perform a "preliminary permanent colostomy… Later the pelvic structures can be removed *en bloc*." For added emphasis he reminded his readers of the difficulty of this surgery: "The removal of an extensive adenomyoma of the rectovaginal septum is infinitely more difficult than a hysterectomy for carcinoma of the cervix."[50] This prudent advice – prudent for the era before antibiotics, safe blood transfusion and better knowledge of body fluid dynamics – was based on personal experience: one patient who developed vesicovaginal and rectovaginal fistulas[51] and two patients with adenomyomas of the sigmoid colon, both of whom died.[52] Cullen had presented his ninth case of adenomyoma of the rectovaginal septum in 1916. In the interim, he had accumulated ten more cases for a total personal experience with 19 cases.[53] In comparison, the Mayo Clinic experience comprised four cases.[54]

Cullen's septum case 10, published as Case 2 in 1920,… illustrates a small adenomyoma of the rectovaginal septum in which the legend describes the lesion thusly: "just posterior to the cervix is a slightly bluish black cystic area about 6 mm. in diameter. This bluish black appearance is, of course, due to the accumulation of old menstrual blood in a small cystic area in the adenomyoma."[55] Cullen also illustrates a sagittal section through the entire uterus, cervix, and a generous portion of the upper vagina, the vaginal cuff.[56] Both illustrations show the adenomyoma high in the posterior vaginal fornix.[57] To emphasize the point, Broedel's illustration unambiguously shows a small lesion in the wall of the posterior vaginal fornix behind the cervix (retrocervical); a location distant from the floor of the rectovaginal pouch of Douglas, distant from the rectum, and distant from the anatomic rectovaginal septum of Denonvilliers.[58] Cullen and Broedel appear to have been unacquainted with the description of the anatomic rectovaginal septum by Denonvilliers in 1836.[59] Cullen described the site of origin of adenomyomatous lesions of the rectovaginal septum. "Adenomyoma of the rectovaginal septum usually starts just behind the cervix, and on bimanual examination, one can feel in this region a small, some-

[45] Cullen TS. Archives of Surgery 1920;1:215–283:222.

[46] Judith Robinson, *Tom Cullen of Baltimore* [London, Toronto, New York: Oxford University Press, 1949], 125. Quotation of Cullen: "Popsy had read von Recklinghausen and he wanted to pull me out. 'You're wrong in your interpretation, Cullen,' he told me, 'von Recklinghausen says…' But I had brought the evidence with me, sectioned and mounted for examination. 'I don't care a hoot what von Recklinghausen says,' I said, 'Look down the barrel of that microscope.' "

[47] Cullen TS. Adenomyoma of the rectovaginal septum. JAMA 1914;62:835–839.

[48] Cullen TS. Adenomyoma of the rectovaginal septum. JAMA 1916;LXVII:401–406.

[49] Cullen TS. The distribution of adenomyomata containing uterine mucosa. Am J Obstetrics Diseases Women and Children 1919;180:130–138.

[50] Cullen TS. The distribution of adenomyomas containing uterine mucosa. Archives of Surgery 1920;1:215–283:225.

[51] Cullen TS. Adenomyoma of the recto-vaginal septum. Johns Hopkins Hospital Bulletin 1917;28:343–349:348.

[52] Cullen TS. The distribution of adenomyomas containing uterine mucosa. Archives of Surgery 1920;1:215–283.

[53] Cullen's total personal experience with adenomyomas of the rectovaginal septum at the time his 1920 paper went to press: 1913 – 2 cases, 1915–1 case, 1916–2 cases, 1917 – 4 cases, 1920 – 10 cases for total of 19 personal cases of adenomyoma of the rectovaginal septum.

[54] Mahle AE, MacCarty WC. Ectopic adenomyoma of uterine type (A report of ten cases). J Lab & Clin Med 1920;5:218–228:226.

[55] Cullen TS. The distribution of adenomyomas containing uterine mucosa. Archives of Surgery 1920;1:215–283. Figure 7, labeled "Adenomyoma of the rectovaginal wall as seen on vaginal inspection."

[56] Cullen TS. The distribution of adenomyomas containing uterine mucosa. Archives of Surgery 1920;1:215–283: Figure 8, labeled "Adenomyoma of the rectovaginal septum. This is a longitudinal section of the uterus and vaginal cuff seen in Figure 7."

[57] Cullen TS. Archives of Surgery. 1920;1:215–283.

[58] Cullen TS. Archives of Surgery. 1920;1:215–283. Page 227, Fig. 8 (case 2). Denonvilliers, CPD. Bull Soc Anatomy of Paris (Series 3) 1836:20:105.

[59] Denonvilliers, CPD. Bull Soc Anatomy of Paris (Series 3) 1836:20:105. This basic anatomic problem was clarified by the research of Nichols and Milley. Nevertheless, the misnomer perpetuated by Cullen, has persisted into the twenty-first century and has created much confusion as has the persistence of Cullen's controversial theory of pathogenesis of these invasive lesions from müllerian embryonic rests.

what moveable nodule scarcely more than a centimeter in diameter."[60] Cullen repeatedly used such phrases as: "a small nodule is felt directly behind the cervix[61]... may break into the vagina[62]...a small nodule directly behind the cervix[63]...in the posterior vaginal wall near the cervix[64]...appears to have begun in the posterior vaginal wall[65]...a small lump was felt in the vaginal wall behind the cervix[66]...behind the cervix was a nodule about 1.5 cm. in diameter."[67] He described endometriotic invasion of the posterior vaginal vault, a lesion associated with deep dyspareunia. "Occasionally, as the growth progresses, the polypoid condition in the vaginal vault directly behind the cervix becomes very prominent, and in those cases in which the growth breaks through the vaginal mucosa, there may be a menstrual flow from the vaginal vault even when a supravaginal hysterectomy has been performed some years before for uterine myomas."[68]

The crucial point to be emphasized is that Cullen relied for diagnosis on detecting a palpable hard lesion that "usually starts just behind the cervix."[69] The nodule distorted the posterior vaginal fornix, was readily palpable vaginally, and sometimes was visible as a bluish lesion in the posterior fornix. Hence, when Cullen had Broedel illustrate adenomyoma of the rectovaginal septum, the illustrations depicted neither rectal involvement nor involvement of the true anatomic rectovaginal septum; instead the illustrations showed, very precisely, an adenomyotic nodule beneath the mucosa of the posterior vaginal fornix, located in the tissue that forms a "septum" between the posterior vaginal fornix and the anterior rectovaginal pouch of Douglas.

Cullen illustrated an adenomyoma that invaded the broad ligament and compressed the right ureter causing partial ureteral obstruction.[70] When the author examined this illustration closely he could understand – for the first time – how Cullen could describe an adenomyoma as "springing from the cervix." By "springing from" Cullen meant the growth of a pedunculated subperitoneal adenomyoma extending well beyond the outer contour of the uterus.[71] Importantly, the accompanying large histologic section of the right broad ligament and adenomyoma demonstrates that *fatty tissue has been invaded and replaced* by connective tissue and adenomyomatous elements. "(Case 10). Discrete adenomyoma of the right broad ligament pressing on and partially obstructing the ureter...At the left, where the nodule was attached to the right side of the cervix, most of the tissue consists of fat. As we pass toward the right the adipose tissue is found to be replaced in part by connective tissue. At the extreme right the tissue consists of nonstriped muscle and fibrous tissue, and scattered throughout it are a moderate number of glands resembling those of the uterine mucosa."[72]

Over the years Cullen constantly equated pathogenesis and morphology.[73] Under the heading "cause of adenomyoma of the rectovaginal septum," Cullen stated in 1916: "The source of origin of their glands is also clear, namely, from the uterine mucosa."[74] Cullen continued: "When discussing cervical adenomyomas, in my work on 'Adenomyoma of the Uterus,' several years ago, I pictured an island of perfectly normal mucosa of the body of the uterus situated near the outer surface of the cervix. Subsequent studies may possibly show that this is no great rarity. If so, this growth might readily become the starting point for those adenomyomas found in the rectovaginal septum."[75]

Nowhere perhaps may Cullen's argument by analogy be more clearly demonstrated than in his statement: "The glands in the adenomyomas of the rectovaginal septum look like, and act exactly like, those of the mucosa of the body of the uterus, and they

[60] Cullen TS. Archives of Surgery. 1920;1:215–283:223.

[61] Cullen TS. Archives of Surgery. 1920;1:215–283:223.

[62] Cullen TS. Archives of Surgery. 1920;1:215–283:223.

[63] Cullen TS. Archives of Surgery. 1920;1:215–283:225.

[64] Cullen TS. Archives of Surgery. 1920;1:215–283:227. Figure 8.

[65] Cullen TS. Archives of Surgery. 1920;1:215–283:229.

[66] Cullen TS. Archives of Surgery. 1920;1:215–283:233.

[67] Cullen TS. Archives of Surgery. 1920;1:215–283:235.

[68] Cullen TS. Archives of Surgery. 1920;1:215–283:223.

[69] Cullen TS. Archives of Surgery 1920;1:215–283:223.

[70] Cullen TS. Archives of Surgery. 1920;1:215–283:250. Figure 27 (Case 10).

[71] Cullen TS. Three cases of subperitoneal pedunculated adenomyoma. Archives Surgery 1921;2:443–454. In this one article alone, Cullen employed the term "springing from" 13 times and "which sprang from" three times. In 1920, he had used the terms 20 times.

[72] Cullen, Thomas S. The distribution of adenomyomas containing uterine mucosa. Archives of Surgery. 1920;1:215–283:252. Figure 29 (Case 10).

[73] Cullen TS. Adenomyoma of the rectovaginal septum. JAMA 1916;LXVII:401–406:405.

[74] Cullen TS. JAMA 1916;LXVII:401–406:404.

[75] Cullen TS. JAMA 1916;LXVII:401–406:404. Thomas Stephen Cullen, *Adenomyoma of the Uterus* [Philadelphia: WB Saunders, 1908], 169, Figure 49.

undoubtedly arise from uterine glands or from remnants of Müller's duct."[76] In this either–or argument, Cullen would not admit the Meyer-Iwanoff heterotopic-coelomic metaplasia theory or the inflammatory theory of Meyer.[77] He was bound to the müllerian origin of all adenomyomas in all locations and demanded their origin from either post-embryonic or embryonic müllerian tissues. Compare the pastoral metaphors that Cullen used to describe adenomyoma of the uterus: "flow, flowing, and rivers"; with the military metaphors with which he described adenomyomas of the rectovaginal septum: "the growth has invaded all parts of the pelvic floor[78]...The mass in question was about 3 cm. long and densely adherent to the side of the rectum, to the posterior vaginal wall, and also to the lateral wall of the pelvis. It really had to be dug out."[79]

In cases where disease obliterated the rectovaginal pouch of Douglas, rectal examination or combined rectal–vaginal examination was preferable to vaginal examination. Cullen believed adenomyomas of the rectovaginal septum originated by "growing from the posterior surface of the cervix" or "springing from the posterior surface of the cervix" [80] Importantly, Cullen's fundamental belief was based on the appearance of small adenomyoma in the surgical specimens. Thanks to the beautiful illustrations of Broedel, we can reconstruct Cullen's reasoning. Thus, when Cullen wanted Broedel to illustrate the "hard nodular" adenomyotic lesion in extensive cases, where the rectovaginal pouch of Douglas was obliterated, he chose to depict the nodule as "springing" from the back of the cervix[81]. Only in Fig. 42 was adenomyoma of the rectovaginal septum depicted as involving the rectum. I believe that the determining factor, in so depicting the adenomyotic "hard nodule," was the operative technique used for its removal. Rather ingeniously, Cullen and his associates overcame the problem of rectal involvement by mobilizing the disease *en bloc*. They exposed the ureters to prevent injury, and then freed the uterus with adherent rectum and cuff of vagina by cutting the vagina anteriorly and laterally. "One can then lift the uterus and vaginal cuff up and with more ease separate the adherent vaginal cuff from the rectum. Sometimes it will be necessary to remove a wedge of the adherent anterior rectal wall with the uterus."[82] In extensive cases of adenomyomata of the rectovaginal septum, this technique facilitated dissecting the rectum from the adenomyoma, which remained adherent to the posterior aspect of the cervix.

Having operated the most difficult cases of deep pelvic endometriosis imaginable, Cullen again gave voice to the difficulty of the surgery for extensive adenomyomas involving the vagina, cervix and uterus, and rectum. He reminded his readers again that excision of an extensive adenomyoma of the rectovaginal septum was, in his experience, "infinitely more difficult than a hysterectomy for carcinoma of the cervix."[83]

Uterosacral Ligament

WW Russell had called Cullen's attention to adenomyoma of the uterosacral ligament "years ago, [which] on histologic examination...presented a typical adenomyomatous picture." Since then, Cullen had seen "a cyst 1.5 cm. in diameter apparently springing from the right uterosacral ligament," a lesion that resembled grossly the adenomyoma of Russell, though the histologic picture "was not very definite."[84] What is particularly interesting is Cullen's phrase expressing pathogenesis, the extrauterine adenomyoma "apparently springing

[76] Cullen TS. JAMA 1916;LXVII:401–406:405.

[77] Cullen TS. Adenomyoma of the rectovaginal septum. JAMA 1916;LXVII:401–406. In an abstract of the discussion to Cullen's paper, Dr. Carey Culbertson stated: "It is not difficult to understand how inflammatory pressure might produce such a squeezing out of the mucosa into the wall of the tube; but in the case of the rectovaginal septum or postcervical space, the distance from the uterine cavity is too great to admit of the presence here of typical uterine mucosa as the result of inflammatory pressure."

[78] Cullen TS. JAMA 1916;LXVII:401–406:403.

[79] Cullen TS. JAMA 1916;LXVII:401–406:401–2.

[80] Cullen TS. The distribution of adenomyomas containing uterine mucosa. Archives of Surgery 1920;1:215–283.

[81] Cullen TS. Archives of Surgery 1920;1:215–283:236. See: Cullen's septum case 14, illustrated in Fig. 16 (Case 6) on page 238. Cullen described this case as "This is the most widespread distribution of an adenomyoma of the rectovaginal septum that I have ever seen." On page 240, Cullen stated this supravaginal (subtotal hysterectomy) "was one of the most difficult hysterectomies I ever attempted."

[82] Cullen TS. The distribution of adenomyomas containing uterine mucosa. Archives of Surgery 1920;1:215–283:225. See also pages 229, 230, 236, 239–40 etc. under operation for each case.

[83] Cullen, Thomas S. Archives of Surgery. 1920;1:215–283:225.

[84] Cullen TS. The distribution of adenomyomas containing uterine mucosa. Archives of Surgery 1920;1:215–283:265. See Case 16, page 272: Septum Case 19; Gyn. No. 23764; Gyn. Path. No. 23891.

from the right uterosacral ligament." Cullen's strength lay in description and synthesis, not analysis or theory.

Sigmoid Colon

Cullen encountered his first case of adenomyoma of the sigmoid colon unexpectedly at laparotomy on a poor risk patient on 4 April 1918, a poor risk patient who also had an adenomyoma that had penetrated the posterior fornix of the vagina.[85] Unfortunately, Lockyer's treatise of 1918 that contained a section on adenomyomas of the sigmoid colon was published too late to alert Cullen to their existence. And from available evidence, though Casler's case of obstruction of the sigmoid colon was successfully operated before Cullen's case, the obstruction was not attributed to adenomyotic invasion of the sigmoid colon.[86] Thus, Cullen was not forewarned. He diagnosed the rectovaginal adenomyoma penetrating into the posterior fornix before surgery. At surgery – completely unaware of the presence of an adenomyoma of the sigmoid colon – Cullen mobilized the rectovaginal septal lesion vaginally before he began the abdominal operation. Only then did he discover the adenomyoma in the sigmoid colon. Thinking it was a carcinoma, Cullen explored the liver and upper abdomen for evidence of metastases. Unexpectedly faced with a possible carcinoma in a poor risk patient, Cullen mobilized the sigmoid colon and displaced it low in the pelvis. Then he exteriorized the sigmoid colon from the peritoneal cavity by sewing the peritoneum over it. Cullen anticipated performing a definitive second stage operation later when the patient was in better condition. Unfortunately the patient died in the interim. Only at autopsy was the true nature of the sigmoid lesion revealed to be a benign adenomyoma.

Cullen consulted Lockyer's book, *Fibroids and Allied Tumors* and observed that Lockyer "gives us the best résumé of the literature on adenomyoma."[87] He also found a case reported by Robert Meyer in 1919.[88] That patient had been operated in 1907 by Professor Mackenrodt, after whom Mackenrodt's ligament was named.

Cullen encountered his second case of adenomyoma of the sigmoid colon at surgery in late June or early July 1919. "On opening the abdomen the first thing which attracted one's attention was a mass the size of a large lemon which was situated in the upper part of the rectum or lower sigmoid colon."[89] He did not attempt to resect the sigmoid lesion. Instead, with considerable difficulty, he performed a total abdominal hysterectomy. In the process he excised a walnut sized adenomyoma located in the posterior vaginal vault that was "intimately connected with the cervix, rectum and broad ligament…It was a difficult operation on account of the fixation of the uterus. In attempting to separate the growth from the rectum, an opening was made in the bowel after which the whole involvement of the rectum by the tumor was cut away and the rectum was sutured."[90] His second patient also died postoperatively.

These were pioneering days in the diagnosis and surgical treatment of adenomyomas of the colon. Again Cullen reviewed the literature. He found the article by Mahle and MacCarty from the Mayo Clinic in which they reported their experience with one case of adenomyoma of the sigmoid colon and cited an earlier case of Leitch.[91] The patient of Mahle and MacCarty had been referred to them for treatment of a tumor of the "lower bowel" found at laparotomy.[92]

[85] Cullen TS. Archives of Surgery 1920;1:215–283. Surgery was performed on 4 April 1918. Analysis of this paper is somewhat frustrating because the illustrations are out of sequence with the text they illustrate. That it was an article in the first volume of a new journal may explain the situation.

[86] Casler DB. A unique, diffuse uterine tumor, really an adenomyoma, with stroma, but no glands. Menstruation after complete hysterectomy due to uterine mucosa in remaining ovary. Transactions of the American Gynecological Society. 1919;44:69–84:76–7. Casler's patient was operated 3 January 1917 with Gyn. Path. No. 22897 ½. Cullen TS. The distribution of adenomyomas containing uterine mucosa. Archives of Surgery 1920;1:215–283:272–3. Cullen's patient was operated 4 April 1918 with Gyn. Path. No. 23891.

[87] Lockyer, Cuthbert. *Fibroids and Allied Tumours.* New York: Macmillan Company, 1918.

[88] Meyer, Robert. Ueber entzündliche heterotope Epithelwucherungen im weiblichen Genitalgebiete und uber eine bis in die Wurzel des Mesocolon ausgedehnte benigne Wucherung des Darmepithels. Virchows Arch. f. path Anat. 1919:195:487.

[89] Cullen TS. The distribution of adenomyomas containing uterine mucosa. Archives of Surgery 1920;1:215–283:276.

[90] Cullen TS. The distribution of adenomyomas containing uterine mucosa. Archives of Surgery 1920;1:215–283:276.

[91] Mahle AE, MacCarty WC. Ectopic adenomyoma of uterine type (A report of ten cases). J Lab & Clin Med 1920;5:218–228:221–225. Leitch A. Migratory adenomyomata f the uterus. Proc Roy Soc Med 1913;vii, Pt. ii, Obst and Gynec Sec: 393–398,

[92] Mahle AE, MacCarty WC. J Lab & Clin Med 1920;5: 218–228:221.

Forewarned, they studied the colon before surgery with an "X-ray of the colon and a proctosigmoidoscopic examination," but both proved negative.[93] This was an example of the early use of diagnostic radiology.[94] At surgery, a "tumor mass was found encircling the sigmoid, involving a segment of the bowel 4 cm. in length. The sigmoid and the bladder were adherent to a mass around the uterus."[95] The sigmoid colon was dissected from the uterine mass and Mahle and MacCarty resected a 12 cm length of sigmoid colon along with "tarry cysts" of both ovaries; they did not perform a hysterectomy.[96] Mahle and MacCarty's patient survived the limited operation apparently without complications. Cullen reported his third and last case of adenomyoma of the sigmoid colon without citing the case of Leitch reported by Mahle and MacCarty.

One's respect for Cullen soars when one realizes that he provided sufficient evidence for the historian to reconstruct his personal learning curve for recognizing and treating adenomyomas containing uterine mucosa. This historical reconstruction is possible only because of Cullen's honesty and his full and meticulous recording of exactly what happened. Early in his career, Cullen recommended reporting all clinical experience, both good and adverse, so that other surgeons could learn from the Johns Hopkins experience and avoid complications when treating their patients.[97]

Rectus Muscle

Cullen presented a fascinating case of adenomyoma in the left rectus muscle, fascinating for its pathogenesis and because it provides a window on the practice of gynecology before widespread use of hospitals for surgery and before rigorous residency training and certification.[98] Following an incomplete abortion, "curettage was performed for retained membranes and the dilator passed through the retroflexed uterus at the cervical uterine junction. The body of the uterus was torn half loose from the cervix before the accident was discovered. The patient evidenced considerable shock, was rushed to the hospital, the abdomen was opened and the damage repaired."[99] Nine and one half years later, the patient noticed a "little soreness in the lower abdomen just to the left of the lower angle of the abdominal scar."[100] The same surgeon, who had saved the patient's life nine and a half years before, was again consulted and he removed the "entire lower end of the left rectus" muscle which contained a tumor without capsule approximately 2.5–3 cm long and 1.5 cm wide and 1.5 cm "thick." Cullen examined sections from the tumor and confirmed the diagnosis of an adenomyoma. Cullen's illustration, does not show the scar, and neither the referring physician nor Cullen mention the type of incision made at the emergency surgery. Nevertheless, based on the patient's localization of the lesion, "just to the left of the lower angle of the abdom-

[93] Mahle AE, MacCarty WC. J Lab & Clin Med 1920;5: 218–228:221.

[94] Had this been a cancer originating in the mucosa of the sigmoid colon, the proctosigmoidoscopy would have been diagnostic, and probably the barium enema study also. However, adenomyomas originate on the serosal or outer surface of the sigmoid colon. While the adenomyomatous mass within the wall of the sigmoid colon might have indented the lumen, the bowel mucosa overlying the adenomyoma would have been smooth and normal appearing.

[95] Mahle AE, MacCarty WC. J Lab. & Clin Med. 1920;5:221. The authors referred to a similar case of adenomyoma of the sigmoid colon observed by Leitch.

[96] Mahle AE, MacCarty WC. Ectopic adenomyoma of uterine type (A report of ten cases). J Lab & Clin Med 1920;5:218–228:221.

[97] Judith Robinson, *Tom Cullen of Baltimore* [London, Toronto, New York: Oxford University Press, 1949], 122–23. The Gynecological Service lost four of five patients from postoperative septic peritonitis in 1 week; one patient was infected before surgery and survived, the four clean cases did not. At the weekly staff meeting in January 1895, Cullen recommended the cases be reported in detail. Kelly assigned the task to Cullen. See Cullen TS. Post-operative septic peritonitis. Johns Hopkins Hospital Reports 1895;IV:411.

[98] Cullen TS. The distribution of adenomyomas containing uterine mucosa. Archives of Surgery 1920;1:215–283:272. See Figure 44, on page 272 an anatomical illustration labeled: "Adenomyoma in the left rectus muscle." See also Figures 45, on page 273, a histologic section labeled: "The nodule consisted of nonstriped muscle and fibrous tissue, and scattered throughout it were areas of typical uterine mucosa." Figure 46, on page 274 (also a microscopic section) shows islands of normal uterine mucosa "scattered throughout the myoma."

[99] Cullen TS. Archives of Surgery 1920;1:215–283:278. Subsequently the patient had a normal pregnancy, normal labor and delivery at term. However, a hematoma of the left broad ligament and left vaginal wall developed postpartum. It was successfully drained vaginally.

[100] Cullen TS. Archives of Surgery 1920;1:215–283:272. Figure 44, Adenomyoma of the left rectus muscle. See Figure 45 on page 273 and Figure 46 on page 274 for the histology.

inal scar, the incision was probably midline."[101] Supporting this assumption, a midline incision is generally employed for emergency laparotomy, especially with a patient in shock.

The case begs for analysis. Apparently, neither Cullen nor the referring surgeon appreciated the pathogenesis of this lesion. The referring surgeon mused that the adenomyoma "did not seem to be associated with the scar of the incision" from the emergency surgery. Cullen reached for an explanation, citing two cases of adenomyoma of the abdominal wall reported by Mahle and MacCarty from the Mayo Clinic.[102] Both cases were examples of iatrogenic transplantation of uterine mucosa. In the first case, the adenomyoma was located in the lower abdominal wall, "under a previous laparotomy scar." In the second case, an 8 cm adenomyoma extended from the uterus to the abdominal wall at the site of a previous ventral uterine suspension. Fortunately, Cullen supplied sufficient data to reconstruct the pathogenesis of the adenomyoma in this unusual case. In all probability a family practitioner, working under trying circumstances in the patient's home around 1909, curetted the uterus to complete the miscarriage, but failed to recognize the retroflexed position of the uterus before curettage. The operator unknowingly perforated the anterior wall of the uterus with the instrument and curetted the lower anterior abdominal wall vigorously. When he pressed the sharp curette upward, thinking the instrument was inside the uterus, the curette engaged and lacerated the abdominal wall. As the operator drew the curette downward and outward, the abdominal wall tissue caught by the curette remained attached at its lower end and the bleeding continued. Undoubtedly, the operator curetted harder and harder in an effort to retrieve all products of conception and stop the bleeding. In the process, he not only lacerated the left rectus muscle with its artery and vein, but also enlarged the uterine perforation tearing the "body of the uterus… half loose from the cervix." The patient bled profusely from lacerated blood vessels in the abdominal wall and uterine wall and went into shock from blood loss. By repeated manipulation of the curette, uterine mucosa was caught in the curette and transferred to the traumatized left rectus muscle where the transplanted tissue developed into an adenomyoma. Many years later Cullen and Broedel wrote an article thoroughly describing the anatomy of the rectus abdominis muscle, an article that adds credence to the traumatic pathogenesis of this adenomyoma of the rectus muscle.[103]

Ovary

In all, Cullen operated one patient and reported five other patients who had uterine mucosa in an ovary.[104] The first patient was reported by Russell from the Johns Hopkins Hospital in 1899.[105] Cullen reported the second case from the archives of Johns Hopkins Pathology Laboratory (GYN. Path. No. 22505, Sept. 19, 1916.) The patient had a myomatous uterus and a small left ovarian cyst "partially filled with blood [and] containing uterine mucosa in its walls."[106] Cullen continued: "The cyst wall is lined by one layer of cylindric epithelium. In places, this lies in direct contact with the ovarian tissue, but here and there is separated by a definite stroma. Near the right, the stroma is very evident, and embedded in it is a gland resembling those of the body of the uterus."[107]

Cullen's third patient was operated by Casler in 1917.[108] Cullen summarized Casler's case. From Cullen's remarks it is obvious that he had reviewed the microscopic slides. The specimen was remarkable because scattered throughout a diffuse myomatous

[101] Cullen TS. Archives of Surgery 1920;1:215–283:272. Figure 44, Adenomyoma of the left rectus muscle. See Figure 45 on page 273 and Figure 46 on page 274 for the histology.

[102] Mahle AE, MacCarty WC. Ectopic adenomyoma of uterine type (A report of ten cases). J Lab. & Clin Med. 1920;5:221.

[103] Cullen TS, Broedel M. Lesions of the rectus abdominis muscle simulating an acute intra-abdominal emergency. Bulletin Johns Hopkins Hospital 1937;lxi:295–315.

[104] Cullen, Thomas S. The distribution of adenomyomas containing uterine mucosa. Archives of Surgery. 1920;1:215–283:258. William Wood Russell was the same man who reconsidered his withdrawal and accepted the residency position that Kelly had offered to Cullen in the interim. This resulted in Cullen spending three precious years in the pathology laboratory.

[105] Russell WW. Aberrant portions of the müllerian duct found in an ovary. Johns Hopkins Hospital Bulletin. 1899;8–10 with an additional three pages labeled Plate I, Plate II, and Plate III each with illustrations of whole-ovary microscopic sections drawn by Max Broedel.

[106] Cullen, Thomas S. Archives of Surgery. 1920;1:215–283: 260, 262.

[107] Cullen, Thomas S. Archives of Surgery. 1920;1:215–283:260, 263, Figure 36 (Case 13).

[108] Cullen, Thomas S. Archives of Surgery. 1920;1:215–283: 259–60.

thickening [of the uterus] "were quantities of stroma identical with that of the uterine mucosa…This stroma however contained no glands. The tumor resembled in every particular the picture of an ordinary adenomyoma of the uterus except for the fact that the glands were missing from the stroma."[109] Cullen examined the ovary and uterus and opined that the histologic sections explained the ectopic menstruation. "On histologic examination great quantities of typical uterine mucosa were found scattered throughout the ovarian tumor, thus clearly explaining why the patient had continued to menstruate without any uterus. The ovary contained all the essential elements, normal ova, and practically normal uterine mucosa, and the small tract left where the uterus had been removed supplied the necessary avenue along which the menstrual flow escaped."[110]

Curiously, Cullen did not elaborate on the difference between the misplaced uterine mucosa within the uterine wall, the uterine polyp, and that found in the ovary. Histologic sections of the adenomyoma near the uterine serosa showed uterine stroma – without glands – "infiltrating and dividing the uterine muscle into a course mesh-work."[111] The large uterine polyp was also composed of aggressively infiltrating uterine stoma with few glands. In contrast, the ovarian cyst was lined by broad-based polyps; some were composed of uterine stroma only, while other polyps were composed of "masses of stroma but with many large atypical uterine glands,[112] many of the glands filled with degenerated blood."[113]

Casler had described within the ovarian cyst other "liver-colored polypi, irregular in size, generally with a broad base, each…made up of uterine tissue, glands, stroma and muscle."[114] In his opening remarks, Casler addressed tangentially Cullen's concept of the pathogenesis of diffuse uterine adenomyoma. "Adenomyoma… has generally been regarded as a benign tumor, characterized in the main by invasion of the muscle columns, or, as some pathologist regard it, by a 'flowing in' of the glandular tissue into the crevices of the muscle bands, the glandular tissue always accompanied by a larger or smaller amount of interglandular stroma."[115] Furthermore Casler questioned Cullen's passive "flowing in" metaphor. "The structure of the tumor and the remarkable way in which the stroma has invaded from the mucosa to the serosal surface of the growth, suggests an active process of an infiltrating character on the part of the stroma and not a passive 'flowing in,' between the muscle columns, and at once brings up the question in cases of adenomyoma as to whether the stroma is not as active an agent in these growths as the glands and possible a more active agent."[116] Referring to his own case, Casler used such active and aggressive words as "exterminated… strangulation… [and] attacked,"[117] to explain the pathogenesis of uterine adenomyomata. However at this late date in his career, Cullen did not deign to respond to Casler's not so subtle challenge regarding the finer points of pathogenesis of diffuse uterine adenomyoma.

Cullen's fourth case consisted of a histologic slide of a "relatively small ovary containing a large island of normal uterine mucosa" sent to him from Philadelphia by Dr. Charles Norris.[118] An "area of typical uterine mucosa [was] embedded in the substance of the ovary…connected with an irregular cyst cavity."[119]

On May 12, 1919, Cullen operated ovarian Case 5, his one and only patient with uterine mucosa in the ovary, also his Septum Case 14.[120] At surgery Cullen found "the most wide-spread distribution of an adenomyoma of the rectovaginal septum that I have ever seen

109 Cullen, Thomas S. Archives of Surgery. 1920;1: 215–283:259.

110 Cullen, Thomas S. Archives of Surgery. 1920;1:215–283: 250–60.

111 Casler DB. A unique, diffuse uterine tumor, really an adenomyoma, with stroma, but no glands. Menstruation after complete hysterectomy due to uterine mucosa in remaining ovary. Transactions of the American Gynecological Society. 1919;44:69–84. See Fig. 5.

112 The glands were atypical only in the sense of being dilated, they resembling Swiss cheese hyperplasia of the uterine endometrium.

113 Casler DB. Transactions of the American Gynecological Society. 1919;44:69–84.

114 Casler DB. Transactions of the American Gynecological Society. 1919;44:69–84. See Figure 7.

115 Casler DB. Transactions of the American Gynecological Society. 1919;44:69–84:69.

116 Casler DB. Transactions of the American Gynecological Society. 1919;44:69–84:70.

117 Casler DB. Transactions of the American Gynecological Society. 1919;44:69–84:74. "The pathological process beginning in the polyp is really an orderly overgrowth of the stroma, which has gradually exterminated the uterine glands by strangulation, and then in the same manner has attacked the uterine musculature."

118 Cullen, Thomas S. The distribution of adenomyomas containing uterine mucosa. Archives of Surgery. 1920;1:215–283: 259–60:258.

119 Cullen TS. Archives of Surgery 1920;1:215–283:259–260. Figures 33 and 34.

120 Cullen TS. Archives of Surgery 1920;1:215–283:237.

[and] it was one of the most difficult hysterectomies I ever attempted."[121] The rectovaginal pouch of Douglas was obliterated completely. However, the pathology of the tube and ovary was the more interesting aspect of the case. Cullen described an: "Extension of an adenomyoma of the rectovaginal septum to the surface of the adherent fallopian tube…On the surface of the tube is an area of typical uterine mucosa…It really looks as if the widespread adenomyoma of the rectovaginal septum has literally flowed over on the surface of the tube."[122] Cullen found histologic proof also of "uterine mucosa on the surface of the ovary…The mucosa of the adenomyoma of the rectovaginal septum seems to have overflowed to the surface of the adherent ovary."[123]

Characteristically, Cullen described minutely the gross as well as microscopic pathology: "The [right] tube and ovary form a conglomerate mass which has been densely adherent to the side of the uterus as well as to the surrounding structures. Notwithstanding this the fimbriated end of the tube is patent and appears relatively normal."[124] In this case Cullen postulated the pathogenesis of uterine mucosa on the tube and ovary. He pictured the extensive adenomyoma of the rectovaginal septum "flowing" onto ovary and tube.[125] Cullen came tantalizingly close to – and yet so far from – Sampson's later observations when he wrote: "One gathers the impression that the uterine mucosa from the diffuse adenomyoma on the posterior surface of the cervix and uterus has overflowed upon the adherent tube [and ovary]."[126] Cullen had the pathogenesis in reverse.

Cullen's sixth and final ovarian case, consisting of a letter and specimen, was sent to him from St. Louis by Dr. Otto Schwarz. Such was Cullen's thoroughness that he later visited St. Louis and reviewed other slides from the case with Dr. Schwarz in the latter's laboratory. So perfect was the analogy that Cullen commented on the microscopic features: "a photomicrograph that I have had made from one of Dr. Schwarz' sections…It is a beautiful example of an ovary containing miniature uterine cavities." In the very next sentence, Cullen repeated his invitation for others to take up the research, an invitation first made in Syracuse in 1919. "From the foregoing it is evident that in due time a sufficient number of cases will undoubtedly be reported, and then we shall possibly be able to give a composite picture of both the clinical course and of the histologic changes that occur in this most unusual group of cases."[127]

By 1920, Cullen was the undisputed North American authority on uterine and extrauterine adenomyomas. He was self confident to the point of being completely self referential in his "bird's eye" review of 1919,[128] and except for three citations, self referential in his major review of 1920.[129] Lack of references to the work of other colleagues, domestic and foreign, also reflected his declining interest in the subject.[130] Cullen was tired when he wrote this final major article on adenomyomata and he did not attempt "to cover the literature on the subject."[131] This is the same man who for years had spent "three afternoons a week in the Surgeon General's

[121] Cullen TS. Archives of Surgery 1920;1:215–283:238–240. See supra-vaginal hysterectomy specimen, amputated through the cervix: Cullen's septum case #14, Figure 16, page 238.

[122] Cullen TS. Archives of Surgery 1920;1:215–283:242. Cullen's septum case #14 See: Fig. 20, page 242. Here, Cullen extended the use of his "flow" metaphor for describing adenomyoma of the tube.

[123] Cullen TS. Archives of Surgery 1920;1:215–283:243. Cullen's septum case #14. Fig. 21, page 243. The legend reads: "Uterine mucosa on the surface of the ovary in a case of adenomyoma of the rectovaginal septum…The miniature uterine cavity on the surface of the right ovary is represented by a. The lining mucosa resembles in every particular that of the body of the uterus. Some of the glands show hypertrophy. The mucosa of the adenomyoma of the rectovaginal septum seems to have overflowed to the surface of the adherent ovary. The same condition was noted on the surface of the corresponding tube."

[124] Cullen TS. Archives of Surgery. 1920;1:215–283: 242.

[125] Cullen TS. Archives of Surgery 1920;1:215–283:262. See Cullen's septum case 14 (Gyn.-Path. No. 25003) on page 237 and endometriosis of the tube: Figure 20 on page 242. See also endometriosis of the ovary: Figure 21 on page 243.

[126] Cullen TS. Archives of Surgery. 1920;1:215–283: 244.

[127] Cullen TS. The distribution of adenomyomas containing uterine mucosa. Archives of Surgery 1920;1:215–283:264,

[128] Cullen TS. The distribution of adenomyomata containing uterine mucosa. American Journal of Obstetrics and Diseases of Women and Children 1919;180:130–138.

[129] Cullen TS. The distribution of adenomyomas containing uterine mucosa. Archives Surgery 1920;1:215–283.

[130] Cullen TS. Thomas S. Cullen, *Henry Mills Hurd, the First Superintendent of the Johns Hopkins Hospital* [Baltimore, MD: Johns Hopkins Press, 1920]. In 1920, Cullen published a small biography honoring Henry Mills Hurd, the first superintendent of the Johns Hopkins Hospital, the man who had so encouraged publication by members of the faculty. Three cases of subperitoneal, pedunculated adenomyoma. Arch Surgery 1921;2:443–454. Cullen TS. Further remarks on diseases of the umbilicus Surg Gynecol Obstet 1922;35:257–283. Cullen TS, Broedel M. Lesions of the rectus abdominis muscle simulating an acute intra-abdominal condition. Bull Johns Hopkins Hospital, November, 1937.

[131] Cullen TS. Archives Surgery 1920;1:215–283:215.

Library."[132] In other circumstances, Cullen would have written a book. In his "fragmentary article" of 1919[133] as well as in this review of 1920,[134] Cullen invited others to study uterine mucosal lesions in the ovary and adenomyoma of the sigmoid colon. After studying adenomyomas for 25 years, he was ready to pass the baton of authority to a successor.[135]

Nonetheless, Cullen managed to write one more short case series in 1921 on a relatively rare condition, subperitoneal pedunculated adenomyoma, a topic he had discussed thoroughly in his monograph on uterine adenomyomas in 1908. Cullen expressed the main reason that he revisited this topic. "These three cases are such beautiful examples of a relative rare condition that we may with profit consider them in detail." What struck the author with considerable force was Cullen's use of the expressions "springing from" and "which sprang from" 20 times to express the origin of uterine adenomyomas. He had used these same expressions elsewhere with extrauterine adenomyomas.[136] Cullen concluded this article with his last formal statement on adenomyomas. "The more we study adenomyomas the more fully are we convinced that they should, if possible, be removed as soon as they have been diagnosed."[137] As a final caveat, recall that Cullen came to the belief that hormone-resistant endometriosis would continue to invade the bowel and cause problems even after hysterectomy and removal of both tubes and ovaries.

***

Chapters 8 and 9 that follow present pure analysis and synthesis of John A. Sampson's scientific articles during his most creative period in a long and productive academic career. To put these chapters in historical context: this was the period when European countries lay devastated by the most ghastly war yet fought in world history, compounded by the further loss of young men and women from the Asian influenza epidemic of 1918 that swept from a military installation in the United States to engulf and kill millions of civilians worldwide. During the post-war years medical research in Europe ground to a snail's pace – a Europe plagued by inflation and loss of a whole generation of young men. Meanwhile relatively unscathed, medical research continued virtually unabated in some former European colonies, especially the United States of America and Canada where the era came to be known as the roaring twenties, a time of economic prosperity. Paradoxically, research into endometriosis at Johns Hopkins seemed to grind to a snail's pace, but for a different reason – loss of interest by its leading investigator, Thomas Cullen.

For John A. Sampson, Professor of Gynecology at Albany Medical College on the eastern end of the Erie Canal in upstate New York – time stood still in those immediate postwar years as he immersed himself totally in endometriosis research. Sampson, with two decades experience studying all aspects of cervical cancer and a budding interest in endometriosis, was inspired initially by an insight derived from DeWitt Casler's case of the menstruating ovary. During the feverish pace of research that followed, Sampson generated the second of three insights, retrograde menstruation and implantation, that would ultimately lead to his mature theory of implantation endometriosis. The third insight, spread by lymphatic and venous metastases, came from his realization that endometriosis shared many characteristics of cervical, endometrial, and ovarian cancer. Such must have been the pace and the exhilaration of discovery that in 1923 Sampson unwittingly expressed the foundation for his success in academic medicine and medical research. In a semi-autobiographical presidential address before the American Gynecological Society, Sampson dis-

[132] Judith Robinson, *Tom Cullen of Baltimore* [London, Toronto, New York: Oxford University Press, 1949], 117.

[133] Cullen TS. The distribution of adenomyomata containing uterine mucosa. Am J Obstetrics Diseases Women and Children 1919;180:130–138.

[134] Cullen TS. The distribution of adenomyomas containing uterine mucosa. Archives of Surgery 1920;1:215–283.

[135] Cullen TS. Archives of Surgery 1920;1:215–283. Cullen began his classification of adenomyomata with adenomyoma of the body of the uterus and ended with adenomyoma of the umbilicus, subjects on which he had written books.

[136] Cullen TS. Archives of Surgery 1920;1:215–283:250. Figure 27 (Case 10). Cullen illustrated an adenomyoma [springing from the cervix] that invaded the broad ligament and compressed the right ureter causing partial ureteral obstruction.

[137] Cullen TS. Three cases of subperitoneal pedunculated adenomyoma. Archives Surgery 1921;2:443–454:454. Mahle AE, MacCarty WC. Ectopic adenomyoma of uterine type (A report of ten cases). J Lab & Clin Med 1920;5: 218–228:218. Cogently, Mahle and MacCarty from the Mayo Clinic had observed in 1920: "It is evident, regardless of the amount of literature which has been written on the subject, that the importance of adenomyoma has not been recognized either clinically or surgically."

closed that his childhood role model was President Theodore Roosevelt and his adult professional role model none other than Howard A. Kelly, his professor at Johns Hopkins Hospital.

Put into medical historical context, Chaps. 8 and 9 represent the first in-depth analysis of Sampson's classic theory for the pathogenesis of external endometriosis. Whereas the theories of pathogenesis from embryonic rests, serosal and coelomic metaplasia, and direct invasion of the uterine and tubal muscle were all derived from observations in the laboratory, Sampson's theory could only have been conceived by a seasoned surgeon steeped in biological field research and cross-trained in human pathology. In sum, Sampson's theory required the composite scientific and creative talents of a field biologist, a master cancer surgeon, and a mature gynecologic pathologist. Chapters 8 and 9 provide the window through which we may observe Sampson's scientific creativity.

Equally important they reveal the first theory of pathogenesis of endometriosis amenable to experimental testing to prove or disprove its validity. Furthermore, Sampson's theory of pathogenesis: by implantation of endometrial tissue shed from ruptured endometrial chocolate ovarian cysts, from endometrial tissue shed directly through the fallopian tubes onto the ovaries and other pelvic organs, and from venous and lymphatic metastases is the only theory that has the power to explain the precise anatomical distribution of all but the most esoteric endometriotic lesions.

Sampson's Theory of Implantation Endometriosis

8

From Cullen to Sampson Via Casler

Cullen, Thomas Stephen.
Three cases of subperitoneal pedunculated adenomyoma.
Archives of Surgery 1921;2:443–454.
Sampson, John Albertson.
Perforating hemorrhagic (chocolate) cysts of the ovary.
Archives of Surgery 1921;3:245–323.

From a cursory examination of the literature, one might conclude that research and authorship on adenomyomas passed seamlessly and directly from Cullen to Sampson in 1921; Cullen's last contribution appearing in Volume two and Sampson's first article in Volume three of the *Archives of Surgery*.[1] Such was not the case. Unlike the clear and seamless continuity from von Recklinghausen to Cullen, the transfer of authority from Cullen to Sampson was mediated and complicated. Cullen remained the undisputed authority on uterine adenomyomas, but not of extrauterine adenomyomas. In the sense that Sampson postulated a novel theory of pathogenesis to explain the many extrauterine adenomyomas described by Cullen – and in that sense only – there was continuity: mutual interest in the same subject, but the torch had not been passed as it had from von Recklinghausen to Cullen. In every other sense, the transition was marked by discontinuity.

Sampson had been casually interested in extrauterine adenomyomas for over a decade. He burst into print in 1921 with his first theory of peritoneal implantation from *internally menstruating ovaries*[2] which was beyond doubt directly inspired by the case of the *externally menstruating ovary* of De Witt Casler.[3] Furthermore his research was facilitated by tissue sections and tissue blocks of hemorrhagic cysts of the ovary that Sampson had requested and received from Emil Novak, instructor in clinical gynecology at Johns Hopkins Medical School.

[1] Cullen TS. Three cases of subperitoneal pedunculated adenomyoma. Archives Surgery 1921;2:443–454. Sampson JA. Perforating hemorrhagic (chocolate) cysts of the ovary: their importance and especially their relation to pelvic adenomas of endometrial type ("Adenomyoma" of the uterus, rectovaginal septum, sigmoid, etc.) Archives of Surgery 1921;3:245–323:245.

[2] Sampson JA. Perforating hemorrhagic (chocolate) cysts of the ovary: their importance and especially their relation to pelvic adenomas of endometrial type ("Adenomyoma" of the uterus, rectovaginal septum, sigmoid, etc.) Archives of Surgery 1921;3:245–323.

[3] Casler DB. A unique, diffuse uterine tumor, really an adenomyoma, with stroma, but no glands. Menstruation after complete hysterectomy due to uterine mucosa in remaining ovary. Transactions of the American Gynecological Society. 1919;44:69–84. It is unknown when Sampson first heard of Casler's case. He could have learned from Cullen's presentation at the annual meeting of the New York State Medical Society at Syracuse, New York on May 7, 1919, or have read Cullen's article in the August 1919 issue of the American Journal of Obstetrics and Diseases of Women and Children. On the other hand Sampson may have heard Casler present at the American Gynecological Society or read Casler's article in the Transactions of the American Gynecological Society, 1919;44:69–84. What is known beyond doubt, Casler's *case of the externally menstruating ovary* directly inspired Sampson's hypothesis of *the internally menstruating ovary*. Casler precipitated an experiment of nature when he placed a cigarette drain in the vaginal cuff after hysterectomy. The drain created a fistula, an artificial channel connecting the left ovary and the vagina. When, 4 years later, an ovarian endometrioma ruptured – it ruptured into the fistulous tract and "menstruated" into the vagina, instead of rupturing into the abdomen and menstruating into the abdomen as perforating hemorrhagic (chocolate) cysts containing endometrial tissue are wont to do. It was Casler's unique case that furnished the critical

R.E. Batt, *A History of Endometriosis*,
DOI 10.1007/978-0-85729-585-9_8,

Some years later, Novak wrote a historical note: "The report of the first case of aberrant ovarian endometrium by Russell in 1899 didn't cause a ripple of general interest, and the case was complacently accepted as representing an interesting but rare instance of misplaced muellerian rests. Following this an occasional instance of this sort was encountered in laboratories of gynecological pathology, but no one appreciated its significance until 1921, when Sampson published his first paper on the subject. I well recall that for a year or two before this I had gotten letters from him asking me to send him sections or blocks of any available hemorrhagic lesions of the ovary, and I wondered what he had in the back of his head. We all found out when he published his first classical paper in 1921, establishing the frequency and importance of endometriosis as both a pathological and clinical entity.– Emil Novak, M.D."[4]

This discontinuity was not a "paradigm shift" of Kuhnian proportions, but a normal scientific progression. The editors of Thomas S. Kuhn's essays, from 1970 to 1998, explain Kuhn's position on normal science, a position that he had arrived at just before his death.[5] "It is only because individuals working in a common research tradition are able to arrive at differing judgments concerning the degree of seriousness of the various difficulties they collectively face that some of them will be moved individually to explore alternative (often - as Kuhn likes to emphasize - seemingly nonsensical) possibilities, while others will attempt doggedly to resolve the problems within the current framework. The fact that the latter are in the majority when such difficulties first arise is essential to the fertility of scientific practices. For, *usually*, the problems can be resolved, and eventually are. In the absence of the requisite persistence to find those solutions, scientists would not be able to home in as they do, on those rarer but crucial cases in which efforts to introduce radical conceptual revision are fully repaid."[6]

Undoubtedly, Cullen's research on extrauterine adenomyomas contributed to the fund of knowledge that Sampson possessed when he grasped the significance of the "case of the menstruating ovary."[7] In one giant intuitive leap, Sampson bounded from Casler's ovarian-uterus that "menstruated externally" into the vagina to perforating hemorrhagic (chocolate) cysts of the ovary that "menstruated internally" into the pelvis and their relation to pelvic adenomas of endometrial type. Inspired, he secured a ready supply of hemorrhagic ovarian cysts from Emil Novak. In less than 2 years, Sampson completed his study and presented his *first theory* of the pathogenesis of pelvic adenomas of endometrial type from perforating hemorrhagic (chocolate) cysts of the ovary in 1921.[8] Two years earlier Cullen had issued an implicit invitation for others to investigate uterine mucosa in the ovary.[9] This released Sampson

data that stimulated Sampson's imagination and allowed him to make the intuitive leap from external ovarian "menstruation" to internal ovarian "menstruation" from a perforated hemorrhagic (chocolate) cyst into the abdomen, and the final intuitive leap to the deposition of endometrial tissue into the pelvis and the formation of pelvic adhesions.

[4] Novak, Emil. A Note on the History of Endometriosis. Undated. Current Medical Digest, page 52. Reference obtained from the Sampson Archives at the Albany Medical College. Year and volume are not available.

[5] James Conant and John Haugeland, "Editor's Introduction." in Kuhn, Thomas S. *The Road Since Structure: Philosophical Essays, 1970–1993, with an Autobiographical Interview* [Chicago, IL: University of Chicago Press, 2000], 3.

[6] James Conant and John Haugeland, "Editor's Introduction." in Kuhn, Thomas S. *The Road Since Structure: Philosophical Essays, 1970–1993, with an Autobiographical Interview* [Chicago, IL: University of Chicago Press, 2000], 1. "In *The Structure of Scientific Revolutions,* as nearly everyone knows, Thomas Kuhn argued that the history of science is not gradual and cumulative but rather punctuated by a series of more or less radical 'paradigm shifts.' What is less well known is that Kuhn's own understanding of how best to characterize these episodes itself underwent a number of significant shifts." Thomas S. Kuhn, "The Natural and the Human Sciences," in Kuhn, Thomas S. *The Road Since Structure: Philosophical Essays, 1970–1993, with an Autobiographical Interview,* edited by James Conant and John Haugeland [Chicago, IL: University of Chicago Press, 2000], 221. In this essay, Kuhn admitted that he seldom uses the term paradigm shift, "having totally lost control of it."

[7] Casler DB. A unique, diffuse uterine tumor, really an adenomyoma, with stroma but no glands. Menstruation after complete hysterectomy due to uterine mucosa in remaining ovary. Transactions American Gynecological Society 1919;44:69–84.

[8] Sampson JA. Perforating hemorrhagic (chocolate) cysts of the ovary: their importance and especially their relation to pelvic adenomas of endometrial type ("Adenomyoma" of the uterus, rectovaginal septum, sigmoid, etc.) Archives of Surgery 1921;3:245–323. See also: Sampson JA. Perforating hemorrhagic (Chocolate) cysts of the ovary: their importance and especially their relation to pelvic adenomas of endometrial type ("Adenomyoma" of the uterus, rectovaginal septum, sigmoid, etc.) Transactions American Gynecological Society 1921;46:162–241.

from all ethical concern that he might be trespassing on the sovereign terrain of his former teacher in medical school and residency at Johns Hopkins University.

In the title of "Perforating hemorrhagic (chocolate) cysts of the ovary: their importance and especially their relation to pelvic adenomas of endometrial type ('Adenomyoma' of the uterus, rectovaginal septum, sigmoid, etc.)," one may discern a definite shift in emphasis from adenomyoma to ovary. The ovary became the organ of primary interest.[10] Terminology changed. Adenoma replaced adenomyoma. The adjective "endometrial" replaced the phrase "of uterine mucosa." Chocolate evoked the commonplace descriptive words introduced into pathology by Rokitansky. Analysis replaced description. Living pathology observed by the surgeon displaced the primacy of morbid pathology in the laboratory. Descriptive pathology gave way to pathogenesis as the prime focus of research.

Sampson recalled in 1921 that it was by observing the pelvic findings in a single case in 1910 that his "attention was first directed to the dense peritoneal adhesions which may result from the escape of the contents of these [perforating hemorrhagic] cysts."[11] He had operated his very first case on May 8, 1910, a patient with a frozen pelvis. Here is how Sampson described Case 1: "Perforating hemorrhagic cysts of both ovaries; multiple leiomyomas of the uterus; dense adhesions in the "cul-de-sac" uniting the anterior rectal wall to the supravaginal portion of the cervix and the lower portion of the uterus. The induration of the anterior rectal wall was so great as to simulate malignancy."[12] Unfortunately, he did not examine the ovarian cysts or the posterior wall of the uterus microscopically.

His second case, operated on March 27, 1912, also presented with a frozen pelvis.[13] This case provided Sampson with a new insight. He recalled that he realized for the first time "the association between these [perforating hemorrhagic (chocolate)] cysts and 'adenomyomas' of the posterior uterine wall with adhesions between it and the rectum."[14] Rephrased, in 1912 Sampson stated he associated chocolate cysts of the ovary with adenomyomas and adhesions of the posterior wall of the uterus, the rectum and the rectovaginal septum. He saw the association, but not the pathophysiologic relationship; he had too little information to postulate pathogenesis.

Sampson operated his third patient with "much less extensive" disease on April 26, 1912.[15] He noted that he

---

[9] Cullen TS. The distribution of adenomyomas containing uterine mucosa. Am J Obstetrics and Diseases of Women and Children 1919;180:130–138:135–6. Cullen commented on cases of uterine mucosa in ovaries reported by Russell, Norris, and Casler and implicitly invited others to investigate these lesions when he stated: "In due time a sufficient number of such cases will undoubtedly be reported and then we shall be able to give a composite picture of both the clinical course and of the histological changes that occur in this most unusual group of cases." Cullen repeated this invitation in 1920. Cullen TS. The distribution of adenomyomas containing uterine mucosa. Archives of Surgery 1920;1:215–283:264. Cullen commented on the microscopic features seen in "a photomicrograph that I have had made from one of Dr. Schwarz's sections…It is a beautiful example of an ovary containing miniature uterine cavities….From the foregoing it is evident that in due time a sufficient number of cases will undoubtedly be reported, and then we shall possibly be able to give a composite picture of both the clinical course and of the histologic changes that occur in this most unusual group of cases."

[10] Sampson JA. Perforating hemorrhagic (chocolate) cysts of the ovary: their importance and especially their relation to pelvic adenomas of endometrial type ("Adenomyoma" of the uterus, rectovaginal septum, sigmoid, etc.) Archives of Surgery 1921;3:245–323:248. "Of physiologic interest, it is to be noted that the adenoma of endometrial type developing in the ovary and arising in the portion of the pelvis as the result of the escape of the hemorrhagic contents of the ovary may be the seat of periodic hemorrhages, i. e., they may be 'menstruating organs'."

[11] Sampson JA. Perforating hemorrhagic (chocolate) cysts of the ovary: their importance and especially their relation to pelvic adenomas of endometrial type ("Adenomyoma" of the uterus, rectovaginal septum, sigmoid, etc.) Archives of Surgery 1921;3:245–323:249. Sampson made a point of recording his early observations in 1910 and 1912, precise to the exact date he operated each of these early cases, May 8, 1910 and March 27, 1912, as well as the exact dates he operated his later patients.

[12] Sampson JA. Perforating hemorrhagic (chocolate) cysts of the ovary. Archives of Surgery 1921;3:245–323:291.

[13] Sampson JA. Perforating hemorrhagic (chocolate) cysts of the ovary. Archives of Surgery 1921;3:245–323:291. Sampson described Case 2. "Perforating hemorrhagic cysts of both ovaries; "adenomyoma" of the posterior wall of the uterus, adherent to and invading the anterior wall of the rectum."

[14] Sampson JA. Perforating hemorrhagic (chocolate) cysts of the ovary. Archives of Surgery 1921;3:245–323:250. "On March 27 of that year [1912] I removed an 'adenomyomatous' uterus in which the 'adenomyoma' had apparently extended through the posterior uterine wall and had invaded the anterior wall of the rectum…On section, the 'adenomyoma' was apparently not connected with the uterine mucosa. Bilateral perforating hemorrhagic cyst of the ovary were present."

[15] Sampson JA. Perforating hemorrhagic (chocolate) cysts of the ovary. Archives of Surgery 1921;3:245–323:292. Sampson described Case 3. "Perforating hemorrhagic cysts of both ovaries; adherent retroflexed uterus; adenoma of endometrial type

would have "overlooked" his third case, had he not operated his second patient just 1 month before.[16] He said he did not "observe another similar case" until June 13, 1918. Sampson confessed he "undoubtedly overlooked many" other cases in the interim.[17] This 1918 case was his first patient with histologic evidence. "The hemorrhagic cyst was lined by low cuboidal and columnar epithelium, the columnar predominating. There was a vascular subepithelial stroma, containing evidence of old and recent hemorrhages and an occasional gland, which resembled a uterine gland."[18] As had Rokitansky in 1860, Sampson reported finding endometrial glands and stroma in the ovary. During 1918 and 1919, Sampson observed perforated hemorrhagic cysts "many times and studied them more from the standpoint of gross pathology, basing the microscopic studies solely on the routine examination of the material in the pathologic laboratory."[19] In 1920, subsequent to his insight from Casler's case and mindful of Casler's microscopic studies, Sampson began systematic microscopic studies in his own laboratory.[20] He stated: "It was only this last year that I fully realized the true relation between these cysts and pelvic adenoma of the endometrial type and that the pelvic adhesions were often associated with or were in large part due to this adenomatous growth."[21]

In 1921, Sampson acknowledged his debt to DeWitt B. Casler when he wrote the following lines: "Of physiologic interest, it is to be noted that the adenoma of the endometrial type developing in the ovary and arising in the portion of the pelvis as the result of the escape of the hemorrhagic contents of the ovary may be the seat of periodic hemorrhage, i.e., they may be '*menstruating organs*.'"[22] Sampson recounted Casler's menstruating ovary: "Casler, in 1919, reported an unusual case in which a patient menstruated through the vagina after a conservative hysterectomy in which one ovary was saved…at the second operation, 4 years later, the enlarged ovary was removed and it was found to contain cavities lined by 'normal uterine mucosa.'"[23]

invading the posterior wall of the uterus and uniting it with the anterior wall of the rectum."

[16] Sampson JA. Perforating hemorrhagic (chocolate) cysts of the ovary. Archives of Surgery 1921;3:245–323:250.

[17] Sampson JA. Perforating hemorrhagic (chocolate) cysts of the ovary Archives of Surgery 1921;3:245–323:250. For some reason Sampson seems to have skipped Case 4, operated October 11, 1917, and Case 5, operated February 7, 1918, in his story, but report them in his chronology of cases on pages 293 and 294, respectively. I believe the explanation lies with absence of satisfactory histology of the ovaries, none was attempted in Case 4, and in Case 5 only one microscopic section was taken from the ovarian cyst which "showed a cyst with its wall lined by low and cuboidal epithelium." No sections were taken from the posterior wall of the uterus. In Case 6 operated June 13, 1918, Sampson observed: "Perforating hemorrhagic cyst of the right ovary; adherent retroflexed uterus; 'adenomyoma' of posterior uterine wall; gall stones."

[18] Sampson JA. Perforating hemorrhagic (chocolate) cysts of the ovary. Archives of Surgery 1921;3:245–323:295.

[19] Sampson JA. Perforating hemorrhagic (chocolate) cysts of the ovary. Archives of Surgery 1921;3:245–323:250–51.

[20] As the title explicitly states, Sampson built this essay around gross pathology of the ovarian hematomas. He realized the full significance of chocolate cysts when he found they were partially or wholly lined by "tissue of the endometrial type" (page 247). Recognizing that ovarian cysts of this type might be "menstruating organs" (page 248), Sampson began systematic microscopic examinations of hemorrhagic ovarian cysts supplied by Emil Novak and then began microscopic examinations of his own material starting with Case 9 operated at the Albany Hospital on March 17, 1920 and continuing to his last case in this report, Case 23 operated on April 18, 1921.

[21] Sampson JA. Perforating hemorrhagic (chocolate) cysts of the ovary. Archives of Surgery 1921;3:245–323:251.

[22] Sampson JA. Perforating hemorrhagic (chocolate) cysts of the ovary. Archives of Surgery 1921;3:245–323:248. See Casler DB. A unique, diffuse uterine tumor, really an adenomyoma, with stroma, but no glands. Menstruation after complete hysterectomy due to uterine mucosa in remaining ovary. Transactions American Gynecological Society 1919;44:69–84. In 1919 Casler provided information decisive to the formation of Sampson's initial theory of pathogenesis of pelvic endometriosis and pelvic endometriotic adhesions. Casler published a case report of an ovarian cyst which on microscopic examination was "made up almost entirely of uterine tissue." Even more emphatically, Casler wrote of: "a large uterine growth of the ovary…the entire cyst, or uterine cavity, as it really is, is lined throughout by a single layer of tall columnar epithelium of the uterine type, and in places cilia can be made out." Then Casler explained how regular "menstruation" could happen every month after total hysterectomy. "It is a natural process then that the uterine glands in the ovarian cyst should take on the active work of the uterus and maintain menstruation regularly." In sum, Casler had presented a case of ovarian menstruation through the vagina: *external ovarian menstruation*. I believe Casler's morphologic description and his physiologic reasoning planted the seed that led Sampson to imagine "internal ovarian menstruation." I believe Sampson's initial theory of the pathogenesis of pelvic endometriosis and pelvic endometriotic adhesions from perforating hemorrhagic (chocolate) cysts of the ovary was inspired by Casler's observations.

[23] Sampson JA. Perforating hemorrhagic (chocolate) cysts of the ovary. Archives of Surgery 1921;3:245–323:255.

Sampson described the living pelvic pathology observed at surgery. He found perforated hemorrhagic cysts of the ovary adherent to adjacent structures. When the ovary was mobilized, the cyst ruptured and spilled its chocolate contents. Sampson reasoned "this rupture arises from reopening a previous perforation which has been sealed by the organ or structure to which the cyst has become adherent at the site of the perforation, or the cyst is torn in freeing it."[24] The ovarian cysts were usually between 2 and 4 cm. in diameter and were often bilateral. In Sampson's experience, the site of perforation was always located on the "lateral surface of the ovary or on its free border; [he had] never found it on the mesial surface."[25] He noted that "adhesions are also found in other portions of the pelvis and especially in the culdesac, and these adhesions are apparently the result of the escape of the contents of the cyst."[26] Sampson found the most extensive development of adenoma of endometrial type in the culdesac. These were variously described as ranging from a "quiescent…localized thickening" to a "diffuse [invasive] growth involving the posterior surface of the supravaginal portion of the cervix, the posterior uterine wall, the floor of the culdesac and the anterior wall of the rectum, all of which may be adherent to one another."[27] The adenomatous disease of "endometrial type" and the associated pelvic adhesions had the same anatomic distribution, except when the endometrial disease invaded beyond the confines of the rectovaginal pouch of Douglas.

Sampson noted that invasion variously occurred posteriorly into the rectum or sigmoid colon; laterally into the broad ligament; anteriorly into the uterus, supravaginal cervix, or vaginal wall; and even through the entire thickness of the vagina into the posterior fornix.[28] In Sampson's own words the disease: "may grow down between the rectum and vagina, forming an 'adenomyoma of the rectovaginal septum' and may penetrate the vagina and appear in the posterior vaginal vault. In other cases, they may extend through the wall of the rectum or sigmoid."[29] What Sampson, Cullen, and other investigators referred to as "adenomyoma of the rectovaginal septum" were lesions formed by the obliteration of the rectovaginal pouch of Douglas. Put more precisely, the adenomyomatous disease obliterated the rectovaginal pouch of Douglas forming a "pseudo-rectovaginal septum" located above or cranial to the true anatomic rectovaginal septum of Denonvilliers. Sampson and Cullen were not referring to invasion of the anatomical rectovaginal septum of Denonvilliers.[30]

Sampson offered a modification of Emil Novak's classification of ovarian hematomas.[31] He suggested that a "fourth variety of ovarian hematoma…one lined wholly or in part by "endometrial tissue" should be added to Novak's ovarian follicular, stromal, and corpus luteum hematomas.[32] Sampson used the terms "tissue of endometrial type"[33] and 'endometrial tissue'"[34] in place of Cullen's term "uterine mucosa." This was the first time that Sampson used the term "endometrial tissue." I believe this was the first step toward his coining the term endometriosis.

One can see Sampson thinking deeply about the pathophysiology of endometrial tissue within the ovary and the histologic standard of comparison. "In the study of ovarian hematomas to determine whether or

---

[24] Sampson JA. Perforating hemorrhagic (chocolate) cysts of the ovary. Archives of Surgery 1921;3:245–323:251–252.

[25] Sampson JA. Perforating hemorrhagic (chocolate) cysts of the ovary. Archives of Surgery 1921;3:245–323:253.

[26] Sampson JA. Perforating hemorrhagic (chocolate) cysts of the ovary. Archives of Surgery 1921;3:245–323:252.

[27] Sampson JA. Perforating hemorrhagic (chocolate) cysts of the ovary. Archives of Surgery 1921;3:245–323:248. I prefer the descriptive anatomical term rectovaginal pouch of Douglas to cul-de-sac which means literally – a blind diverticulum.

[28] Sampson JA. Perforating hemorrhagic (chocolate) cysts of the ovary. Archives of Surgery 1921;3:245–323:249.

[29] Sampson JA. Perforating hemorrhagic (chocolate) cysts of the ovary. Archives of Surgery 1921;3:245–323:249.

[30] Late in the twentieth century, Dr. Dan Martin and Professor Philippe R. Koninckx found that only in about 1 in 450 cases of deeply invasive endometriosis of the rectovaginal pouch of Douglas did the lesion actually invade through the floor of the rectovaginal pouch into the true anatomic rectovaginal septum of Denonvilliers. Personal communication from Dan Martin to Ronald E. Batt, October 20, 2007.

[31] Novak E. Hematomata of the ovary including corpus luteum cysts. Bulletin Johns Hopkins Hospital 1917;28:349–354.

[32] Sampson JA. Perforating hemorrhagic (chocolate) cysts of the ovary: their importance and especially their relation to pelvic adenomas of endometrial type ("Adenomyoma" of the uterus, rectovaginal septum, sigmoid, etc.) Archives of Surgery 1921;3:245–323:254.

[33] Sampson JA. Perforating hemorrhagic (chocolate) cysts of the ovary. Archives of Surgery 1921;3:245–323:247.

[34] Sampson JA. Perforating hemorrhagic (chocolate) cysts of the ovary. Archives of Surgery 1921;3:245–323:254.

not the lining of the hematomas is of endometrial type, it would seem preferable to use as our standard of comparison not normal endometrium but ectopic endometrium in which there is a cyst (hematoma) formation due to the retention of 'menstrual blood,' similar to the condition in ovarian hematomas. We have abundant opportunity to study the variations in the appearance of the uterine mucosa in the hemorrhagic cysts or cavities, so often found in uterine 'adenomyomas.' These should be our standards of comparison in the study of ovarian hematomas because the physical conditions are similar."[35]

By 1921, Sampson had developed his *first* theory of pathogenesis of pelvic adenomas and associated adhesive disease; both resulted from chocolate fluid containing endometrial tissue that spilled into the pelvis from ruptured hemorrhagic ovarian cysts. Next, Sampson pondered the pathogenesis of these perforated ovarian cysts. He cited the research of Runge[36] and Wolf,[37] who made serial sections through the site of rupture and "demonstrated the 'epithelialization' of ovarian hematomas by the invasion of 'surface epithelium of the ovary' through the opening caused by the rupture."[38] In other words, Runge and Wolf postulated *secondary* invasion of ovarian hematomas – be they follicular, stromal, or corpus luteum hematomas. Sampson interpreted their work: "It may be possible that, following the rupture of the hematoma or whatever structure preceded the secondary invasion, misplaced epithelium of endometrial type was present in the periphery of the ovary at this site and this epithelium was stimulated to become invasive and reline the cavity of the hematoma."[39] However, in the sentence just preceding this last statement, Sampson had speculated: "If these cysts are of endometrial type and if their epithelial lining arises from the invasion of the surface epithelium of the ovary through the place of rupture, we must conclude that a metaplasia of the epithelium occurs, by which it may not only assume the histologic picture of endometrial tissue but may even function as such."[40] Without reference to the serosal metaplasia theory of Iwanoff or the peritoneal metaplasia theory of Meyer,[41] Sampson seems to have tentatively accepted metaplasia of the ovarian surface cells as the pathogenesis of perforating hemorrhagic cysts of the ovary, contingent on the validity of his assumptions stated above. Sampson gave us insight into his thoughts

[35] Sampson JA. Perforating hemorrhagic (chocolate) cysts of the ovary. Archives of Surgery 1921;3:245–323:255–256.

[36] Runge E. Ueber die Veranderunger der Ovarien bei Syncytralen Tumoren und Blasenmole; Zugleich ein Beitrag zur Histogenese. Arch f. Gynak. 1903;69:33–70.

[37] Wolf EH. Ueber Haematoma Ovarii. Arch f. Gynak 1908;84:211–243.

[38] Sampson JA. Perforating hemorrhagic (chocolate) cysts of the ovary: their importance and especially their relation to pelvic adenomas of endometrial type ("Adenomyoma" of the uterus, rectovaginal septum, sigmoid, etc.) Archives of Surgery 1921;3:245–323:256–257.

[39] Sampson JA. Perforating hemorrhagic (chocolate) cysts of the ovary. Archives of Surgery 1921;3:245–323:257.

[40] Sampson JA. Perforating hemorrhagic (chocolate) cysts of the ovary. Archives of Surgery 1921;3:245–323:257.

[41] Cuthbert Lockyer, *Fibroids and Allied Tumours (Myoma and Adenomyoma): Their Pathology, Clinical Features and Surgical Treatment* [London: Macmillan and Company, 1918]. In 1898, N.S. Iwanoff published his theory that glandular cystic spaces in fibromyomas originated by an ingrowth of overlying serosa. [Iwanoff NS. "Drusiges cystenhaltiges Uterusfibromyom complicíert durch Sarcom und Carinom." Monatsschr fur Geb und Gynak 1898; Bd. vii: S. 295.] Iwanoff claimed that, in a paper published previously in Russia, he had demonstrated microscopically that glandular structures in an adenomyoma were derived from the serosal epithelium. (Lockyer pp 292–3) Iwanoff also believed the carcinoma he observed within the adenomyoma resulted from malignant changes within the adenomyoma. Accordingly he labeled the lesion *Adeno-fibromyoma cysticum sarcomatodes carcinomatosum.* This important paper of Iwanoff has been accepted as the origin of the theory of coelomic metaplasia. Later, Robert Meyer introduced the analogous concept of "epithelial heterotopy." "Meyer showed as many other observers since have done, that epithelial *heterotopy* or displacement can occur in the serosa as well as in the mucosa." (Lockyer: 293) Lockyer stated his own position [his italics] of the pathogenesis of extrauterine endometriosis: "*Heterotopy of serosal epithelium is the probable explanation of the existence of the epithelial spaces and cysts in most of the extra-uterine swellings found between the rectum and genital tract.*" (Lockyer: 295) Lockyer contended that many reliable observers – without the possibility of doubt – had proved by "repeated investigations" the transformation of flattened "so-called 'endothelium' of the peritoneum" to be transformed into cylindrical and columnar epithelium under the excitation of inflammation or the influence of pregnancy. (Lockyer: 295, 299. Lockyer quotes from Klages R. Zeitschr fur Geb und Gynak 1912; Bd. lxx: S. 858. "that the transition of flat peritoneal epithelium into cubical or cylindrical can occur, has been repeatedly proved, and notably so by Opitz and Robert Meyer." Lockyer states that "Opitz had found that where the peritoneum lies in natural folds, as it does at the tubal angles, the initial condition already exists for the down-growth of epithelial elements.") Such a positive statement from an authority of the caliber of Lockyer serves to demonstrate the strength of the theory of coelomic metaplasia and its hold on medically sophisticated investigators of the World War I era. The theory of coelomic metaplasia was well established before Sampson began his investigations and would remain a powerful alternative to his theory of pathogenesis during his lifetime.

and his reservations. "In most of the specimens which I have examined it has been impossible to determine the exact nature of these cysts before the initial rupture. They may have been endometrial cysts at the start; or they may have resulted from an abnormal condition of a follicle by which a hematoma arose in a graafian, or atretic follicle; or possibly following ovulation, an abnormal corpus luteum developed, due to the invasion of the epithelial tissue as above mentioned. With my present knowledge, I prefer to mention these possibilities rather than made definite statements which later may prove to be incorrect."[42]

Sampson divided 26 cysts that he had examined microscopically into three groups.[43] Groups one and two represent different developmental stages of cysts lined with "misplaced atypical endometrial tissue." The third group consisted of "tissue of endometrial type…present in pockets in the periphery of the ovary about the perforation." He pondered the idea of ovarian cysts lined by "misplaced endometrial tissue" as having a "definite life history" characterized by passage through "various stages of growth or development to be followed by various stages of retrogression by which smaller cysts may 'disappear' as they are apparently rare after the menopause."[44] Once again Sampson avoided premature conclusions: "I hesitate to state what I believe their life history to be because I am not sure that I am correct."[45] But Sampson could not leave the subject without commenting further. "Both the hematoma and the clefts or pockets are apparently part of the same process. The stimulus which causes the epithelial invasion of the hematoma or the development of an 'endometrial' cyst also apparently causes the development of the clefts or pockets."[46] At this point he could not define the stimulus.

Twenty pages into this essay[47], Sampson first employed the word "implanted," an essential element of the ancient seed and soil botanical metaphor that one day would make his theory of retrograde uterine menstruation so compelling and memorable.[48] "The 'menstrual' blood escaping [from the ovary] into the peritoneal cavity may carry with it some of the epithelium lining the cyst cavity, or similar tissue may escape from the endometrial pockets in the periphery of the ovary about the perforation. This epithelium may become implanted in the culdesac or other portions of the pelvis and there give rise to other foci of 'endometrial' tissue."[49]

Sampson then turned to the subject of endometrial pelvic adhesions, the cause of which he began studying in 1918.[50] He described an uncontrolled experiment by Dr. George S. Graham in 1918. Graham injected material "obtained aseptically" from ovarian cysts into the peritoneal cavity of eight rabbits and peritoneal adhesions resulted.[51] Sampson said he had planned to write a paper in 1920 "describing these cysts and the adhesions resulting from them…At the time I believed that these cysts were 'endometrial' hematomas and that the adhesions arose from the escape of 'menstrual' blood into the peritoneal cavity."[52] He still believed so in 1921.

In Sampson's judgment, when endometrial cysts ruptured, the spill was usually small and rarely caused symptoms.[53] However, symptomatic or not, the spilled cystic contents caused irritation and adhesions about the ovary and in recesses in the pelvis. Sampson cited the work of Savage[54] who believed that the adhesions

---

[42] Sampson JA. Perforating hemorrhagic (chocolate) cysts of the ovary: their importance and especially their relation to pelvic adenomas of endometrial type ("Adenomyoma" of the uterus, rectovaginal septum, sigmoid, etc.) Archives of Surgery 1921;3:245–323:258–259.

[43] Sampson JA. Perforating hemorrhagic (chocolate) cysts of the ovary. Archives of Surgery 1921;3:245–323:259–264.

[44] Sampson JA. Perforating hemorrhagic (chocolate) cysts of the ovary. Archives of Surgery 1921;3:245–323:261–262.

[45] Sampson JA. Perforating hemorrhagic (chocolate) cysts of the ovary. Archives of Surgery 1921;3:245–323:262.

[46] Sampson JA. Perforating hemorrhagic (chocolate) cysts of the ovary. Archives of Surgery 1921;3:245–323:263.

[47] Sampson JA. Perforating hemorrhagic (chocolate) cysts of the ovary. Archives of Surgery 1921;3:245–323:263.

[48] Michael Worboys, *Spreading Germs: Disease Theories and Medical Practice in Britain, 1865–1900* [Cambridge, UK: Cambridge University Press, 2000], 6.

[49] Sampson JA. Perforating hemorrhagic (chocolate) cysts of the ovary Archives of Surgery 1921;3:245–323:264.

[50] Sampson JA. Perforating hemorrhagic (chocolate) cysts of the ovary. Archives of Surgery 1921;3:245–323:263.

[51] Sampson JA. Perforating hemorrhagic (chocolate) cysts of the ovary. Archives of Surgery 1921;3:245–323:263.

[52] Sampson JA. Perforating hemorrhagic (chocolate) cysts of the ovary. Archives of Surgery 1921;3:245–323:266.

[53] Sampson JA. Perforating hemorrhagic (chocolate) cysts of the ovary. Archives of Surgery 1921;3:245–323:264.

[54] Savage S. Hematoma of the ovary and its pathological connection with the ripening and retrogression of the graafian follicle. Brit Gynaec J 1906;121:285–305.

"arose from a reactive inflammation due to the escape of the hemorrhagic contents of the cyst [unassociated with any] gross evidence of tubal inflammatory disease."[55] Hedley found similar evidence of inflammation and lack of evidence of tubal inflammatory disease.[56] Sampson described the inflammatory host response to the irritation from spilled cyst contents.[57] Based on 13 cases "in which tissue involved in the adhesions was examined histologically and adenoma was found," Sampson described four adhesion patterns and locations of adenoma resulting from the rupture of endometrial cysts of the ovary and the spilling of their contents into the pelvic cavity.[58]

> Pattern one: "extensive adhesions…obliterating …the culdesac: with adenoma of the endometrial type invading the cervical and uterine tissues and probably also…the rectum."[59]
> Pattern two: "adhesions between the uterus and rectum with multiple discrete invasions of the posterior uterine wall by adenoma of the endometrial type."
> Pattern three: "Adhesions in the normal peritoneal folds associated with the development of adenoma of endometrial type."
> Pattern four: "Discrete nodules of adenoma in the wall of the rectum and sigmoid."[60]

Tellingly, Sampson documented that endometrial adenomas existed without adhesions, but he did not attempt to explain this apparent anomaly.

The crux of Sampson's paper in the *Archives of Surgery* revolves around the answer to his own question: "What is primary?" His answer is interesting – not least – because it has been forgotten by nearly everyone. "The study of my material has convinced me that the ovary is the primary site."[61] By that Sampson meant the ovary was the source of all the pelvic adenoma of endometrial type and of all the associated pelvic adhesive disease. He believed the extension of the disease could be "growth by continuity" from the ovary or by "implantation of epithelial cells carried with the contents of the cyst or from the epithelial clefts and pockets in the ovary."[62] In 1921, Sampson used a powerful analogy to express his conviction that the ovary was the primary source of endometrial implants; he suggested that they were analogous to the implantation of cancer in the cul-de-sac from rupture of cancerous ovarian cysts.[63]

Sampson was particularly interested in "blebs or small peritoneal cysts, some containing blood [which] histologically are cystomas of endometrial type."[64] He offered three modes of pathogenesis to explain the presence of these blebs on the serosa of the uterus; "first, from the deposit of epithelial cells from the ovary on the peritoneum and their subsequent development into a cyst…; second, a small cyst or dilated gland may have been detached from the ovary…and may be implanted on the peritoneum and then increase in size, and third, the 'specific' irritation of the contents of the ovary caused a metaplasia of the peritoneal endothelium giving rise to a cyst of endometrial type."[65] Though not an advocate of the theory of metaplasia, but in fairness to his readers, Sampson quoted Lockyer,

---

55 Sampson JA. Perforating hemorrhagic (chocolate) cysts of the ovary. Archives of Surgery 1921;3:245–323:265.

56 Hedley JP. Hematoma of the ovary with report of 18 cases. J Obstet Gynec Brit Empire 1910;18:293–311.

57 In 1943, James Robert Goodall would describe in detail all the host responses to endometriosis.

58 Sampson JA. Perforating hemorrhagic (chocolate) cysts of the ovary: their importance and especially their relation to pelvic adenomas of endometrial type ("Adenomyoma" of the uterus, rectovaginal septum, sigmoid, etc.) Archives of Surgery 1921;3:245–323:246. Sampson operated 14 cases between May 1, 1920 and May 1, 1921. The incidence was 14 cases in 178 operations. What first drew Sampson's attention to the importance of perforating hemorrhagic (chocolate) cysts of the ovary was not only their frequency (p. 246), but more importantly the "nature of the *adhesions* resulting from the escape [of very irritating … chocolate] contents into the peritoneal cavity." (pp. 245–6) The adhesive pattern reflected the effect of gravity within the pelvis: the "most extensive and densest adhesions [were] usually found in the culdesac uniting the supravaginal portion of the cervix and lower portion of the posterior wall of the uterus to the bottom of the culdesac and the anterior rectal wall." (p. 246.)

59 It is not by accident that Sampson placed the most severe disease in Pattern One. Most cases were severe.

60 Sampson JA. Perforating hemorrhagic (chocolate) cysts of the ovary. Archives of Surgery 1921;3:245–323:268.

61 Sampson JA. Perforating hemorrhagic (chocolate) cysts of the ovary Archives of Surgery 1921;3:245–323:269.

62 Sampson JA. Perforating hemorrhagic (chocolate) cysts of the ovary. Archives of Surgery 1921;3:245–323:269.

63 Sampson JA. Perforating hemorrhagic (chocolate) cysts of the ovary. Archives of Surgery 1921;3:245–323:270.

64 Sampson JA. Perforating hemorrhagic (chocolate) cysts of the ovary. Archives of Surgery 1921;3:245–323:271–272. See Figure 68, page 314 and Figure 70, page 316. Figure 70 (Case 22) is a low power photomicrograph of a bleb "lined by columnar cells resting on a cellular stroma" and filled with menstrual debris.

65 Sampson JA. Perforating hemorrhagic (chocolate) cysts of the ovary. Archives of Surgery 1921;3:245–323:316. Figure 70 (Case 22).

who was an advocate. [66] "Lockyer expresses the following views of the advocates of this theory: 'Heterotopy of serosal epithelium is the probable explanation of the existence of the epithelial spaces and cysts in most of the extra-uterine swellings found between the rectum and genital tract,' and again he states that 'it has also been conclusively shown that the connective tissue which surrounds the 'endothelial' inclusions can be excited to hyperplasia which causes it to assume the characteristic histological features of the stroma of the uterine mucosa.'"[67]

Specifying that "a large percentage, and possibly all, of the ovarian hematomas reported in this paper were of endometrial type,"[68] Sampson postulated the pathogenesis of bowel endometriosis, specifically endometriosis of the sigmoid colon: "Apparently some of the contents escaping from the ovarian hematoma had carried with them some of its epithelium, which was deposited on the surface of the sigmoid and later invaded it."[69] This is an important statement; Sampson essentially believed that living, viable endometrial cells from the ovarian hematoma were capable of implanting on the serosa of the sigmoid colon, invade and cause an "adenoma of endometrial type."[70] So saying, Sampson reinforced the principle message of this essay; that the ovary is the primary source of pelvic adenomas of endometrial type and the associated pelvic adhesions. After saying that "a large percentage… of the ovarian hematomas…were of endometrial type," Sampson seemed to offer a circular argument: "The most important evidence that these ovarian hematomas and clefts or pockets are of endometrial type is the secondary development of adenoma of endometrial type in the tissue or structure which have become 'infected' by material escaping from them."[71]

Sampson considered the pathogenesis of uterine adenomyomas. He accepted "invasion from 'within' the uterus…and…invasion from 'without' the uterus, [because] histologically the two tumors are identical."[72] However, he expressed uncertainty regarding the existence of a third group of uterine adenomyomas. "I do not know whether or not there is a third group of 'adenomyoma' arising from misplaced endometrial tissue in the uterine wall or by invasion from 'without' from other sources than the ovary."[73] Granting that ovarian hematomas may be the source of secondary endometrial adenomas in the pelvis, Sampson asked a provocative question. "Are all ectopic pelvic adenomyomas of endometrial type secondary to a similar condition in the ovary? I cannot answer this question."[74]

Despite the explanatory power of his ovarian theory, Sampson's question indicates he was not satisfied that it gave a comprehensive explanation. For example, Sampson "operated on two patients with pelvic adenoma of endometrial type without gross evidence of hematoma of the ovaries."[75] He considered two possible sources of the endometrial tissue he found on the surface of the ovary; either it represented "remains of an 'endometrial' hematoma in which nearly complete retrogression had occurred or 'endometrial' pockets or clefts which had functioned, namely, had menstruated, and the secondary pelvic adenomas had arisen from them."[76] Then, Sampson made two remarkable statements that reveal that he was thinking deeply of an alternative hypothesis, perhaps to complement rather than replace his theory of the primacy of ovarian hematomas as the source of adhesions and pelvic adenomas of endometrial type. The first statement was that: "It is also possible that their origin was independent of the ovaries."[77] The second statement is the more remarkable: "There is

---

[66] Cuthbert Lockyer, *Fibroids and Allied Tumours (Myoma and Adenomyoma): Their Pathology, Clinical Features and Surgical Treatment* [London: Macmillan and Company, 1918], 295, 296.

[67] Sampson JA. Perforating hemorrhagic (chocolate) cysts of the ovary: their importance and especially their relation to pelvic adenomas of endometrial type ("Adenomyoma" of the uterus, rectovaginal septum, sigmoid, etc.) Archives of Surgery 1921;3:245–323:272.

[68] Sampson JA. Perforating hemorrhagic (chocolate) cysts of the ovary. Archives of Surgery 1921;3:245–323:274.

[69] Sampson JA. Perforating hemorrhagic (chocolate) cysts of the ovary. Archives of Surgery 1921;3:245–323:274.

[70] Sampson JA. Perforating hemorrhagic (chocolate) cysts of the ovary Archives of Surgery 1921;3:245–323:274.

[71] Sampson JA. Perforating hemorrhagic (chocolate) cysts of the ovary. Archives of Surgery 1921;3:245–323:275.

[72] Sampson JA. Perforating hemorrhagic (chocolate) cysts of the ovary. Archives of Surgery 1921;3:245–323:276.

[73] Sampson JA. Perforating hemorrhagic (chocolate) cysts of the ovary. Archives of Surgery 1921;3:245–323:276.

[74] Sampson JA. Perforating hemorrhagic (chocolate) cysts of the ovary. Archives of Surgery 1921;3:245–323:276.

[75] Sampson JA. Perforating hemorrhagic (chocolate) cysts of the ovary. Archives of Surgery 1921;3:245–323:277.

[76] Sampson JA. Perforating hemorrhagic (chocolate) cysts of the ovary. Archives of Surgery 1921;3:245–323:277.

[77] Sampson JA. Perforating hemorrhagic (chocolate) cysts of the ovary. Archives of Surgery 1921;3:245–323:277.

such a great variation both in the invasiveness of the pelvic adenomyomas and also in their finer histologic appearance that one wonders whether they are all the same."[78]

In this first essay, Sampson analyzed the clinical features of his first 23 patients from which he fashioned a durable clinical picture of moderate, severe, and extensive endometriosis. He observed endometriotic disease in women aged 30 years to menopause, which also happens to be the ages at which uterine myomas are prevalent.

Given that Sampson observed mostly moderate, severe, and extensive disease at laparotomy, one can better appreciate the clinical picture he assembled. Sampson's observations gained such an aura of authority that physicians soon came to regard endometriosis as a disease of the fourth and fifth decades of a woman's life. Endometriosis in adolescents was not considered seriously until gynecologists began to investigate pelvic pain in adolescents by laparoscopy in the 1970s and 1980s. Sampson estimated he encountered "perforating hemorrhagic cysts of the ovary" in about 10% of his operations for relief of pelvic disease.[79] He encountered both primary and secondary infertility; "the shortest time that had elapsed since childbirth in any of these cases was 5 years."[80] Sampson believed that the "extent and situation" of the adhesions and other pelvic diseases were the most important factors in "the origin of subjective symptoms."[81] In his cases, adhesions were always present. They resulted from the "irritating action" of spilled material produced during the "menstrual" cycle of the perforated hemorrhagic cysts of the ovary.[82] Sampson specified that these cysts were more common in women with primary infertility, but were "apparently rare in women who have had salpingitis."[83]

Then Sampson made a highly significant observation. "In not a single instance of the 23 cases reported in this paper was there any gross evidence of a recent or an old inflammatory disease of tubal origin; the fimbriated extremities of the tubes in all cases appeared normal and whatever adhesions were present about the tubes were of extratubal origin, that is, from the contents of the cyst."[84] He concluded that "the condition under consideration" was the cause of fixed retroversion or retroflexion of the uterus observed in ten of his cases. The cysts were usually small, often bilateral, and between 2 and 4 cm. in diameter, the largest being 9 cm. Note that Sampson did not consider cysts and adhesions to be invasive disease when he discussed the patients' symptoms.

Twelve of the 17 symptomatic patients sought relief for pain, three for increasing constipation, and one each for uterine bleeding and sterility.[85] The amount of pain and abnormal bleeding were quite variable, and often absent.[86] Sampson concluded: "It is very difficult to decide whether or not these cysts cause profuse or irregular (too frequent) menstruation."[87] As for pelvic pain, he concluded that "there is usually nothing characteristic about the pain present in this condition nor is there necessarily any relation between the extent of the adhesions and the severity of the pain."[88] Later Sampson modified this statement saying, "if painful menstruation results, it is of the acquired variety, of recent development and may be progressive in severity."[89] Constipation is sometimes worse at the menses and "the symptoms of the advanced cases with narrowing of the lumen of the intestine are similar to those of intestinal obstruction due to other causes such as malignancy."[90]

[78] Sampson JA. Perforating hemorrhagic (chocolate) cysts of the ovary. Archives of Surgery 1921;3:245–323:278.

[79] Sampson JA. Perforating hemorrhagic (chocolate) cysts of the ovary. Archives of Surgery 1921;3:245–323:319.

[80] Sampson JA. Perforating hemorrhagic (chocolate) cysts of the ovary: their importance and especially their relation to pelvic adenomas of endometrial type ("Adenomyoma" of the uterus, rectovaginal septum, sigmoid, etc.) Archives of Surgery 1921;3:245–323:279.

[81] Sampson JA. Perforating hemorrhagic (chocolate) cysts of the ovary. Archives of Surgery 1921;3:245–323:280.

[82] Sampson JA. Perforating hemorrhagic (chocolate) cysts of the ovary. Archives of Surgery 1921;3:245–323:319.

[83] Sampson JA. Perforating hemorrhagic (chocolate) cysts of the ovary. Archives of Surgery 1921;3:245–323:280.

[84] Sampson JA. Perforating hemorrhagic (chocolate) cysts of the ovary. Archives of Surgery 1921;3:245–323:281.

[85] Sampson JA. Perforating hemorrhagic (chocolate) cysts of the ovary. Archives of Surgery 1921;3:245–323:284.

[86] Sampson JA. Perforating hemorrhagic (chocolate) cysts of the ovary. Archives of Surgery 1921;3:245–323:281–282.

[87] Sampson JA. Perforating hemorrhagic (chocolate) cysts of the ovary. Archives of Surgery 1921;3:245–323:283.

[88] Sampson JA. Perforating hemorrhagic (chocolate) cysts of the ovary. Archives of Surgery 1921;3:245–323:284.

[89] Sampson JA. Perforating hemorrhagic (chocolate) cysts of the ovary. Archives of Surgery 1921;3:245–323:285.

[90] Sampson JA. Perforating hemorrhagic (chocolate) cysts of the ovary. Archives of Surgery 1921;3:245–323:285.

Within his first 23 cases, Sampson encountered many of the typical presentations of pelvic endometriosis, some of which he illustrated. A transverse section of the pelvic structures and surrounding pelvic and vertebral bones, with an ovarian hematoma adherent to the pelvic side wall.[91] An illustration of a sagittal section of the pelvis depicts a retroflexed uterus adherent to endometriosis of the rectovaginal pouch of Douglas [RVPD] overlying the posterior fornix of the vagina.[92] A sagittal view of the pelvis with complete obliteration of the RVPD showing a large ovarian endometrioma adherent to the rectum posteriorly and the upper posterior uterine fundus anteriorly.[93] The sagittal section of the pelvis with an "adenomyoma" that has invaded the rectum and posterior wall of the uterus with complete obliteration of the RVPD but has not invaded the posterior vaginal fornix.[94] Complete obliteration of the RVPD with the rectum densely adherent to the supravaginal portion of the cervix up to the insertion of the uterosacral ligaments.[95] There are good illustrations of an intact surgical specimen consisting of the complete uterus with both tubes and ovaries showing "perforating hemorrhagic cysts of both ovaries with discrete 'adenomyomas' of the posterior wall of the uterus."[96] A sagittal section of the uterus and posterior vaginal fornix showing an "adenoma of endometrial type" invading the posterior vaginal fornix and the supravaginal portion of the uterine cervix.[97] A cross section of the uterine cervix and ovaries illustrating "centripetal disease" with both ovaries and the rectum densely adherent to the cervix with complete obliteration of the RVPD.[98] "Multiple hemorrhagic peritoneal 'blebs' (adenomyomas)" on the posterior aspect of the uterus.[99] A low power photomicrograph of one of the blebs.[100]

In describing his physical examination of such patients, Sampson stated that "palpatory finding in the culdesac [RVPD], when present, [were] the most characteristic physical signs."[101] Palpatory findings would include nodules in the uterosacral ligaments and rectum, adenomatous lesions penetrating into the posterior fornix of the vagina, as well as fixed retroflexed or retroverted uteri. Paraphrase simply cannot capture the experience of this gifted physician, only his own description of what he felt on examination and of his assessment of those findings will do justice to him. "The physical findings vary greatly...the uterus is often retroflexed or retroverted and adherent and the degree of adenomatous growth in the culdesac varies greatly in character in different cases. When slight, it is impossible to detect it. The involvement may be localized or diffuse. If localized, the area of induration may be flat or nodular, in the median line just behind the cervix, or laterally in the region of the uterosacral ligaments. The induration is usually low down, but occasionally may be higher up. Sometimes it is best detected on vaginal palpation and at other times felt best through the rectum."[102] Sampson commended Lockyer's description of "extensive involvement of the rectogenital space by adenomyoma,"[103] but no one ever described the physical findings better than Sampson.

The clinical picture – both history and physical findings – established by Sampson in 1921, with its analogy to "implantation" and the adhesive pattern of ovarian malignancy, not only captured the visual imagination of physicians but became fixed in textbooks for the next 50 years until modified by the addition of signs and symptoms, found at laparoscopy, that accompanied

[91] Sampson JA. Perforating hemorrhagic (chocolate) cysts of the ovary. Archives of Surgery 1921;3:245–323:247.

[92] Sampson JA. Perforating hemorrhagic (chocolate) cysts of the ovary. Archives of Surgery 1921;3:245–323:253.

[93] Sampson JA. Perforating hemorrhagic (chocolate) cysts of the ovary. Archives of Surgery 1921;3:245–323:259.

[94] Sampson JA. Perforating hemorrhagic (chocolate) cysts of the ovary. Archives of Surgery 1921;3:245–323:272.

[95] Sampson JA. Perforating hemorrhagic (chocolate) cysts of the ovary> Archives of Surgery 1921;3:245–323:279.

[96] Sampson JA. Perforating hemorrhagic (chocolate) cysts of the ovary. Archives of Surgery 1921;3:245–323:289, 300 and 308. See Figure 43 (Case 17) on page 289, Figure 54 (Case 19) on page 300, and Figure 60 (Case 12) on page 306.

[97] Sampson JA. Perforating hemorrhagic (chocolate) cysts of the ovary. Archives of Surgery 1921;3:245–323:298.

[98] Sampson JA. Perforating hemorrhagic (chocolate) cysts of the ovary: their importance and especially their relation to pelvic adenomas of endometrial type ("Adenomyoma" of the uterus, rectovaginal septum, sigmoid, etc.) Archives of Surgery 1921;3:245–323:301.

[99] Sampson JA. Perforating hemorrhagic (chocolate) cysts of the ovary. Archives of Surgery 1921;3:245–323:314.

[100] Sampson JA. Perforating hemorrhagic (chocolate) cysts of the ovary. Archives of Surgery 1921;3:245–323:316.

[101] Sampson JA. Perforating hemorrhagic (chocolate) cysts of the ovary. Archives of Surgery 1921;3:245–323:285.

[102] Sampson JA. Perforating hemorrhagic (chocolate) cysts of the ovary. Archives of Surgery 1921;3:245–323:285–286.

[103] Cuthbert Lockyer, *Fibroids and Allied Tumours (Myoma and Adenomyoma): Their Pathology, Clinical Features and Surgical Treatment* [London: Macmillan and Company, 1918].

earlier stages of the disease. In a subsequent publication Sampson enhanced his argument regarding implantation adenomas of endometrial type originating from ovarian hematomas of endometrial type by analogizing them to pelvic implantations from ovarian carcinoma: "Implantation carcinoma of the various organs and structures of the peritoneal cavity is well recognized both by pathologists and clinicians and likewise the important part played by ovarian carcinoma as a source of these implantations. Implantation adenomas of endometrial type are analogous to those of carcinoma."[104]

In 1921, Sampson believed that there were two pathologic conditions to treat, "the one present in the ovary or ovaries, and the secondary adhesions in the pelvis which are often associated with an adenoma of the endometrial type, the latter varying greatly in the degree to which it has invaded the tissues and organs involved."[105] Note that Sampson emphasized the ovarian cyst(s) and adhesions and that invasion was secondary in his thinking at this point. He believed that, as a rule, albeit with possible exceptions, "tissues of endometrial type" would stop growing and "actually atrophy" once the menopause was established.[106] While Sampson respected the patients' desires and performed conservative surgery, preserving ovarian and reproductive function in some cases, he realized that these patients might require a second surgery. To emphasize the risks involved in conservative surgery, Sampson wrote: "Casler's case…is an extreme example of the possible results of conservative surgery in these cases."[107] By his reference to Casler and his statements that follow one may infer that Sampson believed that removal of the ovaries and the disease was the treatment of choice: "To remove the pelvic adenoma and disregard the ovarian condition would be to leave the original growth behind, and furthermore, the persistence of the ovarian function might increase the growth of secondary pelvic adenomas not removed."[108] Then returning to the analogy to ovarian malignancy, Sampson stated further in italics: "*Certainly we would not sanction the surgical judgment of the operator who removed the secondary peritoneal implantations of ovarian papilloma or cancer and did not remove the primary ovarian tumor.* The conditions are analogous except that fortunately the adenoma of endometrial type is only rarely sufficiently invasive to cause serious damage to the parts involved."[109]

Likely learning from the complications of sigmoid colon and rectal surgery experienced by Cullen, Sampson stated: "I have never resorted to the extremely radical operations, as in cancer of the uterine cervix, and even in these operations it may be impossible to remove all of the adenomatous growth."[110] To put his statement in proper context, one must remember that Sampson had extensive experience in the surgical treatment of cervical cancer.[111] Nonetheless, where possible Sampson avoided operating adenoma of the rectum, stating: "In the radical operations which I have employed, I have removed the entire uterus with both ovaries, and in freeing the uterus from the rectum, I have purposely kept close to the uterus, undoubtedly sometimes leaving adenoma on the rectal wall. In freeing the cervix laterally, I have kept close to it, in one case intentionally leaving adenoma in the broad ligament because it was too extensive to remove (Case 12)."[112] Sampson qualified this statement by saying that only more experience would reveal whether this was the proper choice. Again, one must consider the circumstances under which Sampson operated. The average remaining life expectancy of a

[104] Sampson JA. Intestinal adenomas of endometrial type: their importance and their relation to ovarian hematomas of endometrial type (perforating hemorrhagic cysts of the ovary). Archives of Surgery 1922;5:217–280;224–225.

[105] Sampson JA. Perforating hemorrhagic (chocolate) cysts of the ovary: their importance and especially their relation to pelvic adenomas of endometrial type ("Adenomyoma" of the uterus, rectovaginal septum, sigmoid, etc.) Archives of Surgery 1921;3:245–323:287.

[106] Sampson JA. Perforating hemorrhagic (chocolate) cysts of the ovary. Archives of Surgery 1921;3:245–323:287.

[107] Sampson JA. Perforating hemorrhagic (chocolate) cysts of the ovary. Archives of Surgery 1921;3:245–323:287–288.

[108] Sampson JA. Perforating hemorrhagic (chocolate) cysts of the ovary. Archives of Surgery 1921;3:245–323:287.

[109] Sampson JA. Perforating hemorrhagic (chocolate) cysts of the ovary. Archives of Surgery 1921;3:245–323:287–288.

[110] Sampson JA. Perforating hemorrhagic (chocolate) cysts of the ovary: their importance and especially their relation to pelvic adenomas of endometrial type ("Adenomyoma" of the uterus, rectovaginal septum, sigmoid, etc.) Archives of Surgery 1921;3:245–323:289.

[111] Clement, PB. History of Gynecologic Pathology IX: Dr. John Albertson Sampson. International Journal of Clinical Pathology 2001;20:86–101. In the bibliography of Sampson's works following this scholarly biographical essay, Clement lists many articles of Sampson that pertain to radical surgery for cervical cancer and to the pathology of cervical cancer.

[112] Sampson JA. Perforating hemorrhagic (chocolate) cysts of the ovary. Archives of Surgery 1921;3:245–323:289–290.

30 year-old woman in 1921 was 38.15 years compared to 50.1 years in 2004.[113] In other words, if a woman 30 years of age in 1921 had a hysterectomy and removal of both ovaries, on average she would be menopausal for 38.15 years. Estrogen hormone replacement therapy had not been invented. In fact, the estrogen hormone had not been identified, let alone isolated as a treatment modality. Sampson relied on surgical menopause to atrophy rectal and broad ligament endometriosis and other endometriotic deposits he left behind.

Given that "there seems to be a great variation in the degree of 'invasiveness' of the secondary pelvic deposits which is often evident in the individual case at operation," Sampson did individualize his surgical treatment once the abdomen was open.[114] Unfortunately, he had no reliable means to assess the extent of invasion before operating. Hence, his patients could not know before surgery whether Sampson could be conservative or if he would find it necessary to remove both ovaries. Judging from the following statement, we may assume that Sampson did discuss with his patients how he would proceed at surgery: "My present plan is to employ ovarian conservatism (excising the portion of the ovary or ovaries involved) or removing only the apparently diseased ovary in patients who desire to have the ovarian function maintained but only if the invasion of the pelvic tissues by the adenoma is slight."[115] Then Sampson expressed his reservations about conservative surgery. "I am anxiously waiting to see whether the end-results will justify this stand. I am inclined to believe that ovarian conservatism is a rather dangerous experiment."[116] Sampson summarized his treatment recommendations in 1921: "In all other cases, either when ovarian conservation is not strongly desired or when the pelvic growth is apparently actually invasive, I believe that all ovarian tissues should be removed and as much as possible of the pelvic growth with it."[117]

Sampson summarized his thinking in this classic paper by offering six data as evidence that perforating hemorrhagic cysts of the ovary are hematomas of endometrial type. (1) "These hematomas, as the uterine mucosa, manifest their 'activity' during the menstrual life of the patient. (2) Histologically, the epithelial lining of the ovarian hematomas is similar to that of the uterine hematomas, due to the retention of 'menstrual' blood, often present in 'adenomyoma' of the uterus. (3) Periodic hemorrhages occur in the ovarian hematomas which are similar in gross and histologic appearance to that of menstruating endometrium. (4) The 'chocolate' contents of the ovarian hematomas resemble old menstrual blood. (5) In two patients operated on at the time of the menstrual period, one the day that menstruation was due (Case 13), and the other the last day of menstruation (Case 19), the histologic changes in the ovarian 'endometrial' tissue corresponded to the phase of the menstrual cycle indicated by the menstrual history of the patient. (6) The fact that material escaping from the ovarian hematomas may give rise to the development of adenoma of endometrial type in the tissues thus soiled is further proof that these hematomas contain 'endometrial' tissue."[118]

Having delivered a paper of such importance, Sampson ended with the provocative conclusion: "I cannot state that these ovarian hematomas of endometrial type are the only cause of ectopic pelvic adenomas."[119]

Indeed, when Sampson published that statement, James C. Janney, a gynecologist in Brookline, Massachusetts, was in the process of reviewing 4,853 pathological specimens at the Free Hospital for Women. He found three cases of uterine tissue in the ovary which he explained as rare anomalies of development from embryonic rests.[120] However, prior to publication,

[113] U. S. Department of Health and Human Services Centers for Disease Control and Prevention: National Center for Health Statistics, National Vital Statistics System. United States Life Tables, 2004. National Vital Statistics Reports: Volume 56, Number 8, December 28, 2007, Page 30. Table 11. Life expectancy by age, race, and sex: Death-registration states, 1900–1902 to 1919–1921, and United States, 1929–1931 to 2004.

[114] Sampson JA. Perforating hemorrhagic (chocolate) cysts of the ovary. Archives of Surgery 1921;3:245–323:290.

[115] Sampson JA. Perforating hemorrhagic (chocolate) cysts of the ovary. Archives of Surgery 1921;3:245–323:290.

[116] Sampson JA. Perforating hemorrhagic (chocolate) cysts of the ovary. Archives of Surgery 1921;3:245–323:290–291.

[117] Sampson JA. Perforating hemorrhagic (chocolate) cysts of the ovary. Archives of Surgery 1921;3:245–323:291.

[118] Sampson JA. Perforating hemorrhagic (chocolate) cysts of the ovary: their importance and especially their relation to pelvic adenomas of endometrial type ("Adenomyoma" of the uterus, rectovaginal septum, sigmoid, etc.) Archives of Surgery 1921;3:245–323:322–323.

[119] Sampson JA. Perforating hemorrhagic (chocolate) cysts of the ovary. Archives of Surgery 1921;3:245–323:323. Nowhere in this paper did Sampson mention transtubal menstrual dissemination of endometrial tissue into the peritoneal cavity.

[120] Janney JC. Report of three cases of a rare ovarian anomaly. Am J Obstet Gynecol 1922;Feb:173–187.

Janney read Sampson's article in the *Archives of Surgery* of October 1921. He appended a note referring to a key element of Sampson's article that uterine tissue in the ovary was not a rare phenomenon after all. "Note: Since the preparation of this paper, several cases of the same sort have been reported by Sampson in a paper read before the American Gynecological Society, which appeared in *Archives of Surgery*, October 1921. The discovery of endometrium in the wall of a large proportion of the so-called 'hemorrhagic cysts of the ovary' would seem to bear out the opinion expressed in this [Sampson's] paper that the condition under discussion is not of such rare occurrence as the scarcity of reported cases would suggest."[121]

Sampson presented his *first theory* to the American Gynecological Society on June 3, 1921. In his closing remarks to the discussion that followed this paper Sampson replied: "In answer to the questions which have been asked, I believe the growth is primary in the ovary, and not in the adenomyoma, and that the extension is from the ovary to the uterus and not from the uterus to the ovary."[122]

A Historical Note by Sampson

"When these endometrial hematomas or cysts were described by me in 1921, I was not aware that they had been previously recognized and described. Three years later I found that Pick had described them in 1905 and had designated them adenoma or cystomas endometroides ovarii. Pick suggests that these cysts may be the same as Rokitansky's cystosarcoma adenoids ovarii uterinum, described by the latter in his textbook of pathological anatomy published in 1861. Should anyone's name be attached to these ovarian cysts, it should be Pick's or Rokitansky's, not mine."[123]

Sampson acknowledged that Ludwig Pick had confirmed the likelihood that Rokitansky described ovarian endometriosis in 1861. Pick thought that *Cystadenoma or Adenoma endometroides ovarii* was a good name for chocolate ovarian cysts with the structure of the endometrium of the uterine corpus that he observed. He also thought it likely that *Cystadenoma or Adenoma endometroides ovarii* was identical with *Cystosarcoma adenoids ovarii uterinum* described by Rokitansky in 1861.[124] (Italics added)

After his presentation at the American Gynecological Society, Sampson seized upon his second insight while doing further research; the powerful *second theory* of transtubal retrograde menstruation and implantation. However, in his rush to publish *Perforating hemorrhagic (chocolate) cysts of the ovary*, Sampson had sent the manuscript to the *Archives of Surgery* before he submitted the same manuscript to the editor of the Transactions of the American Gynecological Society. This delay gave him an opportunity to insert a historical note – the announcement of his *second theory.*

A Historical Announcement by Sampson

In a duplicate publication of *Perforating Hemorrhagic (Chocolate) Cysts of the Ovary* published in the Transactions of the American Gynecological Society for the year 1921, Sampson inserted an announcement

121 Janney JC. Report of three cases of a rare ovarian anomaly. Am J Obstet Gynecol 1922;Feb:173–187: 187.

122 Sampson JA. Perforating hemorrhagic (chocolate) cysts of the ovary. Am J Obstet Gynecol 1921: 2:526–33. Note the discussion of his paper delivered at the American Gynecological Society meeting was published in the American Journal of Obstetrics and Gynecology while his paper was published in the Archives of Surgery in 1921 and also in the Transactions of the American Gynecological Society in 1921, in the later instance with the addition of a historical note of great importance.

123 Sampson JA. Heterotopic or misplaced endometrial tissue. Am J Obstet Gynecol 1925;10:649–664:655. Pick L. Arch f Gynaek 1905;lxxvi:251–275. Sampson was referring to Meigs who initiated the use of the term "(Sampson's cyst)," and undoubtedly others. See Meigs JV. Endometrial hematomas of the ovary. Boston Med Surg J 1922;clxxxvii:1–13:10, 12.

124 Pick L. Arch f Gynaek 1905;lxxvi:251–275:261–262. "Ein- oder mehrfache im Ovarium verstreute Cysten mit syruposblutigem, chocoladenbraunem oder rothlichem Inhalt und schleimhautahnlicher pigmentirter Auskleidug weisen makroskopisch auf diese Form des Adenomas, das ein Adenoma oder Cystadenoma ovarii vom Bau des Endometrium corporis uteri darstellt und kaum einen treffenderen Namen erhalten kann als den eines Adenoma endometroides ovarii).1" [Footnote 1] "Vielleicht ist diese Geschwulstform identisch mit dem alten Rokitansky-schen Cystosarcoma adenoides ovarii uterinum. Lehrb. D. pathology. Anatom. III. Aufl. Bd. III. 1861. Wien. S. 423, S431." On examination of a copy of Rokitansky's contribution: Lehrbuch der Pathologischen Anatomie 1855–61. III:475–490, reference to page S 431 is actually a reference to a running heading at the top of page 475 and reads "Rokitansky Uterusdrüsen – Neubildung. 1. c. (S. 431)." Since the copy I possess runs from pp. 475–490, I do not have the earlier pages which would contain the reference to S. 23.

of historic proportions, an announcement that is nowhere else to be found. "Note: Since sending in this paper for publication in the *Archives of Surgery*, I have had the opportunity to study material from more cases and wish to add this note. I described in this paper small hemorrhagic elevations in the ovaries of patients operated upon during the menstrual period which histologically proved to be due to hemorrhage about or into a space lined by tissue of endometrial type. I stated that I believed that they might develop into perforating hemorrhagic cysts and also might furnish the epithelium for the relining of follicular hematomas which might rupture near them. In my later studies I have found that these small ovarian hematomas may develop into larger ones, i.e., they may give rise to perforating hemorrhagic cysts. I have not as yet been able to demonstrate the relining of ruptured follicular hematomas from this source. The presence of ciliated epithelium in both the ovarian hematomas and also in the pelvic adenomas strengthens the implantation theory of the origin of the latter and weakens the serosal theory. The luteal like lining of many of these cysts could be explained as the result of hemorrhage in the walls of an endometrial cyst with consequent loss of the surface epithelium instead of the remains of a follicular hematoma.

Two possible sources of the origin of these small tubules or cysts of endometrial type in the ovary present themselves: first, congenital and second, *acquired from the implantation of epithelium escaping from the tube during menstruation and its subsequent invasion of the ovary. Epithelium escaping from the tubes during menstruation and its subsequent implantation in the pelvis might also be a source of pelvic adenoma of endometrial type other than from perforating hemorrhagic cysts of the ovary.*"[125] (Italics added)

Close on the heels of a full explication of his *first theory*, Sampson had announced his *second theory* of pathogenesis, that of retrograde menstruation; menstrual endometrium escaping through the fallopian tubes to implant and invade the ovary and pelvis. This second theory was not meant to replace the first theory; Sampson presented both theories as valid, as complementary. However, with the second theory Sampson explained the origin of ovarian adenoma of endometrial type and of perforating hemorrhagic cysts of the ovary. Both the first theory and the second theory explained the origin of pelvic adenoma of endometrial type. However, whereas the *first theory* better explained the dense pelvic adhesions as originating from the intensely irritating chocolate contents of the perforating hemorrhagic cysts of the ovary, the *second theory* not only explained the origin of ovarian adenomas of endometrial type and of perforating hemorrhagic cysts of the ovary, it also explained the origin of pelvic adenomas of endometrial type – including deeply invasive adenomas – when both ovaries were normal.

Taken together, Sampson's *first theory* and his *second theory* fulfill the purpose of any scientific theory… explanation and control as explained by K. Codell Carter: "Thus we see that systematic explanations of disease phenomena depend on accepting the Distinguishability Hypothesis. There is another way of making this point. The purposes of any scientific theory are explanation and control. In a theory of disease, achieving either purpose requires universal necessary causes, and such causes depend on etiological characterizations. But etiological characterizations are possible only if the causes, in terms of which different diseases are defined are themselves distinct. Thus the formulation of etiological definitions (and hence the adequacy of any theory of disease) requires distinguishability."[126]

In short, according to Sampson's theories, the proximate cause of pelvic adenomas and adenomyomas of endometrial type was endometrial tissue derived from the ovary – the *first theory* – or from the uterine endometrium – the *second theory*; with the latter being the dominant theory. Again, K. Codell Carter clarifies: "The introduction of etiological definitions simply made what had been specific *remote* causes into new *proximate* causes: whenever possible the essence of each disease became infection by a certain organism (say, tubercle bacilli) [endometrium] instead of a morbid alteration (for example, the formation of tubers) [adenomas and adenomyomas]. And the new proximate

[125] Sampson JA. Perforating hemorrhagic (chocolate) cysts of the ovary: their importance and especially their relation to pelvic adenomas of endometrial type ("Adenomyoma" of the uterus, rectovaginal septum, sigmoid, etc.) Transactions of the American Gynecological Society 1921;46:162–241: 235–6.

[126] K. Codell Carter, *The Rise of Causal Concepts of Disease: Case Histories* [Burlington, VT: Ashgate, 2003], 106. See also pages 199 and 200. "Between about 1830 and 1880, medicine reorganized itself around the concept of universal necessary causes…The etiological research programme [achieved an] enormous increase in explanatory power."

causes achieved *in spades* the same benefits as the old ones. Instead of merely explaining symptoms in terms of lesions (as the pathologists had done), researchers were now able to explain the lesions themselves, (and thereby symptoms and everything else lesions could ever explain) as well as many clinical and epidemiological facts that the pathologists could never begin to account for. ..The new proximate causes also provided much more effective targets for therapy and prophylaxis than did internal lesions".[127]

Explication of Sampson's Second Theory

In a paper presented to the Harvard Medical Society on February 14, 1922, Sampson explained his *second theory* of implantation adenomas of endometrial type, an explanation often overlooked because it was buried within the text of an article whose title only alluded to the treasure within.[128]

Implantation Adenomas of Endometrial Type

On February 14, 1922 Sampson awakened the community of medical scholars at Harvard University to a new disease – ovarian hematomas of endometrial type and implantation adenomas of endometrial type – when he presented a review of the subject at a meeting of the Harvard Medical Society at the Peter Bent Brigham Hospital.[129] The first fruits of that teaching moment came from the pen of Joe Vincent Meigs.[130] Meigs, a gynecologic oncologist inspired by Sampson's scholarship, not only became an authority on endometriosis, but also spearheaded an interest in endometriosis that led to important contributions by him, his students, and his colleagues at Harvard, contributions that have continued without interruption into the twenty-first century.

Sampson opened his lecture praising Lockyer's excellent monograph of 1918 that presented a substantial review of uterine and extrauterine adenomyomas. The first ten pages of this well-illustrated article, printed in the Boston Medical and Surgical Journal, recapitulated much of Sampson's first paper in the *Archives of Surgery* with supplementary historical references.[131] Chiari's salpingitis isthmica nodosa of 1887 was now called "adenomyoma of the tube." Sampson paid tribute to Cullen, his colleague and former professor at Johns Hopkins. "In 1895, Cullen described his first case of adenomyoma, and through his writing on this subject with their superb illustrations, he, more than anyone else, has demonstrated that the generally recognized adenomyoma of the uterus arises from an invasion of the uterine mucosa into the wall of the uterus. The origin of certain forms of adenomyoma of the uterus and the tube by the invasion of the mucosa lining their cavities is an established fact." Sampson credited Baraban in 1891 and Pilliet in 1894 with the observation that adenomyoma resulted from mucosal invasion. Though recorded before Cullen, these observations had rested quietly in the medical literature until Cullen emphasized the importance of mucosal invasion in his 1896 rebuttal to von Recklinghausen's theory of Wolffian rests.[132]

Then Sampson turned his attention briefly to adenomyomas that invaded the sigmoid colon, rectum, and "also those situated between the rectum and vagina; the latter are known as adenomyoma of the rectovaginal septum." He considered the latter "the most interesting ones clinically."[133] This was followed by an excellent review of the theories of pathogenesis in which he singled out Iwanoff's serosal theory as the most interesting, citing Lockyer's review of its many supporters.[134] So said, Sampson distanced himself from Iwanoff's theory. "Cilia may sometimes be found on the epithelium lining the ovarian hematomas of endometrial type and likewise in the implantation adenomas. This latter fact weakens the

[127] K. Codell Carter, *The Rise of Causal Concepts of Disease: Case Histories*, 107.

[128] Sampson JA. Ovarian hematomas of endometrial type (perforating hemorrhagic cysts of the ovary) and implantation adenomas of endometrial type. Boston Medical and Surgical Journal 1922;186:445–56.

[129] Sampson, JA. Ovarian hematomas of endometrial type (perforating hemorrhagic cysts of the ovary) and implantation adenomas of endometrial type. Boston Med Surg J 1922;186:445–456.

[130] Meigs, JV. Endometrial hematomas of the ovary. Boston Med Surg J 1922:187:1–13.

[131] Sampson JA. Boston Med Surg J 1922;186:445–456.

[132] Sampson JA. Ovarian hematomas of endometrial type (perforating hemorrhagic cysts of the ovary) and implantation adenomas of endometrial type. Boston Med Surg J 1922;186:445.

[133] Sampson JA. Boston Med Surg J 1922;186:445–456;445.

[134] Sampson JA. Boston Med Surg J 1922;186:445–456:446.

serosal theory of the origin of ectopic adenomas of endometrial type and strengthens the implantation theory."[135] In a statement designed to raise his audience's expectations, Sampson said: "I consider an ovarian hematoma with perforation as a frequent source of implantation adenoma of endometrial type, but possibly not the only source – as will be discussed later."[136]

"Later" came after seven more pages of audience preparation and 17 magnificent illustrations. "The data which I have been able to obtain suggest that tubal and uterine epithelial cells may, under certain circumstances (*as an abnormal menstruation with a back flow through the tube*), be expelled from the fimbriated end of the tube and lodge on the surface of the ovary. They may become imbedded in the tissues of the ovary and, true to their type, form glands and tubules which actually invade the ovary. The process is analogous to that which results from the implantation of epithelial cells on the peritoneum from the perforation of ovarian hematomas of endometrial type, as described in the previous and also in this communication."[137] (Italics added)

Sampson casually inserted an observation that anticipated by 2 years Josef Halban's theory of lymphatic dissemination of adenomatous tissue.[138] "Adenoma is sometimes found invading the lymph vessels from these implantations (of adenomas of endometrial type), and metastases may occur from this source and explain the origin of similar growths found in the groin. I have seen a similar invasion of a lymph vessel in a primary 'adenomyoma' of the tube and believe that they also may occur in primary 'adenomyoma' of the uterus."[139]

In this, his first presentation to a general academic audience, Sampson wished to leverage acceptance of his *second theory* of retrograde menstruation on acceptance of his more intuitive *first theory* of the pathogenesis of implantation adenomas of endometrial type resulting from perforating hemorrhagic cysts of the ovary. More simply put; Sampson believed his audience could more easily imagine retrograde menstruation through the relatively large perforation in the wall of a hemorrhagic cyst of the ovary than they could envision retrograde menstruation of viable endometrial fragments through the tiny proximal isthmica portion of the fallopian tube. To facilitate his audience's (and later readers') understanding, he presented circumstantial evidence in support of his *second theory*.[140] "It was interesting to note the character of the implantations when there was no gross evidence of an ovarian hematoma with perforation. They were usually smaller and not as widely distributed as those generally found in the pelvis associated with ovarian hematomas with evidence of perforation. They also often presented a little different histological picture. The implantations apparently derived from the perforated ovarian hematoma are usually more active and rapidly growing. I believe that implantations from both sources may have been present in some specimens. These latter observations are, to me, the most convincing evidence that the ovarian hematomas may arise from tubal or uterine epithelium escaping from the tube (*a possible result of internal menstruation*)."[141] (Italics added)

Toward the end of his presentation, Sampson chose the powerful seed and soil metaphor to help his audience to understand that implantation adenomas "may develop wherever this epithelium falls on suitable 'soil'."[142] He concluded his presentation with speculation regarding the origin of benign and malignant serous, endometrial and mucinous cysts of the ovary.[143]

Endometrial Hematomas of the Ovary

Joe Vincent Meigs was a house officer in 1921, the year Sampson published *Perforating hemorrhagic (Chocolate) Cysts of the Ovary* in the *Archives of Surgery*.[144] Meigs considered it the "foremost contribution to gynecology and gynecological pathology in

[135] Sampson JA. Boston Med Surg J 1922;186:445–456:447.

[136] Sampson JA. Boston Med Surg J 1922;186:445–456:448.

[137] Sampson JA. Boston Med Surg J 1922;186:445–456:455.

[138] Halban J. Hysteroadenosis metastatica. (Die lymphogene Genese der sog. Adenofibromatosis heterotopica.) Wiener klinische Wochenschrift 1924;37:1205–6.

[139] Sampson JA. Ovarian hematomas of endometrial type (perforating hemorrhagic cysts of the ovary) and implantation adenomas of endometrial type. Boston Med Surg J 1922;186: 445–456:448.

[140] Sampson JA. Boston Med Surg J 1922;186:445–456:455.

[141] Sampson JA. Boston Medical and Surgical Journal 1922;186:445–456.:456.

[142] Sampson JA. Ovarian hematomas of endometrial type (perforating hemorrhagic cysts of the ovary) and implantation adenomas of endometrial type. Boston Medical and Surgical Journal 1922;186:445–456:456.

[143] Sampson JA. Boston Med Surg J 1922;186:445–456:456.

[144] Sampson JA. Perforating hemorrhagic (chocolate) cysts of the ovary: their importance and especially their relation to pelvic

recent years," a prescient observation that introduced his own first paper on the subject published just 5 months after Sampson spoke to the Harvard Medical Society.[145] In possibly the first endorsement of Sampson's *first theory* of the pathogenesis of adenomas of endometrial type from perforated hemorrhagic cysts of the ovary, Meigs declared:

"Sampson believes, and we believe has proved, that adeno-leiomyomata of the fallopian tube, of the round ligament, of the posterior wall of the uterus, of the posterior surface of the broad ligament, of the sigmoid, and also of the small intestine and appendix, are in some instances the results of implants from these cysts...His article gives an explanation for the many cases of severe pelvic inflammation, the etiology of which has been so obscure and puzzling heretofore."[146]

So said, Meigs wanted to confirm Sampson's work. He searched through the records of William P. Graves of Boston and the records of the Free Hospital for Women on Pond Avenue, in Brookline, Massachusetts for cases of endometrial hematomas of the ovary. Fortunately since 1903 – concurrent with the birth of surgical pathology – both Graves and the Free Hospital preserved "in formalin all gross specimens removed at operation."[147] In this retrospective case series, Meigs identified 16 cases of ovarian endometrial hematomas with pertinent history on each patient. He cut and stained fresh histologic tissue sections from the preserved specimens. To add further credence to his study, Meigs sought confirmation of the microscopic diagnosis of endometrial hematoma of the ovary "in nearly every case" from Frank B. Mallory, pathologist at the Boston City Hospital.[148] Meigs described the histology in some detail with analysis that emphasized the presence and importance of hemorrhage and hemosiderin. "The endometrial-like tissue is found in various places in the ovary and in various forms, but usually it is near the perforation, and may be in the form of glands composed of columnar epithelium with an undifferentiated connective tissue stroma. Other specimens show a cuboidal, columnar, or cylindrical epithelium resting upon a thin layer of cellular tissue containing many blood vessels, and extravasated new and old blood. Still others have one of the above types of epithelium resting upon a thick layer of fibrous tissue, or even directly upon the ovarian tissue itself. The most important finding is the presence of hemorrhage, and especially the signs of old hemorrhage in a cyst wall lined with epithelium, which is not stratified. The sign of old hemorrhage is blood pigment (hemosiderin) chiefly in endothelial leucocytes, the presence of blood pigment, meaning that hemorrhage has occurred at some previous time. The blood remains in the tissue beneath the epithelium, because it cannot escape as does hemorrhage in the uterus or in the kidney, which have a passage to the outside of the body...The blood cannot escape, so it changes to blood pigment, and is later gathered up by endothelial leucocytes whose function it is to remove foreign bodies of this type."[149]

Meigs confirmed all of Sampson's findings except tubal patency. In his series, the fallopian tubes were normal in nine cases [cases 4,5,6,10,11,12,13,15,16]; the condition of the tubes was not described in one case [case 14]; one case had bilateral chronic salpingitis with open fimbriae [case 3]; and in five cases both tubes were closed [cases 1,2,7,8,9].[150]

He listed the various theories describing the etiology of endometrial hematomas. Contrary to his enthusiastic endorsement of Sampson's *first theory,* Meigs did not endorse any of the theories of pathogenesis for endometrial hematomas of the ovary. He enumerated the

adenomas of endometrial type ("Adenomyoma" of the uterus, rectovaginal septum, sigmoid, etc.) Archives of Surgery 1921;3:245–323.

[145] Meigs, JV. Endometrial hematomas of the ovary. Boston Med Surg J 1922:187:1–13:1

[146] Meigs, JV. Boston Med Surg J 1922:187:1–13:2.

[147] Meigs, JV. Boston Med Surg J 1922:187:1–13:2.

[148] Meigs, JV. Boston Med Surg J 1922:187:1–13:6.

[149] Meigs, JV. Boston Med Surg J 1922:187:1–13:1. Endothelial leucocytes are part of the innate immune system operative at birth. See: Richardson AC, Carpenter MW. Inflammatory mediators in gestational diabetes mellitus. Obstet Gynecol Clin N Am 2007;34:213–224:216. "The immune system defends its host against both external threats, such as bacterial infection, viral infection; physical injury, and internal threats such as malignant transformation. The immune system has historically been divided into two parts: the innate and adaptive. They are separated purely for descriptive purposes and are not mutually exclusive of one another. From an evolutionary standpoint, the innate immune system predates the adaptive immune system. The innate immune system is considered to be the 'first-line' of defense against microbes or tissue damage. The adaptive immune system is activated by the innate immune system and responds to antigens to which the organism has already been exposed, thereby providing the ability to mount a more effective response."

[150] Meigs, JV. Endometrial hematomas of the ovary. Boston Med Surg J 1922:187:1–13.

following theories, evidencing no preference: (1) metaplasia of ovarian germinal epithelium; (2) Sampson's *second theory* due to the implantation of endometrium reaching the ovary by way of the Fallopian tube – a theory Meigs heard directly from Sampson at the Peter Bent Brigham Hospital on February 14, 1922; and (3) the embryological theory expressed by WW Russell in 1899. With reference to the latter, Meigs discussed a paper by Janney from the Free Hospital for Women that antedated publication of Sampson's *second theory.* According to Meigs, Janney postulated that:

"Uterine tissue found in the ovaries may be due to a developmental defect. The funnel, the earliest beginning of the müllerian duct, may develop on the medial instead of the lateral side of the tubal area from which the ovary arises. Tissue may become mixed when these two areas are close together and thus tissue capable of forming endometrium may be included in the ovary, later in life."[151]

It is interesting to quote directly from Janney for the details. He reviewed the collection of human embryos at Harvard Medical School and consulted with Drs. Bremer and Begg of the Department of Embryology at Harvard Medical School. Dr. Bremer believed that ovarian tissue in the ovary "might be explained on the supposition of an accessory aberrant müllerian duct bud which was included in the ovary."[152] "Dr. Begg suggested that the proximity of the 'anlagen' of the ovary and tube in embryonic life was so great that there might be some critical period of embryonic development at which it would be possible for a tissue mixture to take place."[153]

Having first consulted Drs. Bremer and Begg, Janney reviewed the Harvard collection of human embryos and made observations pertinent to the developmental theory of müllerian – endometriotic – rests. "In reviewing this series of embryos I have found cases where the funnel, instead of forming on the lateral side of the tubar area, forms on the medial side, and is thereby brought into a position much closer to the sex gland, a fact which is suggestive in view of the supposition advanced by Dr. Begg.

The funnel, which is the earliest beginning of the müllerian duct, is developed usually on the lateral side of the tubar area and separated from the genital areas by a fissure and the whole width of the tubar ridge, a distance of approximately 0.5–0.75 mm. In one case both funnels opened on the median side of the tubar area. In two other embryos one funnel opened on the medial side, and in a fourth the funnel opening seemed to extend from the lateral through to the median side of the tubar area. This unusual median position of the funnel reduces the distance between the genital gland and the müllerian duct very materially. In the cases which showed this variation the actual distances between the funnel and the genital gland at the nearest point were in four cases less than 0.1 mm (about 0.0875 mm) and in the fifth instance less than 0.2 mm (about 0.175). It is not unreasonable to suppose that tissue mixtures between the tubal and ovarian tissue could take place in cases where the distance separating the two tissues is less than 0.1 mm. I must note here that in the cases where this condition was present three of the embryos were too young to distinguish the sex with certainty. The genital glands were still undifferentiated. In the other two cases testes cords were present and the embryo was probably male. I do not feel that it would argue impossibly of such an explanation of uterine tissue in the ovary, had these been definitely male embryos, for there is nothing to show that such variations could not occur in the female. The most it could argue, I think, is that such an anomaly might someday be found in the testis also."[154]

Theorists may wish to recall Janney's caveat featuring Mark Twain. "Embryology may be suggestive but hardly conclusive, for the reason that suggestive appearances in an embryo can never be proved to be the early stages of a condition found in adults unless all of the steps can be demonstrated which seems unlikely in a condition of this rarity. Only if we are favored, like Mark Twain to the extent of seeing St. Peter's skull at the age of seventeen and again in another museum at the time of his death can we hope to bring forth actual proof by the aid of embryology."[155]

[151] Meigs, JV. Boston Med Surg J 1922:187:1–13:3.

[152] Janney JC. Report of three cases of a rare ovarian anomaly. Am J Obstet Gynecol 1922;Feb:173–187:180.

[153] Janney JC. Report of three cases of a rare ovarian anomaly. Am J Obstet Gynecol 1922;Feb:173–187:181.

[154] Janney JC. Am J Obstet Gynecol 1922;Feb:173–187: 182–184.

[155] Janney JC. Am J Obstet Gynecol 1922;Feb:173–187:187.

[156] Faulconer RJ. Observations on the origins of the müllerian groove in human embryos. Contrib Embryol 1951;229: 161–164:161.

[157] Ludwig KS. The Mayer-Rokitansky-Küster syndrome. An analysis of its morphology and embryology. Part II: embryology. Arch Gynecol Obstet 1998;262:27–42.

In 1951, Faulconer confirmed Janney's hypothesis. He demonstrated in specimens from the Department of Embryology of the Carnegie Institution of Washington that the müllerian groove in human embryos "is not constant in relation to the cranial end of the Wolffian body, but is subject to much variation. The specimens examined revealed groove formation on all surfaces of the Wolffian body. These sites of invagination are designated as (1) dorsolateral, (2) lateral, (3) ventral, and (4) ventrolateral."[156] In 1998, Ludwig analyzed the embryology of the müllerian duct with respect to the pathogenesis of the Mayer-Rokitansky-Küster-Hauser [M-R-K-H] syndrome. He found that the müllerian duct develops independently of the coelomic epithelium above the mesonephros.[157] Ludwig's theory explains the pathogenesis of M-R-K-H syndrome as well as the pathogenesis of ectopic endosalpingiosis in the thorax: mediastinal paravertebral müllerian cystic endosalpingiosis, also known as Hattori cysts.[158]

Joe Vincent Meigs, the young clinician from Boston, appears to have been the first investigator to emphasize endometriosis-associated infertility problems. He did so by offering his own theory to explain the preponderance of ovarian endometrial hematomas in nulliparous women 30 years of age and older and their relation to infertility. "Women who bear children usually marry before 30, the age at which these cysts are first found… Provided the cyst has progressed to any extent the woman married after 30 will often be sterile. If, on the other hand, there is a microscopically small or nonadherent cyst present, and the young woman marries and has a child, the cyst may atrophy and perhaps even disappear in the stage of lactation atrophy which the genital tract frequently undergoes during the nursing period…We believe the explanation of …why they do not cause more frequent damage [at the younger age] …to be that the cysts develop very slowly. This is suggested by the fact that they usually do not appear until the patient is over 30 years of age; in other words, they are not found until 13 to 19 years of menstrual life have passed."[159]

Meigs recorded that 5 of his 16 patients were between 20 and 30 years of age; 2 under age 25 years of age.[160] In succeeding years, Meigs would elaborate on his theory. He would influence many young couples to marry at an early age and have children before the threat of sterility from endometrial hematomas of the ovary. Based on his assumption that the growth is probably very slow and seldom endangers life, Meigs recommended conservative surgery; but only "if all the endometrial tissue [could] be removed." If however, all the endometrial tissue could not be removed, he recommended radical surgery; standard radical surgery for benign disease at that time meant supravaginal hysterectomy and removal of both tubes and ovaries. In 1924 Sampson would respond to some of the ideas in Meig's paper when he addressed the life history of ovarian hematomas.[161]

Intestinal Adenomas of Endometrial Type

In this paper, Sampson displayed both his powers of observation and his pedagogical technique. He repeatedly asked questions of his audience and readers in the subtext of his illustrations. Then giving his readers and audience time for reflection, he answered the questions in the main text that followed. Sampson explained the delay in his appreciating the frequency of perforating hemorrhagic cysts of the ovary. He stated that he had

158 Batt RE. Mhawech-Fauceglia P, Odunsi K, Yeh J. Pathogenesis of mediastinal paravertebral müllerian cysts of Hattori: developmental endosalpingiosis-müllerianosis. Int J Gynecol Pathol 2010;29:546–561.

159 Meigs, JV. Endometrial hematomas of the ovary. Boston Med Surg J 1922:187:1–13:4, 3.

160 Meigs, JV. Boston Med Surg J 1922:187:1–13:4.

161 Sampson JA. Benign and malignant endometrial implants in the peritoneal cavity, and their relation to certain ovarian tumors. Surg Gynecol Obstet 1924;38:287–311.

162 Sampson JA. Intestinal adenomas of endometrial type: their importance and their relation to ovarian hematomas of endometrial type (perforating hemorrhagic cysts of the ovary) Archives of Surgery 1922;5:217–280:218.

163 Sampson JA. Intestinal adenomas of endometrial type. Archives of Surgery 1922;5:217–280:261. For the first time Sampson refers to his "theory." "This theory as to the origin of these ovarian hematomas and also their relation to endometrial implantations is based on the following data."

164 Sampson JA. Intestinal adenomas of endometrial type. Archives of Surgery 1922;5:217–280.

165 Sampson JA. Intestinal adenomas of endometrial type. Archives of Surgery 1922;5:217–280:261–262. Regarding size of ovarian hematomas of endometrial type, see pages 217–8. "The size of these hematomas was described in the previous paper as being usually between 2 and 4 cm. in diameter, occasionally less than 2 cm. and also occasionally larger than 4 cm. … I would modify the foregoing statement in regard to the size

failed to recognize the early stages of development and the later stages of regression and so overlooked many cases.[162] Likewise, in a manner reminiscent of Cullen, he experienced a long learning curve before he routinely recognized intestinal adenomas of endometrial type. Sampson described and illustrated various disease patterns associated with intestinal adenomas, their laterality and asymmetry, and the intimate association with ovarian hematomas of endometrial type. However, he did not address so-called adenomyomas of the rectovaginal septum, or endometrial adenomas that penetrated into the posterior vaginal fornix. Nonetheless, interspersed within the text, Sampson provided insights into the pathogenesis of intestinal adenomas as well as the pathogenesis of the obliterated rectovaginal pouch of Douglas.

For the first time Sampson laid out the essential features of his *second theory* – his theory of retrograde menstruation, implantation, and invasion and the origin of ovarian hematomas of endometrial type.[163] I believe Sampson's crucial insight for the *second theory* that he announced in the Transactions of the American Gynecological Society for the year 1921 came when he observed *tubal epithelium* in a minority of his cases of sigmoid adenomas of endometrial type. Invariably, in this paper Sampson gives precedence to tubal epithelium when referring to tubal and uterine epithelium. I believe Sampson's giving precedence to tubal epithelium is important if subtle clue that his observation of tubal epithelium sparked the insight to his *second theory.*[164]

Sampson's second theory as to the origin of these ovarian hematomas and also their relation to endometrial implantation is based on the following data. Sampson specified: "The ovarian hematomas are of endometrial type as shown by their structure, function (reaction to menstruation) and their endometrial implantations. They are rarely found in women under 30 years of age. If of developmental origin, we would expect to find them in younger women. They develop during the menstrual life of the patient in a period when *tubal and uterine epithelium might escape from the fimbriated end of the tube and become deposited on the surface of the ovary* just as peritoneal implantations arise from perforation of ovarian hematomas. (Italics added) In 49 cases of perforated ovarian hematomas which I have studied, the tubes were apparently patent in all, suggesting that this avenue for this source of implantation was open. These hematomas usually develop on the lateral and the under surfaces of the ovary, the portion of the ovary most likely to be soiled by material escaping from the lumen of the tube, as well seen in the ovarian adhesions found in *pelvic inflammatory disease* of gonorrheal origin, and they are also often bilateral. (Italics added) In 37 cases of ovarian hematomas of endometrial type with perforation, in which I have studied microscopically the tissues involved in the adhesions apparently resulting from escape of the contents of the cyst, adenoma of endometrial type was found in all but one specimen. On the other hand, in three cases of typical ovarian hematomas of endometrial type without any evidence of perforation, adhesions were not present in the pelvis and there was not any gross evidence of implantation adenomas; the pelvis was examined very carefully in each instance. In the cases of perforated ovarian hematoma with implantation, the extent of the implantation usually varied with the size of the hematoma and apparent size of the perforation. The larger the hematoma and the greater the size of the perforation the more extensive the distribution of the implantations."[165]

It was not until near the end of my research when I read Sampson's summary paper, *The development of the implantation theory for the origin of peritoneal* endometriosis published in 1940[166] that I realized my analysis of the origin of Sampson's *second theory* was incorrect.[167] Sampson's crucial insight for the *second theory* came not when he observed *tubal epithelium* in a minority of his cases of sigmoid adenomas of endometrial type. In 1940, Sampson recalled the crucial insight: "The detection of peritoneal endometriosis with and without ovarian involvement led to the second step in the development of the implantation theory. This consisted of strong circumstantial evidence indicating that bits of Müllerian tissue, derived from both the uterine and the tubal mucosa and carried by menstrual blood escaping through patent tubes into the peritoneal

by adding that they are often so small and inconspicuous that they may be easily missed both at the time of the operation and in the pathology laboratory."

[166] Sampson JA. The development of the implantation theory for the origin of peritoneal endometriosis. Am J Obstet Gynecol 1940;40:549–557.

[167] The historian analyzing prospectively runs into similar problems encountered by the clinician and scientist analyzing prospectively.

[168] Sampson JA. Am J Obstet Gynecol 1940;40: 549–557:555.

cavity, could become implanted on various pelvic structures including the ovaries, and the resulting perforating hemorrhagic ovarian cysts are only spectacular foci in the secondary spread of endometriosis."[168]

Adenomas of endometrial type [endometriosis] have characteristics of pelvic inflammatory disease and of cancer. Having drawn a first analogy between the location of ovarian adhesions of endometrial type and the location of ovarian adhesions resulting from pelvic inflammatory disease (see italics above), Sampson drew a second analogy; that between implantations of endometrial type and implantations resulting from cancer. "Intestinal adenomas of endometrial type are implantation growths, similar in many ways to those arising from a rupture or perforation of a malignant (carcinomatous) ovarian cyst."[169] Based on his first 12 cases, Sampson made important observations that have stood the test of time and provided further circumstantial evidence to support his theory of implantation adenomas. "The portions of the intestinal tract most frequently involved are those usually found in the pelvis; as the sigmoid,[170] rectum, appendix and terminal loop of the ileum."[171] He noted the asymmetry and laterality exhibited by intestinal adenomas. In six of eight cases of adenomas of the rectum and sigmoid colon the ovarian hematoma, "with evidence of a previous perforation, was situated in the left ovary." In all four cases of appendiceal adenomas "a similar hematoma was situated in the right ovary in all four."[172]

Even from such a small case series, Sampson recognized three characteristic patterns: (1) "Surface and superficial implantations"; (2) "implantations developing between folds of peritoneum and other adherent structures (pocketed implantations), best seen in the culdesac between the posterior wall of the uterus and the rectum, which are often fused together"; and (3) "the deep invasion of the underlying structure or organ. The tubules worm their way into the tissues of the intestine; and this is often associated with a marked hypertrophy of the surrounding connective tissue and muscle."[173] Sampson chose the expressive biological metaphor "worm"[174] instead of the military metaphor "invade" to express the less aggressive nature of benign intestinal adenoma of endometrial type compared to cancer. He continued: "Many varieties of endometrial tissue and its derivatives may be found, including glands and tubules with and without a characteristic endometrial stroma, dilated tubules, miniature uterine cavities,[175] hematomas, and the invasion of lymph vessels by endometrial polyps."[176]

---

[169] Sampson JA. Intestinal adenomas of endometrial type: their importance and their relation to ovarian hematomas of endometrial type (perforating hemorrhagic cysts of the ovary) Archives of Surgery 1922;5:217–280:277.

[170] Sampson JA. Intestinal adenomas of endometrial type: their importance and their relation to ovarian hematomas of endometrial type (perforating hemorrhagic cysts of the ovary) Archives of Surgery 1922;5:217–280:240. See Figure 27 (case 8) on page 240. This is a good illustration of the kinking of the sigmoid colon cause by implantation adenomas of the sigmoid colon.

[171] Sampson JA. Archives of Surgery 1922;5:217–280:277. See also: 218, 225. See Figure 59 (Case 12) This excellent illustration shows the ileum adherent to an adenoma of the posterior uterine fundus. The caption gives Sampson's interpretation of the pathogenesis of the lesion. "My interpretation of the etiology of this condition is as follows. At the previous operation, 4 years ago, some of the epithelium lining the hemorrhagic cyst of the left ovary became implanted on the posterior surface of the uterus and other portions of the pelvic contents and developed into implantation adenomas of endometrial type. The ileum became adherent to the implantation on the posterior surface of the uterus and was superficially invaded by it. The uterine wall was invaded to a much greater extent as indicated."

[172] Sampson JA. Archives of Surgery 1922;5:217–280:278.

[173] Sampson JA. Archives of Surgery 1922;5:217–280:278. Hypertrophy of surrounding tissues is a good example of the host response to the intrusion of the "tubules" of the adenoma.

[174] Sampson JA. Intestinal adenomas of endometrial type: their importance and their relation to ovarian hematomas of endometrial type (perforating hemorrhagic cysts of the ovary) Archives of Surgery 1922;5:217–280. See Figure 42 (Case 2) on page 251. "Section of the wall of the sigmoid which was excised. It shows a typical adenoma of endometrial type. The implantation apparently began on the peritoneal surface, possibly through an epiploic appendage, indicated by the arrow, and invaded the subserosa and then *wormed* its way through the muscularis forming hematomas." See also Figure 46 (Case 1) on page 254. "Section of the wall of the sigmoid showing an adenoma of endometrial type invading it…The adenoma first invaded the subserosa and then *wormed* its way through the muscularis forming a hematoma."

[175] Sampson JA. Intestinal adenomas of endometrial type: their importance and their relation to ovarian hematomas of endometrial type (perforating hemorrhagic cysts of the ovary) Archives of Surgery 1922;5:217–280:252. See Figure 43 (Case 2) "A small uterine cavity found in a section of the wall of the sigmoid."

[176] Sampson JA. Archives of Surgery 1922;5:217–280:278. See Figure 44 (Case 2) on page 252. "Endometrial polyp invading a lymph vessel in the submucosa of the sigmoid. These polyps are frequently found in implantation adenomas of endometrial type." See also Figure 45 (Case 2) on page 253. "Implantation adenoma (a) on the surface of the broad ligament and invading a lymph vessel in the broad ligament. Two endometrial polyps (e, p) are shown, the large one came from the adenoma (b) of this illustration. The invasion of the lymph vessels by these

Sampson fashioned a "syndrome rarely furnished by any other condition," by gathering symptoms and signs of women between the ages of 30 and the menopause who complained of "acquired dysmenorrhea or recent increase in menstrual pain…disturbance of intestinal function during menstruation," and who on examination were found to have "a small adherent ovarian cyst or adherent ovary and palpatory findings [tenderness or nodules] in the culdesac."[177] Sampson noted that the majority of intestinal implants were insignificant but potentially invasive. But some become important when they interfere with the function of the intestine causing "marked constipation, partial obstruction, painful bowel movements and pressure sensations in the rectum during the menstrual period."[178] Sampson described the pathology and pathophysiology that leads to intestinal obstruction, once again analogous to carcinoma. "The disturbance of the function is then a mechanical one, as in carcinoma, namely, that of obstruction, and the obstruction in endometrial adenoma may be due to three factors: first, the constriction of the lumen of the bowel by growth and especially by the marked hypertrophy of the tissues surrounding the adenoma; second, by kinking the intestine, and third, by the accumulation of menstrual blood in the adenoma causing hematomas. The symptoms of obstruction may be more marked during the menstrual period, as at that time more blood may escape into the adenoma situated in the wall of the intestine…The implantation begins with the deposit of epithelium on the peritoneal surface of these structures. This epithelium sinks into the underlying tissues, and, true to its type, forms glands and tubules as shown in the previous communication. In some instances, a localized growth of endometrial mucosa arises like a polyp which may be sessile, or pedunculated, simulating the polyps found in the uterine cavity. In other instances the tubules invade the underlying tissue with very little evidence of the growth on the surface. The epithelium originally implanted may 'die out' or it may be covered with adhesions so that in some of the older lesions it may be impossible to determine the exact site of the original implantation. The tubules often burrow through the tissues in many directions and the portal of entry, if still present, may only be determined by cutting many sections, or better still by cutting serial sections."[179]

Sampson addressed the issue of pathogenesis of intestinal adenomas when he stated that "probably the principal source" of these benign intestinal implantation adenomas of endometrial type was "epithelium escaping from an ovarian hematoma of endometrial type which has perforated": this accorded with his *first theory* of pathogenesis.[180] Affirming that in his experience the "majority" of intestinal adenomas of endometrial type arose from perforated ovarian hematomas, Sampson interjected his *second theory* to explain a minority of cases. "There is the possibility that some of them may have arisen from *tubal and uterine epithelium* escaping through the fimbriated end of the tube, independent of an ovarian hematoma with perforation."[181]

Sampson addressed the issue of pathogenesis a second time when he asked the fundamental question: "How does this epithelium of endometrial type reach the ovary? Is it of developmental origin from the inclusion of epithelium of the müllerian or the Wolffian ducts or is it acquired during adult life?"[182] Note how the debate between von Recklinghausen and Cullen lingered in the background, and had to be acknowledged before Sampson provided his evidence to the contrary. He affirmed that this epithelium of endometrial type was müllerian and acquired during adult life by employing his *second theory*, now expanded to include retrograde shedding of tubal epithelium as well as retrograde shedding of uterine menstrual endometrium. "The evidence which I have, at present, suggests that it is usually (possibly always) acquired from the implantation on the surface of the ovary of *tubal or uterine*

adenomas suggests that they may metastasize through these channels and offers one explanation for the appearance of adenoma in the groin." Here Sampson has identified endometrial invasion of lymph vessels 2 years before Halban published his theory of lymphatic metastases in 1924.

177 Sampson JA. Archives of Surgery 1922;5:217–280:279.

178 Sampson JA. Archives of Surgery 1922;5:217–280:243–4.

179 Sampson JA. Archives of Surgery 1922;5:217–280:227–9.

180 Sampson JA. Archives of Surgery 1922;5:217–280:279.

181 Sampson JA. Archives of Surgery 1922;5:217–280:279.

182 Sampson JA. Intestinal adenomas of endometrial type: their importance and their relation to ovarian hematomas of endometrial type (perforating hemorrhagic cysts of the ovary) Archives of Surgery 1922;5:217–280:280. See also Figure 10 (case 4) page 226. "I believe that this adenoma of the uterus did not arise from the direct invasion of the uterine mucosa of the uterine cavity or from developmental inclusions of müllerian epithelium or from a metaplasia of the peritoneal mesothelium; but I believe it arose from the implantation of epithelium from the lining of a hemorrhagic cyst of the ovary which had perforated."

epithelium escaping through the fimbriated end of the tube and possibly from tubal fimbriae in contact with the ovary….I consider the ovary as an intermediary host, hotbed or incubator, which may impart increased vigor and virulence to this epithelium, so that when it escapes from the ovary it may be more virulent (malignant) and invasive than before the hematoma developed and the perforation occurred. It may not be an essential intermediary host, *for it is possible that pelvic implantations may arise from tubal and uterine epithelium escaping from the tube*; and also implantation from both sources may be present in the same case."[183] (Italics added) Elsewhere, Sampson opined similarly: "The most natural conception of their origin would be that they arise from developmentally misplaced müllerian epithelium (Russell) or from the invasion of tubal epithelium from the fimbriae in contact with the ovary. Tubules are sometimes present in the hilum of the ovary which are apparently of Wolffian duct origin and these might be considered as a source of these hematomas. The data which I have been able to obtain suggest that *tubal and uterine epithelial* cells may, under certain circumstances (as an abnormal menstruation with a backflow), be expelled from the fimbriated end of the tube and lodge on the surface of the ovary."[184]

However, Sampson favored the perforated ovarian adenoma of endometrial type as intermediate host because he believed incubation in the ovarian adenoma imparted added vigor or virulence to the endometrial tissue implanted there from the fallopian tube as well as accounting for the "wideness of distribution" of intestinal implants. Sampson argued: "Implantation carcinoma of the various organs and structures of the peritoneal cavity is well recognized both by pathologists and clinicians and likewise the important part played by ovarian carcinoma as a source of these implantations. Implantations adenomas of endometrial type are analogous to those of carcinoma."[185] Sampson would not credit the serosal/coelomic metaplasia theory.[186]

The operative treatment of intestinal adenomas of endometrial type was unsettled in 1922. At surgery upon detecting an intestinal lesion, Sampson carefully examined all pelvic structures for other evidence of implantation adenomas of endometrial type, especially searching for any signs of a perforated ovarian hematoma of any size. "If evidence found indicates an adenoma of endometrial type [and not carcinoma] I do not disturb the intestinal lesion, except as it may be easily removed for histologic study, but deal with the pelvic organs as their condition requires."[187] When surgical menopause was acceptable to his patients, Sampson preferred to ignore the intestinal lesions and perform a total hysterectomy and remove both tubes and ovaries, believing that the surgical menopause resulting would accomplish the same good results that he had observed with natural menopause.[188] Sampson made no mention of any adverse effects of surgical menopause. We may assume that Sampson believed spontaneous and surgi-

---

[183] Sampson JA. Archives of Surgery 1922;5:217–280:280. Note how often Sampson mentions tubal epithelium. See text page 258. "The data which I have been able to obtain suggest that tubal and uterine epithelial cells may, under certain circumstances (as an abnormal menstruation with a backflow), be expelled from the fimbriated end of the tube and lodge on the surface of the ovary."

[184] Sampson JA. Archives of Surgery 1922;5:217–280:258–9.

[185] Sampson JA. Archives of Surgery 1922;5:217–280:224–225. See also Figure 9 (Case 4) page 226. "Photomicrograph of an implantation adenoma (of endometrial type) on the surface of the left tube…Histologically it resembles normal endometrium. It is analogous to the implantation carcinoma shown in Figure 2." (page 220).

[186] Sampson JA. Archives of Surgery 1922;5:217–280:242. See Figure 29 (Case 8) on page 242. "Implantation adenoma invading the wall of the uterus. Photomicrograph of a portion of the uterine wall through one of the pits. The arrow indicates the bottom of the pit between the adhesions. The adenoma on the surface of the uterus is here shown invading the wall of the uterus." See also Figure 30 (Case 8) page 242. "Implantation adenoma on the surface of the uterus. The photomicrograph shows a polypoid condition of the endometrium lining the bottom of a wide pit which has been exposed by freeing the uterus from the adherent sigmoid colon." Finally, see Figure 60, page 271. "Adenoma of endometrial type of the posterior uterine wall and superficially invading the wall of the ileum which is fused to the uterus at this place…It only superficially invaded the wall of the intestine but has extensively invaded the uterine wall, giving rise to a typical so-called adenomyoma of the uterus, not arising from the direct invasion of the uterine mucosa from the uterine cavity or from the developmental inclusions of müllerian epithelium in the uterine wall or from a metaplasia of the peritoneal mesothelium but from the implantation of endometrial epithelium from the epithelia lining of a perforated hemorrhagic cyst of the ovary (of endometrial type), as probably the majority of the ectopic pelvic adenomyomas (of endometrial type) shown in this and the previous communication arose."

[187] Sampson JA. Archives of Surgery 1922;5:217–280:279. Ibid: 249.

[188] Sampson JA. Intestinal adenomas of endometrial type: their importance and their relation to ovarian hematomas of endometrial type (perforating hemorrhagic cysts of the ovary) Archives of Surgery 1922;5:217–280:279.

cal menopause to be benign physiological states. As of 1922, Sampson had encountered only one postmenopausal patient with evidence of "an undoubted ovarian hematoma of endometrial type, with its associated implantation adenomas."[189]

As had Lockyer, Cullen, and others, Sampson misdiagnosed his first case of adenomyoma of the sigmoid colon (February 10, 1909) as a carcinoma and performed a segmental resection, the first of only two such resections he performed for bowel adenomas between 1909 and 1922.[190] Sampson went on to describe the patterns of pelvic disease associated with intestinal adenomas of endometrial type. He illustrated four cases observed from the point of view of the surgeon: (1) a case of implantation adenoma of endometrial type involving the sigmoid colon with obliteration of the rectovaginal pouch of Douglas,[191] (2) a case of 'left frozen pelvis' associated with partial obliteration of the rectovaginal pouch of Douglas,[192] (3) another case of 'left frozen pelvis,' with sparing of the right tube and ovary,[193] and (4) a case of a completely frozen pelvis, with centripetal adherence of all structure to the uterus.[194] Sampson also illustrated three cases of obliteration of the rectovaginal pouch of Douglas. In each case, giant sagittal sections were cut through the uterus, vagina, and adherent rectum showing obliteration of the rectovaginal pouch of Douglas.[195] Sampson attributed the pathogenesis of obliteration of the rectovaginal pouch of Douglas to implantation adenoma of endometrial type and associated endometrial adhesive disease, not to müllerian rests or uterine mucosa "springing from" the back of the cervix or uterus as Cullen had postulated when describing the pathogenesis of adenomyomas of the rectovaginal septum.

---

[189] Sampson JA. Archives of Surgery 1922;5:217–280:217.

[190] Sampson JA. Archives of Surgery 1922;5:217–280:219–220.

[191] Sampson JA. Archives of Surgery 1922;5:217–280:222. See Figure 4 (Case 4).

[192] Sampson JA. Archives of Surgery 1922;5:217–280:230. See Figure 14 (case 5). See also Ronald E. Batt, "Conservative and complete operations by laparotomy," in *Text and Atlas of Female Infertility Surgery,* ed. Robert B. Hunt, 3rd ed. [St. Louis, MO: Mosby, 1999], 412–439:424–5. "As reproductive surgeons treat increasingly severe cases of endometriosis they encounter the left-frozen pelvis. A large ovarian endometrioma is fused to the broad ligament and ureter, with the oviduct sandwiched between the ovary and broad ligament, or adherent to tubal or antimesenteric border of the ovary, and the whole completely enveloped by sigmoid colon in obliterative adhesive disease."

[193] Sampson JA. Archives of Surgery 1922;5:217–280:239. See Figure 26 (case 8) page 239.

[194] Sampson JA. Intestinal adenomas of endometrial type: their importance and their relation to ovarian hematomas of endometrial type (perforating hemorrhagic cysts of the ovary) Archives of Surgery 1922;5:217–280:234 See Figure 19 (case 10) on page 234. The completely frozen pelvis with centripetal adherence of all pelvic organs to the uterus is the most devastating form of pelvic adenomata of endometrial type from the viewpoint of the infertile couple. Ronald E. Batt, "Abdominopelvic diagnostic laparoscopy," in *Text and Atlas of Female Infertility Surgery,* ed. Robert B. Hunt, 3rd ed. [St. Louis, MO: Mosby, 1999], 372–385:376–377. Complex disease patterns: (1) Partial and complete obliteration of the rectovaginal pouch. "Partial obliteration of the rectovaginal pouch usually indicates deep, nodular, invasive disease of one uterosacral ligament and sometimes of pararectal or rectal tissue adherent to it. Complete obliteration usually is associated with deep, nodular, invasive disease of both uterosacral ligaments, posterior cervix, and rectum…Centrifugal pattern: The predominant pattern of endometriosis is centrifugal, with adnexa adherent laterally to posterior broad ligaments with or without obliterative disease of the rectovaginal pouch … Centripetal: The centripetal pattern is a less common but more severe form of disease. The uterus is retroflexed, retroverted, and adherent to itself and to the rectum, with complete obliteration of the rectovaginal pouch and adherence of both ovaries to the posterior uterus and side of the rectum…Left frozen pelvis: This pattern is characterized by a large ovarian endometrioma fused to the broad ligament over the ureter, with the oviduct adherent between the ovary and broad ligament or adherent to the tubal pole and antimesenteric border of the ovary, and the whole enveloped by the sigmoid colon in dense obliterative adhesions. It develops spontaneously when the sigmoid colon envelops the left adnexa to contain chocolate debris from repeated ruptures of left ovarian endometriomas. It also may develop in response to surgical intervention. In both instances, the left adnexa often is damaged irreparably. Intravenous pyelogram is recommended to detect partial or complete obstruction of the left ureter.,,, Complete frozen pelvis: Frozen pelvis represents the most complex and severe pattern. It is the final expression of aggressive endometriosis, impaired host immune defenses, and often numerous attempts at medical and surgical treatment. The patient's health may be threatened."

[195] Sampson JA. Archives of Surgery 1922;5:217–280. See Figure 18 (Case 5), page 233. Sagittal section of the myomatous uterus and adjacent pelvic structures indicating the condition present prior to the operation. The adenoma of endometrial type is shown fusing the cervix to the rectum and superficially invading these structures. Also illustrated is a sagittal section of a hematoma of the left ovary. See also Figure 25 (Case 10) page 238. "Condition prior to the operation, as seen in sagittal section of the uterus and adjacent structures. The implantation adenoma lodging and growing in the culdesac has invaded both the uterus and the rectum fusing these parts, and has extended downward between the rectum and the vagina to the right of the cervix (the perforated hematoma was in the right ovary) forming a tumor which could be distinctly felt before operation both on vaginal and rectal palpation." See also Figure 41 (Case 2) on page 250.

9 Life History of Ovarian Endometriomas

Life History of Ovarian Hematomas of Endometrial Type

In a powerful opening statement, Sampson compared the prevalence at operation of "the pathologic conditions arising from the implantations of epithelium which escape from the fallopian tubes into the peritoneal cavity" as second in prevalence only to leiomyomas of the uterus in women between the age of 30 years and menopause.[1] Here in the short span of only 2 years after Cullen's last major publication, Sampson spoke of pelvic adenomas and ovarian hematomas of endometrial type as a common disease entity of women in their fourth and fifth decades. He clarified new terminology used in the title of this paper. "I have discarded the term 'perforating hemorrhagic cysts' as applied to this condition, because perforations may occur in other varieties of ovarian hematomas. I now refer to them as hematomas or hemorrhagic cysts of endometrial (müllerian) type."[2]

Sampson addressed the relative virulence of primary and secondary implantations explicitly and in so doing, articulated the active life history, origin, growth, development, and perforation of ovarian hematomas of endometrial type. "The epithelium primarily giving rise to these implantations is derived from or through the fimbriated ends of the fallopian tubes. It lodges either on the surface of the ovaries or on the peritoneal surface of the other pelvic structures, especially those in the cul-desac, or on both the ovaries and the pelvic peritoneum, and develops into glands or tubules (adenomas) of endometrial (müllerian) type.[3] The primary peritoneal implantation adenomas are usually small and insignificant, but may spread and become invasive. The implantations on the ovary invade tissues of that organ, and as a result of their reaction to menstruation develop into superficial or deep hematomas (hemorrhagic or menstruating cysts) of endometrial (müllerian) type, which usually perforate into the peritoneal cavity. Perforation occurs in the superficial ovarian hematomas while they are still small, a few millimeters in diameter. On the other hand, the hematomas developing in the deeper tissues of the ovary may attain a much larger size, from 1 to 9 cm. in diameter before perforation occurs. The material escaping from the perforation of the ovarian hematoma, whether the latter is small or large, may carry with it epithelium which is cast off from its lining by menstruation. This epithelium may give rise to secondary implantations, which are often apparently more invasive, and have a wider distribution than the primary (original) pelvic implants."[4]

In passing, Sampson recognized the ovarian lesions as a possible source of carcinoma.[5] However, he regarded the ovary as a nonessential "intermediary

[1] Sampson, JA. The life history of ovarian hematomas (hemorrhagic cysts) of endometrial (müllerian) type. American Journal of Obstetrics and Gynecology 1922;4:451–512:451.

[2] Sampson, JA. American Journal of Obstetrics and Gynecology 1922;4:451–512:452:454.

[3] Note how unsettled and awkward the terminology at this juncture: glands or tubules (adenomas) of endometrial (müllerian) type.

[4] Sampson, JA. The life history of ovarian hematomas (hemorrhagic cysts) of endometrial (müllerian) type. American Journal of Obstetrics and Gynecology 1922;4:451–512:451–452. Sampson raised the perennial question, how does the surgeon distinguish, which lesions are more likely to become invasive?

[5] Sampson, JA. American Journal of Obstetrics and Gynecology 1922;4:451–512:452.

R.E. Batt, *A History of Endometriosis*,
DOI 10.1007/978-0-85729-585-9_9,

host" for the development of implantation adenoma of müllerian type.[6] If nonessential, then why did Sampson devote this communication to the life history of ovarian hematomas of endometrial type? He labeled the ovarian "intermediary host" model nonessential in his effort to explain the origin of endometrial (müllerian) type tissue on the surface of the ovary and in ovarian hematomas by his *second theory* of transtubal retrograde menstruation. Likely, he then realized that his *second theory*, that of transtubal retrograde menstruation of viable endometrial cells through the narrow and often tortuous lumen of isthmus of the fallopian tubes, would be difficult to prove, let alone easily accepted by the medical profession. Witness Meigs' enthusiastic acceptance of Sampson *first theory,* while merely describing Sampson's *second theory* as one among several others that attempted to explain the origin of ovarian hematomas of endometrial type.[7]

I believe Sampson launched his more controversial *second theory,* the retrograde menstruation and implantation model, to a highly sophisticated audience at the Harvard Medical Society and then let it drift. Meanwhile, he concentrated on gaining acceptance of his *first theory* of pathogenesis, the ovarian "intermediary host" model. Both theories of implantation rested upon the seed and soil metaphor. "Should the cyst rupture, the hemorrhagic contents, including epithelium and stroma cells, would escape into the peritoneal cavity. Should the epithelium fall on suitable soil, implantation adenoma would arise, which I have designated as secondary implantations, in contradistinction to the primary ones arising from the tube."[8]

Sampson was groping for the right terminology. He replaced one awkward and nonspecific term, "perforating hemorrhagic cysts" with the more specific but still imperfect term "hematomas or hemorrhagic cysts of endometrial (müllerian) type."[9] He could not yet decide, which adjective was more correct: endometrial (anatomic term) or müllerian (embryologic term). Sampson explained: "I have used the term ovarian hematomas of endometrial type rather than endometrial hematomas because I believed that in some instances the epithelium lining them may possibly be derived primarily from the tubal mucosa. The term müllerian would be inclusive and a better one."[10]

Sampson hinted at the complexity of the pathogenesis of endometriosis when he asked: "Is it possible to decide whether a given implantation adenoma was primarily derived from tubal or uterine mucosa? I do not think it can be definitely proved in any instance but the histologic structure of some of these adenomas suggests a tubal, and others a uterine, origin. Adenomyoma of the uterus and of the tube may be classified as ether primary or secondary. In primary adenomyoma the adenomatous growth is derived from the direct invasion of the uterine or tubal wall by the mucosa lining their cavities. In the secondary type of growth, which in my experience is the much more frequent variety, the uterine or tubal wall is invaded by epithelium implanted on its peritoneal surface, which is derived from the perforation of an ovarian hematoma of endometrial type or from or through the fimbriated extremity of the tube. It is obviously possible that the epithelium giving rise to a secondary adenomyoma of the uterus might be derived primarily either from the tubal or the uterine mucosa, and the same is true of secondary adenomyoma of the tube."[11]

Yet, Sampson could not bring himself to use the term müllerian, except bracketed by parentheses. He continued his explication of the life history of ovarian hematomas of endometrial type: "the most natural conception of the source of these tubules is from an abnormal

[6] Sampson, JA. American Journal of Obstetrics and Gynecology 1922;4:451–512:452.

[7] Meigs, JV. Endometrial hematomas of the ovary. Boston Med Surg J 1922:187:1–13.

[8] Sampson, JA. The life history of ovarian hematomas (hemorrhagic cysts) of endometrial (müllerian) type. American Journal of Obstetrics and Gynecology 1922;4:451–512:474. See description accompanying Fig. 29. - Plate III (Case 5) on the bottom of page 474. See also the text on page 478, which reads: When "perforation [of the ovarian cyst] occurs and some of the contents of the cyst escapes into the peritoneal cavity carrying with it epithelial cells which apparently give rise to implantation adenomas wherever the epithelium falls on suitable 'soil.'"

[9] Sampson, JA. American Journal of Obstetrics and Gynecology 1922;4:451–512:454. "I have discarded the term "perforating hemorrhagic cysts" as applied to this condition, because the perforations may occur in other varieties of ovarian hematomas. I now refer to them as hematomas or hemorrhagic cysts of endometrial (müllerian) type. Their epithelial lining, where present, is similar to that found in the hematomas due to the retention of "menstrual" blood, which occur in the adenomyomas of the uterus derived from the uterine mucosa, and the blood in the ovarian hematomas is also apparently of menstrual origin."

[10] Sampson, JA. American Journal of Obstetrics and Gynecology 1922;4:451–512:457.

development of the surface epithelium of the ovary [coelomic metaplasia] or from developmentally misplaced epithelium of the müllerian duct [müllerian rests]."[12]

Ruminating on the idea of developmentally misplaced epithelium, Sampson considered the age of minute adenomas he observed.[13] He began questioning the 30 year lower-age boundary. "These hematomas are unusual in women under thirty years of age and if they were developmental and not of acquired origin we would expect them to occur in younger women, soon after puberty."[14] Sampson continued: "They develop during the menstrual life of the patient, when tubal and uterine epithelium would be more likely to escape from or through the fimbriated end of the tube than before puberty and after the menopause."[15] Then, Sampson seemed to contradict himself, allowing the possibility before puberty and after the menopause. "It is possible that the implantation on the ovary of epithelium derived from or through the tube may occur before puberty and after the menopause, and may develop into ovarian cysts or even carcinoma."[16] How can one account for this a seemingly contradictory statement from a careful observer, an observer that Johann Wolfgang von Goethe, Johannes Müller, and Friedrich Wilhelm Karl Heinrich Alexander von Humboldt undoubtedly would embrace? Perhaps, Sampson was attempting to distance himself even further from the embryologic theory of pathogenesis in order to open space for his audience to receive his implantation theory. Realizing the unsettled state of endometriotic theory, *Sampson* presented a cogent argument to level the field of debate: "it is difficult to disprove any of these theories."[17]

Sampson asserted: "We have abundant proof that apparently normal uterine and tubal epithelium may be invasive, as demonstrated in the development of 'adenomyoma' from the invasion of the uterine and tubal wall by the epithelium lining these cavities."[18] He described the experiments of a colleague from Albany Medical College and Albany Hospital, the pathologist Jacobson, who conducted the first experiments to test Sampson's implantation theory.[19] Sampson believed that Jacobson had proved experimentally that rabbit uterine mucosa could be transplanted and "give rise to adenoma of endometrial type resembling those described by me except for the absence of any reaction to menstruation; furthermore some of the transplantations made by him in the ovary developed into 'ovarian cysts.'"[20] Sampson and his audience were aware that the experiment did not address the issue of transtubal retrograde menstruation, but it did support Sampson's theory of secondary peritoneal implantation following perforation of an ovarian cyst of endometrial type.

Satisfied that he had presented substantial clinical, pathological, and experimental evidence in support of his *first theory* of implantation from ruptured ovarian hematomas of endometrial type, Sampson presented circumstantial evidence to support his *second theory*, that of transtubal retrograde menstruation. He demonstrated that under normal circumstances "the fimbriated end of the [fallopian] tube is frequently situated beneath or lateral to the ovary, with the opening directed towards the surface of that organ by the 'tether' like action of the free margin of the mesosalpinx (tubal tether, t.t.) to which the lower fimbriae of the tube are often attached."[21]

[11] Sampson, JA. The life history of ovarian hematomas (hemorrhagic cysts) of endometrial (müllerian) type. American Journal of Obstetrics and Gynecology 1922;4:451–512:457–458.

[12] Sampson, JA. American Journal of Obstetrics and Gynecology 1922;4:451–512:461.

[13] Sampson, JA. American Journal of Obstetrics and Gynecology 1922;4:451–512:462. Ibid: 468, Fig. 16. (Case 16). "Photomicrographs…of the adenomas of endometrial (müllerian) type invading the lateral surface of the right ovary and posterior surface of the uterus…Their histological structure is similar, and I believe that they both have a common origin from epithelium escaping from or through the fallopian tube. It is impossible to decide, from their structure, whether the epithelium was derived from the tubal or the uterine mucosa."

[14] Sampson, JA. American Journal of Obstetrics and Gynecology 1922;4:451–512:462.

[15] Sampson, JA. American Journal of Obstetrics and Gynecology 1922;4:451–512:463.

[16] Sampson, JA. The life history of ovarian hematomas (hemorrhagic cysts) of endometrial (müllerian) type. American Journal of Obstetrics and Gynecology 1922;4:451–512:463.

[17] Sampson, JA. American Journal of Obstetrics and Gynecology 1922;4:451–512:462.

[18] Sampson, JA. American Journal of Obstetrics and Gynecology 1922;4:451–512:465.

[19] Jacobson VC. The autotransplantation of endometrial tissue in the rabbit. Archives Surgery 1922;5:281–300.

[20] Sampson, JA. American Journal of Obstetrics and Gynecology 1922;4:451–512:465–466.

[21] Sampson, JA. The life history of ovarian hematomas (hemorrhagic cysts) of endometrial (müllerian) type. American Journal of Obstetrics and Gynecology 1922;4:451–512:453. Quotation from the legend under Figure 1.

Sampson described in detail his *second theory* of pathogenesis of primary ovarian and pelvic adenomas of endometrial (müllerian) type. "This mechanism of the 'tubal tether' would facilitate the ovum's escape into the lumen of the tube in ovulation: this same close anatomical relation between the fimbriated end of the tube and the surface of the ovary would also permit epithelium, escaping from the fimbriated end of the tube or through its lumen, to become implanted on the surface of the ovary. The various physiologic changes in the pelvic contents would also cause the fimbriated end of the tube to brush against the structures in the culdesac. Should implantation adenoma arise from the epithelium escaping from the tube, we should expect to find these implantations most frequently on the lateral and under surface of the ovaries, and on the posterior surface of the lower portions of the broad ligament, the uterus and in the bottom of the culdesac; especially about the uterine attachments of the uterosacral ligaments. It is in these situations that the early implantation adenomas are most often found."[22]

Sampson did not include adenomas of endometrial type, which involved the intestinal tract as early lesions, nor did he attribute them to spilled endometrial epithelium from the fallopian tubes. Rather, he believed they "could have arisen from epithelium escaping from a perforated ovarian hematoma."[23] Then, as if he intended to deemphasize the role of the perforated ovarian hematoma and reemphasize the role of the fallopian tube, Sampson recalled explicitly: "On February 14, 1922, before the Harvard Medical Society at Boston, Mass., I reviewed in a general way the entire subject of ovarian hematomas and implantation adenomas of endometrial type. As stated at that meeting my interpretation of the origin and development of these implantations adenomas was as follows: Tubal and uterine epithelium at times escapes into the peritoneal cavity from or through the fimbriated end of the tube."[24]

He reviewed data, which he believed supported his *second theory of* implantation theory. The uterus is often retroflexed; the fallopian tubes "were apparently patent in all" cases;[25] he stressed the effect of the tubal tether, the fimbriated end of the tube "is usually found behind the ovary or below and mesial to it[26];" and finally Sampson noted that "as women spend the greater portion of the 24 h of the day with the body in the upright posture, whether sitting down or standing, the tendency for the fimbriated end of the tube to be tucked beneath, or lateral to, the ovary would be increased, and 'sediment' escaping from the tube would naturally settle on the lateral and the under surface of the ovary and in the bottom of the culdesac, *especially its anterior portion.*"[27] (Italics added)

By explaining that the preferential implantation of shed endometrial and tubal epithelium on the anterior portion of the rectovaginal pouch of Douglas (culdesac) resulted from the combined effects of gravity and female anatomy – the lowest portion of the culdesac being *its anterior portion*, Sampson provided a forceful and concise explanation for Cullen's observation that the anterior or retrocervical portion was the very location in which adenomyomas of the so-called rectovaginal septum originated. From that initial retrocervical location, adenomyomas might stay localized, or penetrate anteriorly into the vagina, or grow posteriorly to invade the rectum, or both; in the latter situation resulting in a frozen pelvis with the rectum firmly fused by dense adhesions to the uterus and the pelvic portion of the cervix.

Continuing the image of "upright posture," Sampson stressed that the distribution of pelvic implantation adenomas of endometrial type arising from the perforation of benign ovarian hematomas corresponded with the distribution of "implantations of carcinoma from the perforation of a malignant ovarian cyst."[28] To complete the correspondence between malignant and benign ovarian cysts and to add emphasis to the extensive pelvic adhesive

[22] Sampson, JA. American Journal of Obstetrics and Gynecology 1922;4:451–512:453. Quotation from the legend under Figure 1.

[23] Sampson, JA. The life history of ovarian hematomas (hemorrhagic cysts) of endometrial (müllerian) type. American Journal of Obstetrics and Gynecology 1922;4:451–512:455. See also Sampson JA. Intestinal adenomas of endometrial type: their importance and their relation to ovarian hematomas of endometrial type (perforating hemorrhagic cysts of the ovary). Archives of Surgery 1922;5:217–280.

[24] Sampson, JA. American Journal of Obstetrics and Gynecology 1922;4:451–512:456.

[25] Sampson, JA. American Journal of Obstetrics and Gynecology 1922;4:451–512:463.

[26] Sampson, JA. American Journal of Obstetrics and Gynecology 1922;4:451–512:466.

[27] Sampson, JA. American Journal of Obstetrics and Gynecology 1922;4:451–512:467.

disease associated with ovarian carcinoma, Sampson made a particularly cogent observation. "All specimens of extensive implantation adenomas which I have studied have been associated with an ovarian hematoma of endometrial type, with evidence of perforation."[29]

Still holding the image of "upright posture," Sampson discussed the distribution of pelvic lesions involving 15 cases formed in the absence of "gross evidence of an ovarian hematoma with perforation."[30] His study suggested "that the epithelium from which the implantation arose was derived from the tubal mucosa in some, and from the uterine mucosa (menstruation with a back flow through the tube) in others."[31] Sampson continued: "It was interesting to note the character of the implantations when there was no gross evidence of an ovarian hematoma with perforation. They were usually smaller, less invasive, and not as widely distributed as those generally found in the pelvis associated with an ovarian hematoma with evidence of perforation."[32] Not only did Sampson discern a difference in the distribution pattern, he also observed a histological difference. "Many of them also presented a little different histologic picture; they usually did not resemble typical endometrium as closely as did the implantations which were associated with an ovarian hematoma with perforation."[33]

Recall that this, his third case series, represented early stages of the disease.[34] Sampson was taking great pains to describe the appearance and distribution of peritoneal and ovarian adenomas of endometrial and tubal type and he needed to see these implants in the early stage of their life history. Did Sampson use a proctoscope inserted through a small incision in the abdomen to detect early implants in the rectovaginal pouch of Douglas? In other words, instead of observing through a large laparotomy incision, did Sampson use a large-bore proctoscope to examine the pelvis in patients he suspected had early implantation adenomas of endometrial and tubal type, as gynecologists would use a laparoscope later in the twentieth century? I suspect he may have done so. By inserting a proctoscope – a round rectal speculum – through a small incision in the lower abdomen and then by placing the patient in head down steep Trendelenburg position, a position that would allow the intestines to slide up toward the diaphragms, Sampson could have obtained a clear visualization of the pelvis. But to attribute such foresight to Sampson is speculative and anachronistic without evidence that Sampson used a large-bore proctoscope.

In fact, there is indirect circumstantial evidence. While a resident at Johns Hopkins in 1903, Sampson published a method of controlling hemorrhage following pelvic surgery by packing the pelvis with gauze inserted through a proctoscope and maintaining counter pressure by packing the vagina with gauze.[35] The caption under Figure 3 of that paper reads: "Figure 3. Introduction of proctoscope into pelvis. The lower end of the abdominal incision has been opened, and the proctoscope has been inserted through the opening into the abdominal cavity, taking care to direct the end well forward against the bladder, so that the coils of the intestines will be displaced backwards. In this instance the uterus with appendages, have been removed leaving in the cervix. By removing the obturator the various portions of the pelvis may be inspected, and here one can see that there is a small accumulation of fluid in the pelvis."[36]

[28] Sampson, JA. The life history of ovarian hematomas (hemorrhagic cysts) of endometrial (müllerian) type. American Journal of Obstetrics and Gynecology 1922;4:451–512:468.

[29] Sampson, JA. American Journal of Obstetrics and Gynecology 1922;4:451–512:469.

[30] Sampson, JA. American Journal of Obstetrics and Gynecology 1922;4:451–512:469.

[31] Sampson, JA. American Journal of Obstetrics and Gynecology 1922;4:451–512:469–70.

[32] Sampson, JA. The life history of ovarian hematomas (hemorrhagic cysts) of endometrial (müllerian) type. American Journal of Obstetrics and Gynecology 1922;4:451–512:469.

[33] Sampson, JA. American Journal of Obstetrics and Gynecology 1922;4:451–512:469.

[34] Sampson, JA. American Journal of Obstetrics and Gynecology 1922;4:451–512:485. By early stage, Sampson meant an early stage of ovarian hematomas of endometrial type, ovarian hematomas that had not perforated. Specifically Sampson stated: "The cases reported in the present [third] series were chosen from those demonstrating the origin and development of ovarian hematomas of endometrial type and ovarian hematomas without perforation rather than from those with perforation and extensive implantations."

[35] Sampson JA. Control of hemorrhage following pelvic operations by packing the pelvis with gauze through a proctoscope and maintaining counter pressure by packing the vagina. Johns Hopkins Hosp Bull 1903;14:237–42.

[36] Fitzgerald WJ. John Albertson Sampson, MD: pioneer gynecologist, teacher, and researcher. NY State J Med 1966;66:-1244–7: 1246. Dr. Fitzgerald was a clinical instructor in the Department of Obstetrics and Gynecology, The Albany Medical College of Union University at the time of Sampson's death.

Fitzgerald wrote the historical note, with the quotation cited above, on the twentieth anniversary of Sampson's death. Of all of Sampson's publications, he cited only six, four related to cervical cancer, one to endometriosis, and the one concerning pelvic packing through a proctoscope. This would indicate to this writer that the proctoscopic packing procedure had been used in Albany since 1905 when Sampson became Professor of Gynecology and possibly was still used 20 years after Sampson's death. It is not difficult to imagine Sampson directing reflected light from a head-mirror, down the short but large-bore proctoscope to visualize early implants on the ovaries and pelvic peritoneum. Howard Kelly had devised such a head-mirror in 1883 for use in gynecology.[37]

Sampson returned to the life history of ovarian hematomas of endometrial type. He addressed the development and regression of superficial and deep ovarian hematomas of endometrial type, noting that "the early stages of development of the deeper hematomas are the same as the early stages in the development of superficial hematomas."[38] He postulated that in superficial hematomas, "if all the epithelial lining is cast off by menstruation the life of the hemorrhagic cyst is ended, and all evidence of it may disappear."[39] With respect to deep ovarian hematomas of endometrial type, Sampson stated that "it was impossible in every instance to determine the source of the tubules from which the hematomas arose, but in many specimens it was evident that the hematoma had developed from a gland or tubule which had invaded the ovarian tissue from its surface…enough sections were made from some specimens to demonstrate that multiple small hematomas may arise in the tortuous course of a tubule, just as multiple ponds and lakes may arise in the course of a stream."[40] The life history of a deep ovarian hematoma may be prolonged by repeated rupture into the peritoneal cavity,[41] or it may grow so slowly that it remains quietly within the ovary without perforating and regresses after the menopause, [42] and lastly, "Some of these hemorrhagic cysts or hematomas lose all of their epithelial lining and 'die' before they reach the surface of the ovary and perforate."[43]

Sampson had only one opportunity to observe the effects of pregnancy on an ovarian hematoma of endometrial type. At hysterectomy and removal of both ovaries for uterine fibroids in a 37-year-old woman, he opened the uterus and found an early pregnancy.[44] From

[37] Kelly HA. An improved attachment for the head-mirror. Med News Philadelphia 1883:xliii:390.

[38] Sampson, JA. The life history of ovarian hematomas (hemorrhagic cysts) of endometrial (müllerian) type. American Journal of Obstetrics and Gynecology 1922;4:451–512:473.

[39] Sampson, JA. American Journal of Obstetrics and Gynecology 1922;4:451–512:472.

[40] Sampson, JA. American Journal of Obstetrics and Gynecology 1922;4:451–512:473.

[41] Sampson, JA. American Journal of Obstetrics and Gynecology 1922;4:451–512:478. Sampson believed "the escape of the contents of the cyst probably prolongs its life. It relieves tension and thus favors repair until the next reaction to menstruation." See page 510. "The hematomas developing in the deeper tissues of the ovary may attain a large size, several centimeters in diameter, before perforation occurs. As the menstrual blood is retained in the cavity of the hemorrhagic cyst and in the stroma of the lining for a long time, many interesting histologic changes occur in the wall of the cyst in the attempt to absorb the menstrual blood, and to reline the denuded surface by epithelium from that which had not been removed by menstruation. The development and activities of the endothelial leucocytes, which act as scavengers, play an important part in the absorption of the menstrual blood and the deposit of the pigment, derived from this blood, in the walls of the hematoma. Perforation permits the contents of the hematomas to escape into the peritoneal cavity, and may temporarily relieve the embarrassment caused by its retention. The perforation is sealed by the ovary or cyst becoming adherent to adjacent structures at the site of its perforation. The hematoma again fills up with blood at its next reaction to menstruation, and repeated perforations may occur. As the reaction to menstruation is destructive, and as the repair and regeneration of the epithelial lining is accomplished under great difficulties (due to the retention of the menstrual blood), the ultimate tendency of the hemorrhagic cyst is one of retrogression."

[42] Sampson, JA. American Journal of Obstetrics and Gynecology 1922;4:451–512:473. Sampson described the mechanism in detail on page 473–474.

[43] Sampson, JA. The life history of ovarian hematomas (hemorrhagic cysts) of endometrial (müllerian) type. American Journal of Obstetrics and Gynecology 1922;4:451–512:475.

[44] Sampson, JA. American Journal of Obstetrics and Gynecology 1922;4:451–512:504. See Fig. 66.-(Case 14) on page 504 entitled: Sagittal section of the uterus shown in the preceding illustration, demonstrating the early pregnancy (embryo 14 mm long) (x 3/5). You might ask, how could Sampson miss diagnosing this early pregnancy and avoid the hysterectomy? After all he describes the 37 year old woman as sterile and having wanted children. The answer is two-fold. First this was before pregnancy tests were available, moreover her periods or uterine bleeding was regular. Secondly, from examination of the illustration, there was a large intramural fibroid anteriorly, a smaller subserous fibroid protruding as a knob from the top of the uterus, and a large fibroid protruding from the posterior uterus. From my own clinical experience, the strategic position of the fibroids, which by their name reveals their fibrous nature, precludes any appreciation of softening of the underlying uterus associated with pregnancy.

this, it was obvious that the corpus luteum in the right ovary was a corpus luteum of pregnancy. He found "the hematoma of the left ovary was lined by typical decidual tissue, with the surface epithelium still present in the depressions. Histologically it was identical with that of the compact layer in the decidua vera of the pregnant uterus. Glands were not present in the lining of the ovarian hematoma."[45] Recall that while Sampson was still a resident at Johns Hopkins, J. Whitridge Williams had demonstrated decidual reaction in an adenomatous uterus at the autopsy of a woman who died shortly after delivery.[46] In Williams' case, the decidual reaction occurred in internal (uterine) endometriosis, whereas in Sampson's case, decidual reaction was observed in external (ovarian) endometriosis.

Once again Sampson addressed the differing ages of the small superficial lesions; indicating the implants represented different generations, indicative of the chronicity of the disease process. "If they have recently reacted to menstruation they are red in color, later bluish black. They are usually multiple, and are often found in various stages of development and retrogression in the same specimen, suggesting that they are not all of the same age."[47] This observation is perfectly compatible with his theory of repeated retrograde menstruation and implantation producing different generations of peritoneal disease.

Lastly, Sampson addressed the influence of menopause and old age on "ovarian hematomas (hemorrhagic cysts) of endometrial (müllerian) type." He based his comments on the two cases he had seen. In the first case, he found "caked" menstrual blood within the cavity of an ovarian hematoma "lined by a wavy hyaline membrane deeply pigmented with hemosiderin. The epithelial lining had completely disappeared."[48] The blood serum within the ovarian hematoma had been absorbed leaving behind the more solid "caked" residue. However, in the same menopausal women, he observed "implantation adenoma was present invading the posterior uterine wall, which histologically resembled the mucosa of the uterine cavity."[49] Sampson had not had time to thoroughly study the second case, but he did comment that an "epithelial lining was present" in two ovarian hematomas in a 59-year-old woman with endometrial carcinoma.[50]

Sampson presented the following evidence that the "hematomas or hemorrhagic cysts [were] of endometrial (müllerian) type."[51] First, he argued similar structure and function: "they develop from glands or tubules in the ovary which are lined by cuboidal or columnar epithelium (often ciliated) resembling tubal and uterine epithelium. Hemorrhage occurs in the ovarian tissue about the glands or tubules at the time of menstruation."[52] Second, he argued for histological similarity between these secondary ovarian lesions and primary adenomyomas of the uterus and fallopian tubes: "Histologically, the epithelial lining of the ovarian hematomas is similar to that of the hematomas and dilated cavities found in primary adenomyoma of the uterus and of the tube...Every variation in the histologic structure of the lining of the ovarian hematomas (often seen in different portions of the same hematoma) is due to different phases in its reaction to menstruation."[53] He concluded that "perforation of the hematoma is but a result of menstruation...but their reaction to menstruation, pregnancy, and old age is similar to that of the mucosa of the uterine cavity."[54]

Before he presented the 20 case reports, Sampson reminded his readers that his first case series published in 1921 and the second published in 1922, for the most part, represented "long standing [or] advanced stages of the disease."[55] In the 1921 case series, all the ovarian

[45] Sampson, JA. American Journal of Obstetrics and Gynecology 1922;4:451–512:481-482.

[46] J. Whitridge Williams. Decidual formation through the uterine muscularis: a contribution to the origin of adenomyoma of the uterus. Transactions of the Southern Surgical Association 1904;17:119.

[47] Sampson, JA. The life history of ovarian hematomas (hemorrhagic cysts) of endometrial (müllerian) type. American Journal of Obstetrics and Gynecology 1922;4:451–512:472.

[48] Sampson, JA. American Journal of Obstetrics and Gynecology 1922;4:451–512:583.

[49] Sampson, JA. American Journal of Obstetrics and Gynecology 1922;4:451–512:483.

[50] Sampson, JA. American Journal of Obstetrics and Gynecology 1922;4:451–512:483.

[51] Sampson, JA. American Journal of Obstetrics and Gynecology 1922;4:451–512:483.

[52] Sampson, JA. The life history of ovarian hematomas (hemorrhagic cysts) of endometrial (müllerian) type. American Journal of Obstetrics and Gynecology 1922;4:451–512:483.

[53] Sampson, JA. American Journal of Obstetrics and Gynecology 1922;4:451–512:483.

[54] Sampson, JA. American Journal of Obstetrics and Gynecology 1922;4:451–512:483–484.

[55] Sampson, JA. American Journal of Obstetrics and Gynecology 1922;4:451–512:485.

hematomas had evidence of perforation.[56] His second case series, published in 1922, included cases with implantation adenoma of endometrial type involving the intestinal tract.[57] This, his third case series, represented early stages of the disease. By early stage, Sampson meant an early stage of ovarian hematomas of endometrial type; ovarian hematomas that had not perforated. Sampson stated: "The cases reported in the present [third] series were chosen from those demonstrating the origin and development of ovarian hematomas of endometrial type and ovarian hematomas without perforation rather than from those with perforation and extensive implantations."[58]

However, on close examination of the cases, it is evident that, while they may well have represented the earliest cases Sampson could gather by 1922, they were not sufficient for his purposes. In cases 1, 6, 7, 9, and 14, the ovaries had perforated. In cases 10 and 11, Sampson indicated "? perforated."[59] In other instances such as cases 4, 5, 8, 13, 16, and 17, Sampson used such qualifiers as "probably arose from…could have arisen from…may have arisen from…suggested that…could have had a common origin."[60] In only four cases, cases 12, 15, 18 and 19, did Sampson have material that substantiated the opening statement in his conclusion: "Next to leiomyomas of the uterus, the pathologic conditions arising from the implantation of epithelium which escapes from the fallopian tubes into the peritoneal cavity probably furnish the most frequent pelvis lesions found in woman between the ages of 30 and the menopause."[61] I believe Sampson realized he needed more evidence. To his concluding rhetorical query of whether "the primary ovarian and peritoneal implantation (those developing from epithelium escaping from the fallopian tube) arise from both tubal and uterine epithelium," Sampson answered "the specimens which I have studied would suggest that they may."[62] He answered in the passive voice, and the operative word in his answer was "suggest." Nonetheless, he seems to have been convinced, as witnessed by a preview of work in progress. "I believe that the implantation adenomas in the ovary derived from tubal and uterine epithelium are the source of many ovarian cysts and carcinomas, and am convinced that two of the latter, which I am studying at the present time, arose from this source."[63]

[56] Sampson JA. Perforating hemorrhagic (chocolate) cysts of the ovary: their importance and especially their relation to pelvic adenomas of endometrial type ("Adenomyoma" of the uterus, rectovaginal septum, sigmoid, etc.) Archives of Surgery 1921;3:245–323.

[57] Sampson JA. Intestinal adenomas of endometrial type: their importance and their relation to ovarian hematomas of endometrial type (perforating hemorrhagic cysts of the ovary). Archives of Surgery 1922;5:217–280.

[58] Sampson, JA. The life history of ovarian hematomas (hemorrhagic cysts) of endometrial (müllerian) type. American Journal of Obstetrics and Gynecology 1922;4:451–512:485.

[59] Sampson, JA. American Journal of Obstetrics and Gynecology 1922;4:451–512:495–496.

[60] Sampson, JA. American Journal of Obstetrics and Gynecology 1922;4:451–512:488, 489, 493, 500, 503, 505.

[61] Sampson, JA. American Journal of Obstetrics and Gynecology 1922;4:451–512:509. See pages 497–498. Case 12: 41-year-old woman with "bilateral hematosalpinx and 'adenomyoma' of the distal ends of both tubes with extension through to their peritoneal surface, implantation adenoma of endometrial type on the posterior surface of the uterus, small intramural leiomyomas of the uterus (no evidence found of hematomas of endometrial type in the ovaries)." Sampson believed "that the adenoma on the posterior surface of the uterus arose from this source…miniature endometrial hematomas" in the distal end of both fallopian tubes.

See pages 501–502. Case 15: 36-year-old woman with implantation adenoma of endometrial type on the mesial surface of the right ovary and on the anterior surface of the uterus just below the attachment of the right round ligament. Sampson believed "that the implantations on the ovary and on the anterior surface of the uterus probably arose from epithelium escaping from the tube."

See page 506–507. Case 18: 22-year-old woman with implantation adenoma (of endometrial type) of the posterior uterine wall, culdesac, and posterior surface of the right broad ligament; retroflexion of the uterus. Sampson noted: "the uterus was found to be retroflexed and after replacing it a pigmented (hemorrhagic) elevation about 2 mm. in diameter was noticed on the posterior surface of the right uterine cornu, and a similar but broader elevation (implantation) was detected in the culdesac, at place which exactly came in contact with the implantation on the uterus when the latter was replaced in retroflexion. A similar implantation (but not hemorrhagic) was found on the posterior surface of the right broad ligament. Both tubes and ovaries appeared normal, and the latter were examined very carefully for implantation… These implantations were in situations which at times could have been in contact with the fimbriated end of the right fallopian tube, and I believe arose from epithelium escaping from the tube. The implantation on the surface of the uterus might have been a contact implantation from the one in the culdesac, or vise versa."

See page 507–509. Case 19: 32-year-old woman with implantation adenoma (of endometrial type) of the mesial surface of the right ovary, the right broad ligament between the tube and the ovary and on the suspensory ligament of the ovary; retroflexion of the uterus. "The situation of the implantation, especially the one directly in front of the fimbriated end of the tube, on the suspensory ligament of the ovary, would indicate that they arose from epithelium escaping from or through the fimbriated end of the tube."

In sum, Sampson had two theories of pathogenesis of implantation endometriosis: the *ovarian* and the *tubal* theories. He thought the *tubal* theory was in a preliminary state in 1922 and had to be presented guardedly even to as sophisticated an audience as the American Gynecological Society. There were still a lot of unknowns and Sampson's terminology reflected his state of partial understanding as he emphasized "The Life History of Ovarian Hematomas (Hemorrhagic Cysts) of Endometrial (Müllerian) Type."

President's Address: An Autobiographical Essay

John Albertson Sampson had been elected by unanimous vote to membership in the prestigious and excusive American Gynecological Society in 1906, 1 year after completing his residency in Gynecology at Johns Hopkins Hospital and 1 year after his appointment as Clinical Professor of Gynecology at Albany Medical College. Cullen, then emeritus Professor of Gynecology at Johns Hopkins, recorded in an obituary that "a letter has been preserved from Dr. Howard A. Kelly saying this [Sampson's case] is the only case where anyone ever received all the votes."[64] Such was the popularity and academic prowess of Sampson in 1906, already the author of 17 papers on gynecologic subjects.

On the occasion of his election to the presidency of the American Gynecological Society in 1923, Sampson chose to honor Theodore Roosevelt and Howard A. Kelly, role models of his youth and professional life, respectively.[65] In essence, this was an autobiographical essay that revealed the formative elements of Sampson; the botanist, the biologist, the surgeon, the investigator, the professor.

From Roosevelt, his youthful hero, he learned the importance of two hobbies as formative for a career in medicine, reading and the study of natural history. As a boy, Sampson, like Roosevelt, studied ornithology.[66] Both learned to observe and record observations, to apply themselves in mastering the subject and to draw their own conclusions. Sampson enumerated four qualities that he believed were largely responsible for Roosevelt's success in life: "first, his personality; second, his energy and persistence; third, the training in learning how to acquire knowledge derived in large part from his pursuit of ornithology; and fourth, his ability to impress people with his thoughts by his convincing speaking and forceful writing, i.e., his ability to use the English language. The hobbies of Roosevelt were of great value to him as a statesman; the same ones would likewise be of great value to a physician, for the habits and methods of observation, of recording observations, and arriving at a diagnosis in the study of ornithology could easily be applied to the study of medicine, both ornithology and medicine being branches of biology. Physicians, as well as statesmen, should know how to use the English language."[67]

Sampson recognized a fellow naturalist when he encountered Howard Kelly in medical school.[68] From Kelly the biologist, herpetologist, and consummate pelvic and abdominal surgeon, Sampson learned the fundamentals and fine points of his lifelong professional hobby, investigation of the malignant invasive disease – cervical cancer, and the benign invasive disease – endometriosis. Like Kelly, Sampson loved the out-of-doors. Whereas Kelly vacationed with Cullen every summer on the rivers and lakes in the bush country of Ontario, Canada; Sampson spent his leisure feeding wild animals and enjoying his woods, pond, and Adirondack-style Hawthorne Lodge in Grafton, New York. Employing a biological analogy,

---

[62] Sampson, JA. The life history of ovarian hematomas (hemorrhagic cysts) of endometrial (müllerian) type. American Journal of Obstetrics and Gynecology 1922;4:451–512:511.

[63] Sampson, JA. American Journal of Obstetrics and Gynecology 1922;4:451–512:512.

[64] Cullen TS. In Memoriam: John Albertson Sampson: 1873–1946. Trans Am Gynecol Society 1947:70:273–4.

[65] Cullen TS. In Memoriam. Trans Am Gynecol Society 1947:70:273–4. "Especially to Dr. Howard Kelly was Dr. Sampson indebted for the stimulating example of a great surgeon and God-loving man."

[66] Cullen TS. In Memoriam Trans Am Gynecol Society 1947:70:273–4. In 1890, at the age 17, Sampson "wrote a report on the evening grosbeak for *Forest and Stream*."

[67] Sampson JA. President's Address. Fundamental elements in the advancement of medicine. Am J Obstet Gynecol 1923;6:1–11:2–3.

[68] Sampson JA. President's Address. Am J Obstet Gynecol 1923;6:1–11:4, Kelly had a lifelong interest in botany and from this interest wrote a book entitled "Some American Medical Botanists." Kelly was also interested in poisonous snakes. Kelly HA. Poisonous snakes. Johns Hopkins Hosp Bull 1900;xi:73.

Sampson said: "Biology is the study of living beings, both plant and animal, including man, and medicine is but one of its many branches…There are two varieties of naturalists, the collector and the investigator. One answers the question *what* and the other the question *why.*[69] The botanist who collects answers the question *what* – and can always remain a botanist, but the one who studies the life history of plants and their struggle for existence, who answers the question *why,* must become a naturalist in the broadest sense of the word."[70]

Sampson spoke of premedical education and the basic sciences so important to the education of physicians: anatomy, physiology, chemistry, and pathology. "They are all indispensable for a better foundation in the study, diagnosis, treatment and prevention of disease, but they are inseparable from each other and from clinical medicine.[71] Of these basic sciences pathology is the most important, as it furnishes a definite understanding for the clinical study of disease, namely living pathology; and the two are inseparable."[72] Sampson then elucidated the theme of "living pathology" that guided his scientific research as it had that of Howard Kelly. "The clinician, especially the surgeon, has a wonderful opportunity to study living pathology, which the laboratory worker unfortunately rarely sees, except in experimental work on the lower animals. To do their best work and make their greatest contributions, clinicians should be fundamentally and eternally pathologists, and pathologists should, at least occasionally, be clinicians."[73]

By stressing the clinical aspects of disease and living pathology that naturally led to explanatory theory and therapeutic innovation,[74] Sampson reversed the reciprocal relationship between laboratory and clinic that Rokitansky had emphasized in mid-nineteenth century. The Danish physician and nosographers, Knud Faber, expressed Rokitansky's position clearly. "Rokitansky…in his textbook of 1846, drew the oft-cited conclusion 'that pathological anatomy should be the base not only of the knowledge of physicians but also of their practice, as it contains all there is in medicine of positive knowledge and the foundation of it!' With such views scientists had wandered far from the nosography of the English [Sydenham] and French [Bichat and Laennec], and landed in anatomical diagnosis of the purest and driest sort. Is it to be wondered that it brought with it a complete therapeutic nihilism in internal medicine."[75]

Having revealed his modus operandi, we can better appreciate Sampson's careful observations expressed in the title of his classic contribution to the pathogenesis of pelvic endometriosis:[76] *Peritoneal endometriosis due to the menstrual dissemination of endometrial tissue into the peritoneal cavity*, published in 1927.[77]

[69] Sampson JA. President's Address. Am J Obstet Gynecol 1923;6:1–11:5.

[70] Sampson JA. President's Address. Am J Obstet Gynecol 1923;6:1–11:4.

[71] Sampson JA. President's Address. Am J Obstet Gynecol 1923;6:1–11:8–9.

[72] Sampson JA. President's Address. Am J Obstet Gynecol 1923;6:1–11:11.

[73] Sampson JA. President's Address. Am J Obstet Gynecol 1923;6:1–11:9.

[74] T.K.A.B. Eskes and L.D. Longo, eds. *Classics in Obstetrics and Gynecology: Innovative Papers that Have Contributed to Current Clinical Practice* [Pearl River, NY: Parthenon Publishing Group, 1994], 277–236.

[75] Knud Faber, *Nosography in Modern Internal Medicine* [New York: Paul B. Hoeber, Inc., 1923], 57.

[76] T.K.A.B. Eskes and L.D. Longo, eds. *Classics in Obstetrics and Gynecology: Innovative Papers that Have Contributed to Current Clinical Practice* [Pearl River, NY: Parthenon Publishing Group, 1994], 277–236. The editors reprinted Sampson's paper. Editorial comments followed on pp. 327–337.

[77] Peritoneal endometriosis due to the menstrual dissemination of endometrial tissue into the peritoneal cavity. Am J Obstet Gynecol 1927;14:422–469.

Explication and Defense of Sampson's Theory of Pathogenesis

10

Peritoneal Endometriosis Due to Menstrual Dissemination

In May 1927, at the 52nd annual meeting of the American Gynecological Society at Hot Springs, Virginia, Sampson stated: "At the meeting of the American Gynecological Society in 1921, the writer presented a paper[1] on perforating hemorrhagic cysts of the ovary and their relation to pelvic adenomas of endometrial type…In view of the theories which have arisen to explain the origin of the peritoneal endometriosis associated with these cysts, the following quotation from that paper may be of interest."[2] "The question naturally arises: in what way do the contents of the cyst or ovary cause the development of these adenomas? Is it due to some specific irritant present in the cyst contents which stimulates the peritoneal endothelium to a metaplasia with the development of endometrial tissue typical both in structure and function? Some may assert that dormant endometrial epithelium may be present in the tissues soiled by the contents of the cyst and this is stimulated to further growth. It seems to me that the conditions found in many of these specimens are analogous to the implantation of ovarian papilloma or cancer on the peritoneal surfaces of the pelvis from the rupture of an ovarian tumor containing these growths."[3]

Immediately, Sampson made a critical statement, critical to medical historiography. "At that time I believed that the ovary was the principal, if not the only source of the peritoneal implantations which arose from endometrial tissue disseminated by the menstrual perforation of an endometrial cyst or by menstrual reaction of endometrial tissue on the surface of the ovary."[4]

While Sampson's theory of implantation endometriosis was intuitively reasonable and dramatically different from embryonic rests and coelomic metaplasia, he could not prove it. Furthermore, pathologists had demonstrated metaplasia in many tissues in the human body. One must remember the power of pathology in gynecology; pathology was the basic science – *sine qua non* – of gynecology before World War II. Among all of the theories put forth to explain the pathogenesis of extrauterine endometriosis, it seems that by 1927 the theory of serosal–coelomic metaplasia of Iwanoff and Meyer had gained increased acceptance,[5] though the stimulus for metaplasia – inflammation

[1] Sampson JA. Perforating hemorrhagic (chocolate) cysts of the ovary: their importance and especially their relation to pelvic adenomas of endometrial type ("Adenomyoma" of the uterus, rectovaginal septum, sigmoid, etc.) Archives of Surgery 1921;3:245–323.

[2] Sampson JA. Peritoneal endometriosis due to the menstrual dissemination of endometrial tissue into the peritoneal cavity. Am J Obstet Gynecol 1927;14:422–469:422.

[3] Sampson JA. Am J Obstet Gynecol 1927;14:422–469:422.

[4] Sampson JA. Peritoneal endometriosis due to the menstrual dissemination of endometrial tissue into the peritoneal cavity. Am J Obstet Gynecol 1927;14:422–469:422.

[5] Sampson JA. Am J Obstet Gynecol 1927;l4:422–469:435. See also Bailey KV. The etiology, classification, and life history of tumors of the ovary and other female pelvic organs containing aberrant müllerian elements, with suggested nomenclature. J Obstet Gynaecol Brit Emp 1924;xxxi:539–573:541. "This serosal theory held good until quite recently for all known extra-uterine "adenomyomata" and also the sub-peritoneal variety… although Cullen stuck to his view…from congenital Müllerian relics." Bailey believed that the serosal theory held good until Sampson's revolutionary theory of 1921. By way of explanation, to demonstrate coelomic metaplasia, histologic observations can be made under high-power magnification and potentially ultra-

R.E. Batt, *A History of Endometriosis*,
DOI 10.1007/978-0-85729-585-9_10, © Springer-Verlag London Limited 2011

or hormonal – was debated. Sampson believed the stimulus was hormonal, Meyer believed it was inflammation.[6] Clinicians as well as gynecologic pathologists or for that matter anyone skilled in microscopy could see the transition from normal germinal layer to endometriosis and back to normal ovarian germinal epithelium. In uterine specimens, they could see also invasion of normal endometrium into underlying uterine myometrium. Cullen's observation of direct invasion of the myometrium by endometrial mucosa was accepted virtually without criticism to explain the pathogenesis of diffuse adenomyosis – uterine endometriosis.[7] In both microscopic demonstrations, seeing was synonymous with believing. The same held true, when in 1925, Sampson presented evidence for the malignant transformation of benign into malignant ovarian endometriosis.[8] Every experienced microscopist could see the transition from benign to malignant. Both gynecologic surgeons and gynecologic pathologists were in complete agreement; there was no debate.[9]

However, in the case of Sampson's original ruptured ovarian endometrioma theory and his second and refined retrograde menstruation theory to explain the pathogenesis of pelvic endometriosis, seeing and believing were not related to looking down the barrel of a microscope. Seeing and believing required active observation at surgery and pattern recognition skills honed by years of surgical experience. Seeing also required imagination to visualize, as a Goethe might have done, the transition from intact endometrium to living shed endometrium to transtubal transport to attachment to implantation and invasion of pelvic organs by the same living shed endometrium.[10] Sampson's first theory[11] of peritoneal implantation, implantation of endometrial fragments shed from ruptured hemorrhagic chocolate cysts of the ovary seemed

high magnification at leisure in the laboratory on specimens that can be cut into serial sections for further study. Tissue could be treated with differential stains derived from bacteriological studies. In sharp contrast, clinical observations are made on living pathology in surgery. Observations are limited several ways: by the time that the patient is under anesthesia; by the intensity of illumination of surface lesions, time for observation is limited by the ethics of prolonged anesthesia for research purposes, and finally observation is limited to surface of the living lesion under observation.

[6] Bailey KV. The etiology, classification, and life history of tumors of the ovary and other female pelvic organs containing aberrant müllerian elements, with suggested nomenclature. J Obstet Gynaecol Brit Emp 1924;xxxi:539–573:540. "Meyer later upheld this serosal –coelomic metaplasia theory [of Iwanoff], and attributed the process to a primary inflammation with secondary epithelial heterotopy or displacement." Sampson JA. Peritoneal endometriosis due to the menstrual dissemination of endometrial tissue into the peritoneal cavity. Am J Obstet Gynecol 1927;l4:422–469:443. See caption under Figure 25, page 443. For additional references to age differential, see Figure 19, page 439; Figure 15, page 443; Figures 27 and 28 on page 445; and Figure 30, page 447.

[7] Bailey KV. The etiology, classification, and life history of tumors of the ovary and other female pelvic organs containing aberrant müllerian elements, with suggested nomenclature. J Obstet Gynaecol Brit Emp 1924;xxxi:539–573:540.

[8] Sampson JA. Endometrial carcinoma of the ovary, arising in endometrial tissue in that organ. Arch Surg 1925; 10:1–72.

[9] Where Sampson produced microscopic evidence of transformation – benign to malignant endometriosis, escape of endometrial fragments into the adjacent vein (at least, the first step in metastasis, he did not show the end organ that received the metastasis) to support his theory of venous metastases, he received support and not criticism.

[10] Daston, Lorraine and Peter Galison. *Objectivity.* New York, NY: Zone Books, 2007:44. As Daston and Galison described "exemplary personas," Sampson was an intuitive expert with trained judgment. He was an "intuitive expert, who depends on unconscious judgment to organize experience into patterns in the very act of perception." See also page 69. "The acute observer can intuit from cumulative experience, as Goethe 'saw' the *Urpflanze*," the archetype of all flowers. Like Goethe, from cumulative experience, Sampson "saw" the archetypical theory of pathogenesis of extrauterine pelvic endometriosis; retrograde transtubal menstruation, and implantation.

[11] Sampson JA. Peritoneal endometriosis due to the menstrual dissemination of endometrial tissue into the peritoneal cavity. Am J Obstet Gynecol 1927;l4:422–469:422. Sampson's first theory of pathogenesis of peritoneal endometriosis was centered on the ovary; inspired by Casler's unique case that had been presented by invitation before the American Gynecological Society. Shortly after he articulated his first theory, Sampson presented transtubal retrograde menstruation as his second theory of pathogenesis for endometriosis and endosalpingiosis. Sampson stated explicitly: "At the meeting of the American Gynecological Society in 1921, the writer presented a paper on perforating hemorrhagic cysts of the ovary and their relation to pelvic adenomas of endometrial type…[Sampson JA. Arch Surg 1921;iii, 245–323]…At that time I believed that the ovary was the principal, if not the only, source of the peritoneal implantations which arose from endometrial tissue disseminated by the menstrual perforation of an endometrial cyst or by the menstrual reaction of endometrial tissue on the surface of that organ."

[12] Meigs JV. Endometrial hematomas of the ovary. Boston Medical and Surgical Journal 1922;clxxvii:1–13:1. "In the *Archives of Surgery* for September 1921, Dr. John A. Sampson, of Albany, N.Y., published a paper which is the foremost contribution to gynecology and gynecological pathology in recent years."

to have been accepted by many clinicians if we can judge by the comments of Meigs[12] in 1922, Bailey[13] in 1924, and Cullen[14] in 1925. Investigators generally and rather rapidly accepted the term endometriosis. Hitherto, Cullen and the investigators, who were his contemporaries and predecessors, tended to see endometriosis as a tumor, an adenomy*oma*, an adenofibromy*oma*, or a cyst*oma*. W. Blair Bell of London coined the terms endometriomy*oma* and endometri*oma*.[15] The suffix "*oma*" denotes a neoplasm or tumor, an unfortunate designation for a benign disease process. This may explain the ready acceptance of the more general term "endometriosis" suggested by Sampson.[16]

Others acknowledged Sampson's contribution toward defining the importance of endometrial cysts, but did not subscribe to his theory of implantation by cellular material spilled from chocolate cysts.[17] Sampson's first and second theories of implantation endometriosis seemed logical and were supported by circumstantial evidence but he could not prove them.[18] By 1927, the lines of debate were visible and palpable: some gynecologic surgeons saw and believed as Sampson did; most if not all gynecologic pathologists and embryologists – and some gynecologic surgeons – saw and believed as Robert Meyer and Emil Novak did. In short, the former favored one or both of Sampson's theories of implantation; the latter chose to believe the evidence for the Iwanoff-Meyer theory of coelomic metaplasia was stronger.

By 1927, the honeymoon was over; Sampson was on the defensive. He could only continue to explain and defend his theory against mounting criticism from respected gynecologic pathologists, especially Robert Meyer and Emil Novak,[19] who espoused the theory of coelomic metaplasia. Sampson defended his theories by employing inferences,[20] questions,[21] "must" assertions,[22] and qualifications such as "suggest…might escape…it might be assumed…not definitely demonstrated…but I believe…probably came from…if it can be shown…might infer…might become…should it be shown…we would have strong presumptive evidence…apparently did…may carry with it bits of endometrium."[23] Sampson argued tirelessly and buttressed his arguments with carefully selected and annotated photomicrographic evidence. There are recurring glimpses of what in the following decade would be Sampson's increasing reliance on analogy with uterine and ovarian endometrial cancer to support his implantation theory of the pathogenesis of endometriosis. The cancer analogy, though powerful and persuasive, was still argument by analogy and not proof.

---

[13] Bailey KV. The etiology, classification, and life history of tumors of the ovary and other female pelvic organs containing aberrant müllerian elements, with suggested nomenclature. J Obstet Gynaecol Brit Emp 1924;xxxi:539–573:541. "Sampson in 1921 revolutionized all preexisting theories as to the etiology of pelvic growths of "adenomyomatous" nature by pointing out their obvious relationship to the so-called "chocolate cysts" found in the ovaries, and described the gross and histological appearance of this ovarian condition. His work, which is well known, undoubtedly set the pathology of this pelvic condition on a sound basis."

[14] Cullen TS. Discussion following a Symposium on Misplaced Endometrial Tissue. Am J Obstet Gynecol 1925;10:732–733:733. "We are under a great debt to Sampson for the careful, painstaking, and brilliant work that he has done toward establishing the modes of origin of peritoneal adenomyomata."

[15] Bell WB. Endometrioma and endometriomyoma of the ovary. J Obstet Gynaecol Brit Emp 1922;xxix:443–446.

[16] Sampson JA. Inguinal endometriosis (often reported as endometrial tissue in the groin, adenomyoma in the groin, and adenomyoma of the round ligament). Am J Obstet Gynecol 1925:462–503.

[17] Bell WB. Endometrioma and Endometriomyoma of the ovary. J Obstet Gynaecol Brit Emp 1922;xxix:443–446:444–445. Referring to ovarian endometriomas, Bell states: "The credit for the discovery of this interesting pathological condition and its clinical importance is, however, entirely due to American investigators, and in particular to Sampson." Sampson observed "that endometrium in the ovary is the cause of the so-called 'chocolate cysts." Bell continues: "It has been suggested, also, that the 'cellular spill' from such a cyst might become implanted in the pouch of Douglas."

[18] Sampson JA. Peritoneal endometriosis due to the menstrual dissemination of endometrial tissue into the peritoneal cavity. Am J Obstet Gynecol 1927;14:422–469. Sampson did not mention the Casler case, which I believe was the *proof case* for his first theory of peritoneal implantation of endometriosis from ruptured ovarian endometriotic cysts.

[19] Novak was a model critic; not only did he respect Sampson; he also offered constructive suggestions to Sampson that would strengthen his theory of implantation.

[20] Sampson JA. Peritoneal endometriosis due to the menstrual dissemination of endometrial tissue into the peritoneal cavity. Am J Obstet Gynecol 1927;14:422–469:437. "We might infer… might also".

[21] Sampson JA. Am J Obstet Gynecol 1927;14:422–469. See pages 430, 432, and 439.

[22] Sampson JA. Am J Obstet Gynecol 1927;14:422–469. See pages 425, 433, and 439.

[23] Sampson JA. Peritoneal endometriosis due to the menstrual dissemination of endometrial tissue into the peritoneal cavity. Am J Obstet Gynecol 1927;14:422–469:428–431, 434, 436, 437; 458.

One can sense Sampson's frustration as he faced increasing acceptance of the theory of coelomic metaplasia.[24] He was open to the possible validity of the theory of coelomic metaplasia.[25] "I fully realize that the implantation theory does not account for all instances of ectopic endometrium-like tissue in the pelvis and that menstruation is only one means of disseminating that tissue."[26] Sampson was a clinician, a skilled cancer surgeon, a natural scientist and a theorist, but not an experimentalist. And experimentation was needed, not analogy. True, animal experiments had been performed on rabbits and monkeys.[27] At this juncture in 1927, no one seems to have been able to conceive of an experiment other than transplantation of human shed menstrual endometrium into an animal or a human as Novak suggested. The needed clinical and laboratory experiments with human tissue would not be performed until after World War II, after Sampson's death. Compared to Cullen's simple demonstration of the pathogenesis of uterine endometriosis, proof of Sampson's implantation theory for the pathogenesis extrauterine endometriosis would turn out to be unbelievably difficult. It would require a small army of basic scientists with sophisticated laboratory techniques; such was the brilliance of Sampson's intuition and imagination.

Sampson stated explicitly that his purpose in writing this article was to present evidence in support of his theory of implantation.[28] In the very first photomicrograph, he presented an "endometrial cavity" filled with menstrual blood, situated within deeply invasive endometriosis of the vaginal vault. The ectopic endometrial cavity was "about" to rupture and menstruate into the vagina.[29] In the same case, Sampson had observed two similar endometrial cavities in the posterior vaginal fornix that actually ruptured into veins with "the embolic implantation of endometrial tissue."[30] Sampson would refer to this case over and over again; it was his *proof case* of venous metastases.[31] Sampson seems to have adopted the term "endometrial

[24] Sampson JA. Am J Obstet Gynecol 1927;14:422–469:425.

[25] Sampson JA. Am J Obstet Gynecol 1927;14:422–469:448. Sampson repeatedly left space for the theory of coelomic metaplasia as he argued for his implantation theory. See figure 7, page 429; page 431; figure 31, page 448; figure 34, page 451; figure 35, page 452; figure 58, page 467. See also figure 31, page 448; this is the first instance where Sampson juxtaposed the theories of coelomic metaplasia and implantation to explain *invasion* of a structure (uterosacral ligament) by endometriosis. Hitherto, Sampson used coelomic metaplasia merely as an alternative explanatory model for the pathogenesis of endometriosis.

[26] Sampson JA. Am J Obstet Gynecol 1927;14:422–469:425.

[27] Jacobson VC. The autotransplantation of endometrial tissue in the rabbit. Arch Surg 1922;5:281–300. Jacobson VC. Further studies in autotransplantation of endometrial tissue in the rabbit. Am J Obstet Gynecol 1923;6:257–262. Jacobson VC. The intraperitoneal transplantation of endometrial tissue. Arch Path Lab Med 1926:1:169–174.

[28] Sampson JA. Peritoneal endometriosis due to the menstrual dissemination of endometrial tissue into the peritoneal cavity. Am J Obstet Gynecol 1927;14:422–469:424. "The purpose of this paper is to present the evidence indicating the origin of peritoneal endometriosis from the implantation of endometrial tissue disseminated by menstruation."

[29] Sampson JA. Am J Obstet Gynecol 1927;14:422–469:432. "Many interesting endometrial lesions were present in an endometriosis of the posterior vaginal wall of the second case. An endometrial cavity filled with menstrual blood and containing bits of endometrial tissue had almost eroded the overlying vaginal mucosa and was about to rapture and discharge its menstrual contents into the vagina. From the study of this lesion, one could readily understand how a similar endometrial cavity in the ovary [Casler] or any other pelvic structure might rupture and disseminate its menstrual contents into the peritoneal cavity." Interestingly, the only other time that Sampson addressed endometriosis in this area (the so-called rectovaginal septum) was in his first article on endometriosis published in 1921. Sampson JA. Perforating hemorrhagic (chocolate) cysts of the ovary: their importance and especially their relation to pelvic adenomas of endometrial type ("Adenomyoma" of the uterus, rectovaginal septum, sigmoid, etc.) Archives of Surgery 1921;3:245–323:245. See also: Bailey KV. The etiology, classification, and life history of tumors of the ovary and other female pelvic organs containing aberrant müllerian elements, with suggested nomenclature. J Obstet Gynaecol Brit Emp 1924;xxxi:539–573. See also Bailey KV. The etiology, classification, and life history of tumors of the ovary and other female pelvic organs containing aberrant müllerian elements, with suggested nomenclature. J Obstet Gynaecol Brit Emp 1924;xxxi:539–573:541. Bailey cites Lockyer work of 1917: "The prevailing view at the present time…is to regard adenomyoma of the recto-genital space as an inflammatory product and not a true neoplasm."

[30] Sampson JA. Peritoneal endometriosis due to the menstrual dissemination of endometrial tissue into the peritoneal cavity. Am J Obstet Gynecol 1927;14:422–469:423. See Figure 1.

[31] Sampson JA. Am J Obstet Gynecol 1927;14:422–469:433. "I can see only one correct interpretation of the etiology of the embolic endometrial lesions in the veins about these endometrial cavities and that is they arose from the implantation of endometrial tissue, disseminated into the veins from the menstrual rupture of the walls of the endometrial cavities into these vessels. If so endometrial issue disseminated by menstruation in this instance must have been alive and capable of growing, when transferred to suitable situations." See also page 437. See another reference to the proof case on page 443.

cavity of the ovary" from Casler.[32] As mentioned earlier, I believe Casler's unique case influenced Sampson profoundly. In Casler's case, a woman who had had a complete hysterectomy, with preservation of one ovary, menstruated from an endometrial cyst of that ovary through an ovarian–vaginal fistula into the vagina each month. The term "endometrial cavity of the ovary," used as a metaphor for any ectopic endometrial cyst was heavily freighted with meaning favorable to Sampson's theory and implied that ectopic endometrial cavities recapitulated the structure and function of uterine endometrial cavities. Clearly demonstrated in a series of photomicrographs,[33] many ectopic endometrial cavities were filled with menstrual detritus, blood, and fragments of endometrial tissue; powerful visual arguments working in Sampson's favor. He used the term endometrial cavity repeatedly to describe cystic endometriotic lesions in various ectopic locations such as the posterior vaginal fornix, the broad ligament,[34] and the ovary.[35] In fact, he often labeled ovarian endometriomas within the actual photomicrographs "Endometrial Cavity."[36] Clearly, Sampson was a master of the English language and used it skillfully to promote his theory.[37]

Novak, in particular, challenged Sampson's thesis that shed endometrial tissue was alive; he believed it was either "dead or dying."[38] Novak suggested two experiments where positive results would bolster Sampson's theory: first, successful growth of menstrual endometrium in tissue culture and a second experiment to prove the capacity of menstrual endometrium to grow in the peritoneal cavity or on the ovary of "the human being or perhaps even one of the lower animals."[39] Sampson immediately referred to his *proof-case* of the ectopic endometrial cavity in the posterior fornix to argue that shed ectopic endometrium that metastasized into the surrounding veins "must have been alive."[40] Following his *proof-case* argument, Sampson argued

[32] Casler DB. A unique, diffuse uterine tumor, really an adenomyoma, with stroma, but no glands. Menstruation after complete hysterectomy due to uterine mucosa in remaining ovary. Trans Am Gynecol Soc. 1919;44:69–84:78–79. "Microscopic examination at once reveals that we are dealing here with an ovarian cyst made up almost entirely of uterine tissue, the interior of the cyst corresponding to the uterine cavity and filled with blood while the walls contain many normal glands and others which show glandular dilatation. A pathological change has also occurred and we have an overgrowth of the interglandular stroma, much resembling that seen four years previously in the uterus....The entire cyst, or uterine cavity, as it really is, is lined throughout by a single layer of tall columnar epithelium of the uterine type, and in places cilia can be made out."

[33] Sampson used photomicrographs to serve as objective evidence. See Daston, Lorraine, and Peter Galison. *Objectivity.* New York, NY: Zone Books, 2007:164. Daston and Galison quoted Wilhelm His, the embryologist from Leipzig who held that drawings and photographs were complementary. His stated: "The photograph reproduces the object with all its particularities, including those that are accidental, in a certain sense as raw material, but which guarantees absolute fidelity." As a youth, Sampson had trained himself to draw and it was he who drew the drawings in this paper. Again His: "In every sensible drawing, the essential is consciously separated from the inessential and the connection of the depicted forms is shown in the correct light, according to the view of the draftsman." In other words, drawings were subjective and unretouched photographs were objective.

[34] Sampson JA. Peritoneal endometriosis due to the menstrual dissemination of endometrial tissue into the peritoneal cavity. Am J Obstet Gynecol 1927;14:422–469:431. See Figure 9.

[35] Sampson JA. Am J Obstet Gynecol 1927;14:422–469. For references to ectopic endometrial cavities, See Figure 1, page 423 for an example of "submucous endometrial cavity." See also Figure 8, page 430; Figure 11, page 433, figure 13, page 435; and Figure 20, page 440 for examples of "endometrial cavity of the ovary."

[36] Sampson JA. Am J Obstet Gynecol 1927;14:422–469:430. For an excellent example, see Figure 8, page 430.

[37] Sampson JA. President's Address before the American Gynecological Society, Hot Springs, Va., May 22, 1923. Fundamental elements in the advancement of medicine. Am J Obstet Gynecol 1923;6:1–11. This address is an autobiographical statement.

[38] Novak E. The significance of uterine mucosa in the fallopian tube, with a discussion of the origin of aberrant endometrium. Am J Obstet Gynecol 1926;xii:501, 503. See also Sampson JA. Peritoneal endometriosis due to the menstrual dissemination of endometrial tissue into the peritoneal cavity. Am J Obstet Gynecol 1927;14:422–469:430.

[39] Sampson JA. Peritoneal endometriosis due to the menstrual dissemination of endometrial tissue into the peritoneal cavity. Am J Obstet Gynecol 1927;14:422–469:443. Emil Novak was a model critic. Not only did he respect Sampson, he also offered constructive suggestions that would strengthen Sampson theory of implantation. Late in the twentieth century, investigators tested the viability of cast off endometrium in tissue culture. See: Willemsen WNP, Mungyer G, Smets H, Rolland R, Vemer H, Jap, P. Behavior of cultured glandular cells obtained by flushing of the uterine cavity. Fertil Steril 1985;44:92. Kruitwagen RFPM, Poels IG, Willemsen WNP, de Ronde IJY, Jap PHK, Rolland R. Endometrial epithelial cells in peritoneal fluid during the early follicular phase. Fertil Steril 1991;55:297.

[40] Sampson JA. Peritoneal endometriosis due to the menstrual dissemination of endometrial tissue into the peritoneal cavity. Am J Obstet Gynecol 1927;14:422–469:433. See footnote 9 for the quotation.

against coelomic metaplasia. He drew attention to two photomicrographs, right ovary[41] and left ovary, surgical specimens from the same patient.[42] The endometrial lesions were located on the *lateral* and *under surfaces* of the left ovary and on the *lateral surface* of the right ovary.[43] Sampson explained. "The lateral surface of the ovary normally lies against the posterior layer of the broad ligament or side of the pelvis and thus a crevice is formed which would retain any material lodging in it. The lesions are situated on the dependent portion of the ovary, namely, the bottom of the crevice."[44] He repeated his "geographical distribution" argument for implantation endometriosis of the ovary.[45]

Sampson followed with his "age differential" argument; the endometrial lesion on the right ovary was "evidently of more recent origin" than those on the left ovary. The difference in age favored the implantation theory and worked against the coelomic theory. "Should the endometrial tissue in this case have arisen from the differentiation of coelomic epithelium due to its stimulation by an ovarian hormone, we should expect that these lesions would all be of the same age."[46] Earlier in this paper, Sampson had argued against differentiation of coelomic epithelium due to its stimulation by bacterial or malignant inflammation as the pathogenesis of endometriosis; here he accepted the differentiation of coelomic epithelium due to its stimulation by an ovarian hormone.

Still examining evidence for endometrial implantation or coelomic metaplasia, Sampson questioned the origin of an endometrial lesion situated in the floor of a peritoneal pocket beneath the ostium of an adherent left fallopian tube. "Is it an implantation of endometrial tissue or a metaplasia of the peritoneum arising from stimulation of the latter by some specific material escaping from the tube?"[47] Examining an "older" lesion removed from the culdesac, older compared to the lesion in the peritoneal pocket, Sampson stated: "It must have arisen from an earlier implantation of endometrial tissue or an earlier specific stimulation of the peritoneal mesothelium."[48] Sampson repeatedly left space for the theory of coelomic metaplasia all the while arguing for his implantation theory. Then, he switched back to the geographical distribution argument. In the very next illustration of a "patch" of peritoneal endometriosis situated "very close to the ostium of the patent left tube and directly over the ureter" and a similar patch involving the left uterosacral ligament, Sampson noted that both tubes were patent and both ovaries were normal.[49] To explain the pathogenesis of the patches of peritoneal endometriosis, Sampson asserted the seed and soil metaphor: "It is an implantation-like lesion in a situation easily soiled by material escaping from the patent left tube."[50] He defended his first and second theories of endometrial implantation: "Peritoneal endometriosis occurs most frequently in

[41] Sampson JA. Am J Obstet Gynecol 1927;14:422–469:443. Figure 25.

[42] Sampson JA. Am J Obstet Gynecol 1927;14:422–469:439. Figure 19.

[43] Sampson JA. Am J Obstet Gynecol 1927;14:422–469. For Geographic arguments that consistently located endometrial lesions of the ovary on the lateral and undersurface of the ovary see: See Figure 2, page 424; Figure 18, pages 438; Figure 19, page 439; Page 440; Figures 23 and 24 on page 442; Figure 25, page 443; Figure 26, page 444; Figure 29, page 446; Figure 32, page 449; Figure 43, page 458; Page 462; and Figure 54 on page 465.

[44] Sampson JA. Am J Obstet Gynecol 1927;14:422–469:446. See Figure 29, page 446.

[45] Sampson JA. Am J Obstet Gynecol 1927;14:422–469:462.

[46] Sampson JA. Am J Obstet Gynecol 1927;14:422–469:443. See caption under Figure 25, page 443. For additional references to age differential, see Figure 19, page 439; Figure 15, page 443; Figures 27 and 28 on page 445; and Figure 30, page 447.

[47] Sampson JA. Peritoneal endometriosis due to the menstrual dissemination of endometrial tissue into the peritoneal cavity. Am J Obstet Gynecol 1927;14:422–469:451. See legend under Figure 34. See page 461. "It would seem that during the menstrual life of women some substance escapes from the tubes into the pelvis which plays an important role in the etiology of pelvic peritoneal endometriosis, including the development of endometrial tissue in the ovaries. This substance may be menstrual blood in some instances and tubal secretions in others. In either case epithelium may be present."

[48] Sampson JA. Am J Obstet Gynecol 1927;14:422–469:452. See Figure 35.

[49] Sampson JA. Am J Obstet Gynecol 1927;14:422–469:452. See Figure 36.

[50] Sampson JA. Peritoneal endometriosis due to the menstrual dissemination of endometrial tissue into the peritoneal cavity. Am J Obstet Gynecol 1927;14:422–469:452. See Figure 36. See also Figures 48 and 49. Implants of endometriosis on ovary and uterus "are in a situation readily 'soiled' by material escaping from the abdominal ostium of the patent left tube." I believe I am familiar with the trees, soil, and landscapes from which Sampson drew his metaphors. For I have hiked, camped, or hunted the woodlands and meadows of New York State from the Adirondack State Park to the ravines that feed the Finger Lakes; and from the Great Bear Swamp in Western New York to the Mohawk and Hudson Rivers near Sampson's Albany.

situations in the pelvis easily soiled by material escaping from the tubes and ovaries. It would seem the tubes and ovaries are the chief distributing agents for the cause of pelvic peritoneal endometriosis. It is not peculiar to the pelvic peritoneum, as the appendix, cecum, small intestine and their mesenteries may be involved. The posture of mankind, whether standing, sitting, or lying down appears to be an important factor in determining the distribution of these lesions."[51]

Gravity was as pivotal for Sampson's theory of implantation endometriosis as it was for Galileo's experiments at the Tower of Pisa or Newton's apocryphal apple.[52] The geographic distribution of intestinal endometriosis: on the appendix, the cecum, small intestine, rectum, sigmoid, and their mesenteries presented a strong argument for gravitational distribution of endometrial tissue shed from the fallopian tubes and ruptured ovarian endometrial cysts.[53] Except for the supine and knee–chest positions, the retrocervical area in the anterior rectovaginal pouch of Douglas is always the most dependent portion of the pelvic cavity in females and the ultimate repository for endometrial tissue shed retrograde through the fallopian tubes or from a ruptured ovarian endometrial cyst.

Next, Sampson asked the quintessential question; could shed endometrial fragments pass through the narrow caliber of the interstitial portion of the fallopian tube in order to gain access to the ovary, peritoneum, and other structures in the pelvis? Critics claimed the passage was too narrow and the transit time too long for retrograde menstrual fragments to pass and still be viable to implant. Sampson had already addressed the question of viability to the best of his ability. So, he addressed the problem of the diameter of the fallopian tube at its narrowest by returning to his uterine injection experiments published in 1918.[54] The diameter of the isthmus of the fallopian tubes, as viewed on roentgenograms, hysterosalpingographic x-rays of the uterus, and fallopian tubes of surgical specimens hardened by fixatives, varied so as to appear as a "mere thread" or "a relatively large canal."[55] Sampson compared the diameter of the isthmus of fallopian tubes in two hysterosalpingograms. In the first, "the interstitial portions of the tubes appear as mere threads, but even so, small bits of endometrial tissue might be carried into the tubes by blood escaping from the uterine cavity during curettage and menstruation."[56] In the second, he argued "The lumen of the interstitial portion of the tube is much greater than that of the preceding specimen, and therefore, larger bits of endometrial tissue could pass from the uterine cavity into the tubes than in the former."[57] Sampson referred to an earlier publication of a Figure, in 1918, and stated that in the legend accompanying the figure, he had "suggested that menstrual blood, at times, might escape through the tubes into the peritoneal cavity."[58] Sampson compared photomicrographs (10×) of a section of menstrual blood from the uterine cavity of one surgical specimen with the (10×) enlargement of "the very narrow threadlike interstitial portion of the tube" in a hysterosalpingogram x-ray. He concluded: "The smaller bits of the uterine mucosa in this blood would easily pass through the lumen of the tube and the larger pieces would readily pass through a tube of greater caliber as the tube of the roentgenogram. Blood escaping from the uterine cavity into the tubes during curettage and menstruation, at times, might carry with it bits of the uterine mucosa suspended in that blood."[59]

Thus far, Sampson had not demonstrated endometrial fragments within the interstitial portion or the ampullary portion of a fallopian tube; instead he compared the diameter of endometrial fragments and the diameter of fallopian tubes and concluded that small endometrial fragments might pass through the narrower isthmus and larger fragments though the tubes with a larger diameter isthmus. In other words, based on comparative measurements of passage and passen-

[51] Sampson JA. Am J Obstet Gynecol 1927;14:422–469:462.

[52] This is a mixed metaphor; Galileo's experiments at Pisa were real, Newton's apple is an allegorical story.

[53] Sampson JA. Am J Obstet Gynecol 1927;14:422–469. See pages 434–435; page 440 and page 462.

[54] Sampson JA. The escape of foreign material from the uterine cavity into uterine veins. Am J Obstet Diseases of Women and Children 1918;lxxxii:161–175.

[55] Sampson JA. Peritoneal endometriosis due to the menstrual dissemination of endometrial tissue into the peritoneal cavity. Am J Obstet Gynecol 1927;14:422–469:444.

[56] Sampson JA. Am J Obstet Gynecol 1927;14:422–469:456. Figure 40.

[57] Sampson JA. Am J Obstet Gynecol 1927;14:422–469:456. Figure 41.

[58] Sampson JA. Am J Obstet Gynecol 1927;14:422–469:456. Figures 40 and 41.

[59] Sampson JA. Peritoneal endometriosis due to the menstrual dissemination of endometrial tissue into the peritoneal cavity. Am J Obstet Gynecol 1927;14:422–469:457. Figure 42.

ger, retrograde menstruation onto the ovary and pelvic peritoneum might be possible. The operative word was "might." Based on the visual images so presented, the endometrial fragments were smaller than the diameter of the tube and seemingly could readily pass retrograde into the pelvis. Sampson presented photomicrographic evidence of endometrial fragments and fibrin "moulded" into a curvilinear "cast of the lumen of a narrow portion of the tube," which he contended was formed during passage through the narrow tubal isthmus and constituted further evidence that the fragments originated in the endometrial cavity.[60] In five photomicrographs of the "healthiest" appearing shed endometrium from the vagina, uterus, and the aforementioned tubal "cast," all at 250× magnification, Sampson contended that the tissue "seemed" alive based on histologic appearance, except perhaps for the central portion of the tubal "cast" specimen.[61]

Sampson recalled eight patients in whom he saw menstrual blood dripping from the fimbriated extremity of the tubes and in which he found endometrial tissue in the histologic sections of the same tubes removed surgically. He also observed the blood dripping from the tubal ostia at laparotomy in non-menstruating patients.[62] "Bits of endometrial tissue, apparently set free by the curette, were found in the lumina of tubes which had been removed and some of these pieces were larger than similar pieces of endometrial tissue set free by menstruation."[63] He supported his clinical observations with solid comparative histologic evidence. A photomicrograph of a cross section of the ampulla of a fallopian tube excised following uterine curettage demonstrated endometrial fragments of larger diameter than found in cross section of the ampulla of a fallopian tube removed during menstruation.[64] On the basis of finding endometrial fragments in the fallopian tubes in the short time between uterine curettage and immediate laparotomy, Sampson deduced that the transit time from endometrium into the tubes "might be very short, not several days but a few moments."[65]

Spurred by the critique of Novak, Sampson considered five ways that endometrial fragments might be found in fallopian tubes removed at surgery. The endometrial fragments could be: (1) artifacts; (2) carried along with blood shed at curettage; (3) from menstruation of uterine mucosa "forming a part of the tubal mucosa"; (4) from entrapment of ectopic pelvic endometrial tissue by the tubal fimbriae[66] similar to ovum pickup at ovulation time; and lastly, the endometrial fragments could be from retrograde transtubal menstruation.[67] Sampson eliminated the artifact possibility when observations were restricted to tubal contents of patients operated while menstruating.[68] Analogous to Janney's critique of embryologic evidence, Sampson demonstrated the possibility for retrograde menstruation through human fallopian tubes, but he had not demonstrated all steps in the chain of evidence from uterine endometrium to endometrial implant nor had he proved the viability of shed human endometrial fragments.

Recall Janney's critique of embryologic evidence. "Embryology may be suggestive but hardly conclusive, for the reason that suggestive appearances in an embryo can never be proved to be the early stages of a condition found in adults unless all of the steps can be demonstrated, which seems unlikely in a condition of this

60 Sampson JA. Am J Obstet Gynecol 1927;14:422–469:460. Figure 46. "Should the endometrial tissue in the photomicrograph above it be forced into a narrow, curved tube, it would be moulded or fashioned into a mass like this. I believe that this moulded mass represents a cast of the lumen of a narrow portion of the tube and adds to the evidence already presented that the endometrial tissue in the tube or tubes was derived from the uterine cavity." Again, Sampson qualified his statements that the evidence suggests but does not prove.

61 Sampson JA. Peritoneal endometriosis due to the menstrual dissemination of endometrial tissue into the peritoneal cavity. Am J Obstet Gynecol 1927;14:422–469:461. See Figure 47.

62 Sampson JA. Am J Obstet Gynecol 1927;14:422–469:446. "I have often observed blood dripping from the abdominal ostia of the tubes in abdominal operations which had been preceded by a curettage of the uterus." Sampson also observed the same phenomenon when he operated during the patient's menstruation. See also page 458. "I fully realize that it is impossible definitely to state the origin of the blood in the lumen of the tubes in these eight cases."

63 Sampson JA. Am J Obstet Gynecol 1927;14:422–469:446.

64 Sampson JA. Am J Obstet Gynecol 1927;14:422–469:459. See Figures 44 and 45.

65 Sampson JA. Am J Obstet Gynecol 1927;14:422–469:446.

66 Sampson JA. Peritoneal endometriosis due to the menstrual dissemination of endometrial tissue into the peritoneal cavity. Am J Obstet Gynecol 1927;14:422–469:449. "Novak has published photomicrographs of sections of tube showing endometrial tissue in their lumina and offers the theory that this tissue might have come from ectopic endometrial tissue in the pelvis and entered the tube through the abdominal ostium, just as the ovum and particles of cancer in peritoneal carcinosis are known to enter the tubes."

67 Sampson JA. Am J Obstet Gynecol 1927;14:422–469:447.

68 Sampson JA. Am J Obstet Gynecol 1927;14:422–469:451.

rarity."[69] Unlike embryonic rests; ovarian, peritoneal, and bowel endometriosis are common lesions. Given time, financing, sophisticated investigational tools, and resourceful laboratory scientists, Sampson's theories of pathogenesis could be put to experimental proof.

Sampson stressed the presence of patent fallopian tubes in patients with endometriosis.[70] He demonstrated to his satisfaction that peritoneal irritation and exudate associated with gonococcal infection and malignancy did not induce metaplasia of the germinal epithelium of the ovary or of the pelvic peritoneum subsequently resulting in endometriosis. Placing three photomicrographs in juxtaposition, he demonstrated the reaction of germinal epithelium of the ovary to gonorrheal infection and argued that it never develops "into peritoneal carcinosis or true peritoneal endometriosis" under such circumstances.[71] Furthermore, exudative reaction to malignant implants did not induce metaplastic transformation of parietal peritoneum into endometriosis. Instead, based on his comparative study of peritoneal endometriosis and peritoneal carcinosis, Sampson "demonstrated the peritoneal reaction is the same in both instances."[72] He also presented photomicrographs of peritoneal carcinosis implants resulting from spill of ovarian cancer into the peritoneal cavity.[73] To further emphasize their similarity, Sampson drew the parallel between cancer and benign endometrial tissue. Both metastasize through vascular channels.[74] The third photomicrograph showed an endometrial implant, one of several, on the *lateral surface* of an ovary. The implant "is enmeshed in an exudate somewhat similar" to that in the two photomicrographs shown in juxtaposition.[75] The surface epithelium [of the ovary] is intact on either side of the endometrial implant but otherwise has disappeared beneath the endometrial implant. Sampson concluded: "The endometrial tissue...may have been derived either from the implantation of similar tissue from other endometrial lesions of the ovary, from endometrial or tubal tissue escaping through the tubes (both were patent) or from localized metaplasia of the surface epithelium of the ovary."[76] His conclusion diluted what seemed, at first reading, a strong argument in favor of his theory.

Sampson demonstrated by microphotographs that peritoneal endometriosis had "apparently" invaded the uterine musculature "causing a so-called adenomyoma" of the uterus (adenomyosis uteri interna).[77] While Cullen had only to demonstrate continuity between uterine endometrium and underlying uterine adenomyoma, Sampson had the additional burden of convincing his peers that shed endometrium, transported through the fallopian tubes, had implanted on the uterine serosa and then invaded to produce the same adenomyoma as that produced by direct invasion of the endometrium from the endometrial cavity. Furthermore, Sampson was explicitly arguing that secondary endometriosis could invade the uterus and produce lesions identical with direct or primary endometriosis. In short, he was arguing that external implantation endometriosis could cause internal endometriosis, albeit in the periphery of the uterine musculature. Implicitly, Sampson was arguing for the identity of pathogenesis of primary (uterine) endometriosis and secondary (extrauterine) endometriosis. For the moment, all he had to do was to convince his peers to accept his theory of implantation endometriosis as a viable alternative to coelomic metaplasia. Sampson knew that, ultimately, general acceptance of his theory by the scientific world depended on experimental proof, not on circumstantial evidence no matter how compelling.

---

[69] Janney JC. Report of three cases of a rare ovarian anomaly. Am J Obstet Gynecol 1922;Feb:173–187:187.

[70] Sampson JA. Peritoneal endometriosis due to the menstrual dissemination of endometrial tissue into the peritoneal cavity. Am J Obstet Gynecol 1927;14:422–469:449. For example of the association of endometriosis with patent fallopian tubes, see Figure 32, page 449. See also page 459. "One of the outstanding features of patients with peritoneal endometriosis is that the tubes are usually patent." In a five year period, Sampson operated 293 patients with peritoneal endometriosis; both tubes "appeared to be patent" in 284 patients. In Sampson's series, most patients were over 30 years old. Three patients had a unilateral hematosalpinx, four had a bilateral hematosalpinx, and only two had bilateral pyosalpinx.

[71] Sampson JA. Am J Obstet Gynecol 1927;14:422–469:438. See Figure 16.

[72] Sampson JA. Am J Obstet Gynecol 1927;14:422–469:462–463.

[73] Sampson JA. Am J Obstet Gynecol 1927;14:422–469. See Figures 21 and 22, page 441. See also Page 436: "cancer escaping into the peritoneal cavity sometimes becomes implanted on the surface of the peritoneum, causing lesions of peritoneal carcinosis."

[74] Sampson JA. Am J Obstet Gynecol 1927;14:422–469:437.

[75] Sampson JA. Peritoneal endometriosis due to the menstrual dissemination of endometrial tissue into the peritoneal cavity. Am J Obstet Gynecol 1927;14:422–469:438–439. Fig. 18.

[76] Sampson JA. Am J Obstet Gynecol 1927;14:422–469:438–439. Fig. 18.

[77] Sampson JA. Am J Obstet Gynecol 1927;14:422–469:453. See Figure 37.

But not all circumstantial evidence was compelling. In the very next photomicrograph of the same specimen by which Sampson had argued that implantation endometriosis on the uterine serosa could invade and "apparently cause" a typical adenomyoma,[78] he pointed out "dead cells" and a "necrotic mass" of dead cells on the peritoneal surface of the uterus.[79] Adjacent to the necrotic mass, Sampson indicated a surface endometriosis and an underlying endometrial lesion embedded deeply in the uterine musculature. Sampson noted that "the greater portion of the tissue in this photomicrograph is dead, but some lived (that in contact with the surface of the uterus) with a resulting endometriosis."[80]

After presenting an impressive amount of circumstantial evidence, ardent assertions, and arguments; all with due deference to the principal competing theory of coelomic metaplasia, Sampson got to the crux of this paper: the integration of his first and second theories of pathogenesis of implantation endometriosis. Recall that his first theory, presented in 1921, explained the etiology of peritoneal endometriosis and accompanying endometriotic adhesive disease from perforating hemorrhagic (chocolate) cysts of the ovary.[81] His second theory, initially presented in Boston in 1922, explained the etiology of ovarian endometriomas and some peritoneal endometriosis from implantation of endometrial fragments shed retrograde through the fallopian tubes during menstruation.[82]

In explaining the etiology of endometrial-like tissue in the ovary, Sampson made reference to the variety of lesions of uterine and tubal origin characteristic of direct or primary endometriosis, which were his standard of comparison for both ovarian and peritoneal endometriosis. The spectrum of uterine lesions ranged from "typical endometrium with glands and stroma identical with that of the müllerian mucosa from which it came," to dilated endometrial glands with little or no supporting endometrial stroma, to "extreme cases" that resembled mesothelium.[83]

Sampson explained in detail. "Marked changes in the mucosa lining the uterine cavity often occur. Of particular interest are those in the mucosa over a submucous leiomyoma. This mucosa becomes thin, the glands disappear, the stroma becomes less and less and in extreme cases the submucous leiomyoma is covered by a mucosa not unlike the mesothelium covering of a subserous leiomyomas. The endometrial epithelium in unfavorable conditions may be very similar to the peritoneal mesothelium and the surface epithelium of the ovary. Both the peritoneal epithelium and the surface epithelium of the ovary, under the stimulation of any irritant, may become hypertrophied and resemble the epithelium of the uterine mucosa. We recognize the mucosal covering of a submucous leiomyoma to be of endometrial origin, even though it simulates the peritoneal mesothelium and the epithelial lining of a follicular cyst of the ovary. When we find patches of typical endometrial tissue in an ovarian cyst with a lining similar to the mucosal covering of a submucous leiomyoma, can it be truthfully said that the typical endometrial tissue represents a metaplasia of the epithelium of a follicular cyst of the ovary, just because the cyst is situated in the ovary and portions of its lining resemble that of a follicular cyst? Is it not more logical to claim that the entire cyst is lined by one kind of tissue and that the endometrial portions of which have failed to attain their full growth, and thus present a histologic picture identical with the linings of some of the atypical endometrial cavities of a direct endometriosis and mucosal covering of submucous

[78] Sampson JA. Peritoneal endometriosis due to the menstrual dissemination of endometrial tissue into the peritoneal cavity. Am J Obstet Gynecol 1927;14:422–469:453. Fig. 37.

[79] Sampson JA. Am J Obstet Gynecol 1927;14:422–469.:454. Fig. 38.

[80] Sampson JA. Am J Obstet Gynecol 1927;14:422–469. See Fig. 38, page 454 and Fig. 39 on page 455.

[81] Sampson JA. Perforating hemorrhagic (chocolate) cysts of the ovary: their importance and especially their relation to pelvic adenomas of endometrial type ("Adenomyoma" of the uterus, rectovaginal septum, sigmoid, etc.) Archives of Surgery 1921;3:245–323.

[82] Sampson JA. Ovarian hematomas of endometrial type (perforating hemorrhagic cysts of the ovary) and implantation adenomas of endometrial type. Boston Medical and Surgical Journal 1922;186:445–456. After Sampson published his first theory in the American Journal of Obstetrics and Gynecology in 1921 and before he published his second theory in the Boston Medical and Surgical Journal in 1922, he annotated his first theory to announce the second, which was published separately in the Proceedings of the American Gynecological Society in 1921.

[83] Sampson JA. Peritoneal endometriosis due to the menstrual dissemination of endometrial tissue into the peritoneal cavity. Am J Obstet Gynecol 1927;14:422–469:463.

[84] Sampson JA. Am J Obstet Gynecol 1927;14:422–469:463–464. Sampson reproduced two photomicrographs objectively illustrating his argument. See Figures 59 and 60 on page 468.

leiomyomas?"[84] Sampson concluded his argument. "On account of the faculty of known endometrial epithelium to simulate peritoneal mesothelium and the surface epithelium of the ovary, it is often difficult to determine the origin of all misplaced endometrium-like tissue in the ovary."[85] Sampson believed in his implantation theory and argued for its acceptance, but he did not believe it was the only mode of pathogenesis of ovarian endometriosis.[86] The hormone-driven theory of coelomic metaplasia provided considerable explanatory power and Sampson left ample room for it.

Sampson began his explanation of the etiology of peritoneal endometriosis with a disclaimer. He could not prove that all lesions of peritoneal endometriosis that he had encountered in the past 5 years had been "instances of true peritoneal endometriosis."[87] Nevertheless, I do believe he had faith that his implantation theories provided the best explanation for peritoneal endometriosis but not necessarily the more persuasive explanation for ovarian endometriosis. Consequently, he spent more time defending the etiology of ovarian endometriosis from tubal spill of shed endometrial tissue. He spent little time discussing the etiology of peritoneal endometriosis, commenting mostly on the histological standards for diagnosis.

Sampson held that typical endometrial histology provided the ideal standard of comparison for younger and more superficial peritoneal implants, while atypical endometrial histology characteristic of Cullen's primary endometriosis (adenomyosis) provided the practical standard of comparison for older and deeper endometriotic lesions.[88]

Realizing that his evidence was insufficient to convince skeptics, Sampson ended his explanation for the pathogenesis of peritoneal endometriosis with a second disclaimer. "These studies indicate that peritoneal endometriosis sometimes arises from the implantation of endometrial tissue disseminated by menstrual blood escaping into the peritoneal cavity." The operative word in this qualified conclusion was "sometimes." This disclaimer suggested a retreat from his earlier strong position, a loss of ground to coelomic metaplasia, and the need for further study.

In sum, when the gynecologic pathologists Robert Meyer, Emil Novak, and others scrutinized his implantation theories, Sampson realized objective circumstantial evidence garnered through his trained judgment[89] did not rise to the level of objective scientific proof, the benchmark for acceptance as fact.[90] He recognized the need for objective experimental studies using animal models as well as human subjects. Though he retreated from his earlier affirmative position, Sampson's belief in the validity of his theories was undimmed as he continued his observational clinical research.

Sampson's Implantation Theory

From 1928 until his death in 1946, Sampson wrote 13 papers, 1 related to medical education, 5 to cancer, and 6 to endometriosis with special emphasis on the fallopian tubes.[91] Though interested in the pathogenesis and life history of all types of endometriosis, he realized he left many problems unsolved.[92] In 1940, 1 year after he retired as Professor of Gynecology, Sampson distilled the observations of his scientific work on endometriosis in a memorable self-critical review entitled: *The development of the implantation theory for the origin of peritoneal endometriosis.*[93] Eighteen years had

[85] Sampson JA. Peritoneal endometriosis due to the menstrual dissemination of endometrial tissue into the peritoneal cavity. Am J Obstet Gynecol 1927;14:422–469:464.

[86] Sampson JA. Am J Obstet Gynecol 1927;14:422–469:465.

[87] Sampson JA. Am J Obstet Gynecol 1927;14:422–469:465.

[88] Sampson JA. Am J Obstet Gynecol 1927;14:422–469:466.

[89] Daston, Lorraine, and Peter Galison. *Objectivity*. New York, NY: Zone Books, 2007:344–346.

[90] Daston, Lorraine, and Peter Galison. *Objectivity*, 36. "What is the nature of objectivity? First and foremost, objectivity is the suppression of some aspect of the self, the countering of subjectivity. Objectivity and subjectivity define each other, like left and right or up and down." See also page 51. "Objective knowledge," understood as "a systematized theoretical account of how the world really is, comes as close to truth as today's timorous metaphysics will permit."

[91] Clement PB. History of gynecological pathology. IX. Dr. John Albertson Sampson. Int J Gynecol Pathol 2001;20:86–101. See pp. 99–100 references. References 2 through 68 all refer to Sampson's articles arranged chronologically from 1902 to 1945.

[92] Sampson JA. The development of the implantation theory for the origin of peritoneal endometriosis. Am J Obstet Gynecol 1940:40:549–557:557.

[93] Sampson JA. The development of the implantation theory for the origin of peritoneal endometriosis. Am J Obstet Gynecol 1940:40:549–557:557. See also p. 549. "I greatly appreciate the appraisals of my observations and interpretations which have been made by others, However, it is my own critical evaluation of these observations and interpretations which I shall attempt to present in this review."

elapsed since Sampson had published the essentials of the implantation theory. Without stating the specific publication, Sampson must have been thinking of his presentation to the Harvard Medical Society at the Peter Bent Brigham Hospital in February of 1922 entitled: *Ovarian hematomas of endometrial type (perforating hemorrhagic cysts of the ovary) and implantation adenomas of endometrial type*, published that same year in *The Boston Medical and Surgical Journal*.[94] He elaborated on what he meant by the essentials of the implantation theory. What this writer has labeled Sampson's first theory and second theory of implantation endometriosis, Sampson called his "first step [and] second step" in the development of the implantation theory.[95] What Sampson called "the third and final step" referred to his observations that a "secondary spread of endometriosis also could arise from foci in other situations than the ovary."[96]

In short, by approaching the history of endometriosis prospectively from early nineteenth century, the writer concluded that Sampson had developed two separate but complementary "theories" and did not recognize a third "theory." However, to Sampson these were merely three steps in the development of his implantation theory of peritoneal endometriosis, not three separate theories.

In the introduction to this invited paper, Sampson wrote an autobiographical sketch that summarized the methodology and intellectual excitement as well as the integration of years of experience with cancer that characterized 10 years of intensive study of peritoneal endometriosis. "For over ten years I studied peritoneal endometriosis constantly and intensively, and since then intermittently according to the operative findings in individual cases. During the intensive study of this subject the distribution and character of its lesions were carefully noted at operation. Sketches were frequently made at that time. Great attention was paid to small implants. When feasible these were excised. Drawings, many in color, were made of all specimens of endometriosis before they left the operating room floor. All material was fixed intact in formalin. After fixation, I selected the exact portions of the specimens which I wished to study histologically. This tissue was embedded in celloidin, since it causes less unequal tissue shrinkage than paraffin. I supervised the mounting of the embedded tissue and instructed the technician how it should be cut. A small notebook was carried, in which I jotted down 'inspirations' before they vanished. Studies of the peritoneal implantation of cancer cells escaping from carcinoma of the ovary and of the body of the uterus and also studies of the spread of these tumors in other ways, were initiated by my desire to investigate more intelligently the spread of benign Müllerian mucosa. I enjoyed every bit of the study of endometriosis; there were an abundance of fresh material, excellent laboratory facilities, including well-trained technicians, an artist whose illustrations speak for themselves better than any words I might employ, a cooperative and skilled microphotographer and interested associates. My chief contribution was an insatiable curiosity which, stirred by difficulties and opportunities which were constantly arising, perpetuated my interest."[97]

Sampson chose the name endometriosis – which he intended to be an all inclusive term – because endometriosis expressed his conviction that uterine endometrial mucosa was the principal source of both internal and external endometriosis. Nevertheless, throughout this paper, as he had many times before, Sampson often reverted to the term müllerianosis – with its embryological implications that made it inclusive of all benign and malignant müllerian diseases – those identified such as adenomyosis, endosalpingiosis, and endometriosis, and those yet to be identified such as endocervicosis and developmental endometriosis.

[94] Sampson JA. Ovarian hematomas of endometrial type (perforating hemorrhagic cysts of the ovary) and implantation adenomas of endometrial type. Boston Med Surg J 1922;186:445–456. See p. 448 where Sampson casually inserted an observation about lymphatic dissemination of adenomatous tissue, anticipating Halban's publication by 2 years.

[95] Sampson JA. The development of the implantation theory for the origin of peritoneal endometriosis. Am J Obstet Gynecol 1940:40:549–557:550, 553.

[96] Sampson JA. Am J Obstet Gynecol 1940:40:549–557:555.

[97] Sampson JA. The development of the implantation theory for the origin of peritoneal endometriosis. Am J Obstet Gynecol 1940:40:549–557:549.

[98] Sampson JA. Heterotopic or misplaced endometrial tissue. Am J Obstet Gynecol 1925;10:649–664:649.

[99] Sampson JA. The development of the implantation theory for the origin of peritoneal endometriosis. Am J Obstet Gynecol 1940:40:549–557:549.

[100] Sampson JA. Am J Obstet Gynecol 1940:40:549–557:555.

In 1925, Sampson had described his dilemma regarding terminology and the reason for his choice of the term endometriosis. "The nomenclature of misplaced endometrial or müllerian lesions is a difficult one to decide upon. As they arise from tubal as well as uterine mucosa (probably much more frequently from the latter), the term müllerian would be inclusive and correct, but unfortunately it suggests an embryonic origin. A variety of lesions is produced by misplaced endometrial or müllerian tissue and it is difficult to classify all of them as true tumors. The term endometriosis müllerianosis would possibly be more correct, as applied to the entire subject, than 'endometrioma and endometriomyoma,' as suggested by Blair Bell, or 'müllerianoma,' as more recently suggested by Bailey. The term endometriosis is more descriptive than müllerianosis and is correct in the majority of instances, because we believe that the uterine mucosa is the chief source of these lesions."[98]

Sampson waited till his retirement before he defined the disease he had been studying for two decades: "The term endometriosis was introduced to indicate the presence of ectopic tissue which possesses the histologic structure and function of the uterine mucosa. It also includes the abnormal conditions which may result not only from the invasion of organs and other structures by this tissue, but also from its reaction to menstruation."[99]

At the end of his professional career, Sampson knew that he had provided "*no positive proof*" that epithelium escaping from endometriotic cysts or from the fallopian tubes implanted on the peritoneum to cause endometriosis."[100] He had strong circumstantial evidence for his three-step implantation theory of peritoneal endometriosis, but not scientific proof.[101] Sampson concluded this paper and his active academic career with an elegant disclaimer that expresses the ideal of scientific inquiry. "If bits of Müllerian mucosa carried by menstrual blood escaping into the peritoneal cavity are always dead, the implantation theory, as presented by me, also is dead and should be buried and forgotten. If some of these bits are even occasionally alive, the implantation theory also is alive. The viability of this theory is of secondary importance to me as compared with the pleasure and the increased knowledge of this and kindred subjects which I have gained in these studies and the resulting more intelligent treatment of patients who have peritoneal endometriosis."[102]

In 1943, James Robert Goodall, emeritus Professor of Clinical Gynecology and Obstetrics, McGill University, published a slender volume entitled *A Study of Endometriosis, Endosalpingiosis, Endocervicosis, and Peritoneo-ovarian Sclerosis: A Clinical and Pathologic Study*, which he dedicated to Dr. John A. Sampson "in recognition of his work as a pioneer in this field and as a token of gratitude for his generosity."[103] In this volume, Goodall reported what he believed was a new benign müllerian disease, which he named endocervicosis.

---

[101] Sampson JA. Am J Obstet Gynecol 1940:40:549–557: 555–556. Henry Campbell Black, *Black's Law Dictionary: Definitions of the Terms and Phrases of America and English Jurisprudence, Ancient and Modern.* Sixth Edition by the Publisher's Editorial Staff. [St. Paul, MN: West Publishing Co., 1990], 243. "Circumstantial evidence. Testimony not based on actual personal knowledge or observation of the facts in controversy, but of other facts from which deductions are drawn, showing indirectly the facts sought to be proved. People v. Yokum, 145 C.A.2n 245, 302 P.2d 406, 410. The proof of certain facts and circumstances in a given case, from which jury may infer other connected facts which, usually and reasonably follow according to the common experience of mankind. Foster v. Union Starch & Refining Co., 11 Ill.App.2d 346, 137 N.E.2d 499, 502. Evidence of facts or circumstances from which the existence or nonexistence of fact in issue may be inferred. Inferences drawn from facts proved. Process of decision by which court or jury may reason from circumstances known or proved, to establish by inference the principal fact. It means that existence of principal facts is only inferred from circumstances. Twin City Fire Ins. Co. v. Lonas, 255 Ky. 717, 75 S.W.2n 348, 350. The proof of various facts or circumstances which usually attend the main fact in dispute, and therefore tend to prove its existence, or to sustain, by their consistency, the hypothesis claimed. Or as otherwise defined, it consists in reasoning from facts which are known or proved to establish such as are conjectured to exist." See also: Robert S. Hunter, *Federal Trial Handbook: Civil.* 4th ed. [Danvers, MA:Thomson West, 2003], 29–1. "Admissibility of circumstantial evidence generally. Circumstantial evidence is evidence which tends to prove a disputed fact by proof of other facts which have a legitimate tendency to lead the mind to a conclusion that the fact exists which is sought to be established. It is legal evidence and the jury must act upon it as if it were direct when it is satisfactory beyond a reasonable doubt. *Rumely v. U.S.*, 293 F. 532 (C.C.A. 2n Cir. 1923). As a legal matter, there is no distinction between direct and circumstantial evidence. Circumstantial evidence has probative value equal to that of testimonial evidence. The law does not belittle the value of circumstantial evidence by making a relative distinction between it and direct evidence. *Rodella v. U.S.*, 286 F.2d 306 (9th Cir. 1960)."

[102] Sampson JA. The development of the implantation theory for the origin of peritoneal endometriosis. Am J Obstet Gynecol 1940:40:549–557:557.

[103] James Robert Goodall, *A Study of Endometriosis, Endosalpingiosis, Endocervicosis, and Peritoneo-ovarian Sclerosis: A Clinical and Pathologic Study* [Philadelphia: JB Lippincott, 1943].

"Endocervicosis is a new disease, a recent discovery. It is characterized by a nonmalignant invasion of the deep cervical and paracervical tissues by the mucosa of the cervix uteri. Just as the endometrium may penetrate deeply into the uterine myometrium, and even extend into the parametrial tissues, so can the cervical mucosa under abnormal stimulation take on similar invasive properties, causing distortion and fixation of the organs involved. Only two cases have come under my observation, both in the past year. Doubtless others will be found when surgeons are familiar with the signs. The true nature of the disease was never suspected prior to operation, but at intervention the multiplicity of the cysts, their diminutive size, their opalescent tenacious contents, and their rigid walls led one to suspect their true nature."[104]

In 1992, Clement and Young acknowledged that Goodall was the first to use the term endocervicosis "to refer to two cases in which there was deep infiltration of the cervical wall and paracervical tissues by benign-appearing endocervical glands." Though Goodall had not illustrated his lesions, Clement and Young noted that, by the standards of late twentieth century pathology, "they would probably be interpreted as examples of minimal deviation adenocarcinoma ("adenoma malignum")." Clement and Young then presented, for the first time, six cases of endocervicosis of the urinary bladder.[105]

In 1925, Sampson had enumerated four benign müllerian diseases, three of which he had seen: adenomyosis, endosalpingiosis, and endometriosis; and he postulated a fourth, developmentally misplaced endometrial tissue, which he had not seen.[106] Why did Sampson include developmentally misplaced endometrium in his classification of the theories of pathogenesis for endometriosis? It was not like him to report that which he had not personally observed, nor include such as a possible mode of pathogenesis of the disease process he was studying so intently.

Although Sampson gave no reference to support inclusion of developmentally misplaced endometrial tissue, I believe he was referring to the case reported by W. W. Russell in 1899 as "aberrant portions of the müllerian duct found in an ovary."[107] Russell had died in 1924 while Sampson was preparing this article: Heterotopic or misplaced endometrial tissue.[108] Russell's case was forcibly

---

[104] James Robert Goodall, *A Study of Endometriosis, Endosalpingiosis, Endocervicosis, and Peritoneo-ovarian Sclerosis*, 89. In 1982, the writer dedicated a monograph to James Robert Goodall. Ronald E. Batt, and John D. Naples, *Conservative Surgery for Endometriosis in the Infertile Couple*. Current Problems in Obstetrics and Gynecology, Vol. VI [Chicago: Year Book Medical Publishers, 1982], 1-98. See Leitch. Proc. R. Soc Med (Obst and Gyn Sect), July 1914:389. Cited by Cuthbert Lockyer, *Fibroids and Allied Tumours (Myoma and Adenomyoma): Their Pathology, Clinical Features, and Surgical Treatment* [London: Macmillan and Company, 1918], 330–331. Archibald Leitch described a "migratory adenomyoma" of the cervix that spread into the base of the left broad ligament. "The cervical epithelium had invaded the musculature of the cervix very deeply." This description sounds like endocervicosis, a lesion that was not described and named as such until 1943 by Goodall. Leitch anticipated Cullen but did not recognize the significance of his observation. See Clement PB, Young RH. Endocervicosis of the urinary bladder. A report of six cases of a benign müllerian lesion that may mimic adenocarcinoma. Am J Surg Pathol 1992;16:633–42. On page 538 in a footnote, the authors' noted: "The term "endocervicosis" was first used in 1943 by Goodall to refer to two cases in which there was deep infiltration of the cervical wall and paracervical tissues by benign-appearing endocervical glands. The pathology of the lesions was not illustrated, but by current criteria they would probably be interpreted as examples of minimal deviation adenocarcinoma ("adenoma malignum"). See also, Young RH, Clement PB. Endocervicosis involving the uterine cervix: a report of four cases of a benign process that may be confused with deeply invasive endocervical adenocarcinoma. Int J Gynecol Pathol 2000;19:322–8. "In adenoma malignum, the lesional glands originate from the mucosa and grow downward, whereas in cases of endocervicosis, the glands usually are confined to the outer aspect of the cervix. When there is a clear demarcation between normal endocervical glands and the more deeply seated glands of endocervicosis, with a zone of uninvolved cervical wall, it should be readily apparent that the deep glands cannot represent glands that have spread from the mucosa."

[105] Clement PB, Young RH. Endocervicosis of the urinary bladder. A report of six cases of a benign müllerian lesion that may mimic adenocarcinoma. Am J Surg Pathol 1992;16:533–542.

[106] Sampson JA. Heterotopic or misplaced endometrial tissue. Am J Obstet Gynecol 1925;10:649–664:649–650. Of historical interest, in this publication, Sampson equated the following terms for adenomyosis: adenomyosis = direct endometriosis = primary endometriosis = müllerianosis. Thereafter, Sampson abandoned such usage for müllerianosis. The writer appropriated the abandoned term müllerianosis in 1990 and thereafter, to designate Sampson's developmentally misplaced endometrial, endosalpingeal, and endocervical tissue. Ronald E. Batt, Richard A. Smith, Germaine M. Buck, Mark F. Severino, and John D. Naples, "Müllerianosis," In *Current Concepts in Endometriosis. Progress in Clinical and Biological Research*, edited by D. Chadha and V. Buttram. [New York: Alan R. Liss, 1990], 323:413–426. (Proceedings of the Second International Symposium on Endometriosis, Houston, Texas, 1-3 May 1989). Ronald E. Batt, Smith RA, Buck Louis GM, Martin DC, Chapron C, Koninckx PR, Yeh J. Müllerianosis. Histology and Histopathology 2007; 22:1161–1166.

[107] Russell WW. Aberrant portions of the müllerian duct found in an ovary. Bull Johns Hopkins Hospital 1899;10:8–10 plus 3 plates. Russell was the physician who displaced Cullen from the residency position promised by Howard Kelly; a displacement that lead to Cullen's spending 3 years in pathology before he entered the gynecological residency.

brought to Sampson's attention by the obituary for Russell written by his old chief and role model, Howard Kelly. In the last sentence of the obituary, Kelly wrote: "Without any doubt, his most important contribution was a carefully made objective study of a case, the first reported, of endometrial tissue in the ovary, far reaching in its consequences in view of the later studies of Thomas S. Cullen and John A. Sampson."[109]

By 1943, while Cullen and Sampson were still alive, three of the five benign müllerian diseases had been described. Rokitansky had described uterine endometriosis (adenomyosis) and extrauterine (ovarian) endometriosis in 1860 and Chiari had identified endosalpingiosis (salpingitis isthmica nodosa) in 1887. Possibly four of the five benign müllerian diseases had been identified, if one will allow that the demonstration by Robert Meyer of a developmental müllerian choristoma, "islands of endometrium in the uterine wall of a fetus of nine months," constituted developmentally misplaced endometrial tissue, developmental adenomyosis;[110] or the case report of Russell, or if one will accept the case report of endometriosis of the kidney in the absence of pelvic endometriosis reported by Victor F. Marshall.[111]

In 1897 and 1898, Robert Meyer had demonstrated non-müllerian choristomas, adrenal rests – developmentally misplaced adrenal tissue – in "the broad ligament of both fetus and adult."[112] Recall also that in 1901, William Welch had diagnosed a non-müllerian choristoma, a developmental anomaly: bone and embryonic connective tissue in a uterus, i.e., developmentally misplaced non-müllerian tissue within the musculature of the uterus.[113] While the above are all examples suggesting developmentally misplaced tissue, in all likelihood, Sampson was aware only of Russell's report – from conversations with Russell at Johns Hopkins during his residency years or later at the American Gynecological Society.

Having observed the historical emergence of acquired adenomyosis, endometriosis, endosalpingiosis, and developmentally misplaced endometrium by mid-twentieth century, we return to the question posed earlier in this work. Are they separate and distinct diseases or different phenotypic expressions of the same disease process? The answer to the question is both yes and no. It seems that all acquired benign müllerian tissues, normally associated with the mature human reproductive organs, possess a latent tendency to invade. Such is the case with benign endometrial and endosalpingeal mucosa, the human blastocyst, the placenta, as well as the hydatidiform mole. In contrast, all developmental benign müllerian choristomas – normal embryonic endocervical, endometrial, and/or endosalpingeal tissue: the developmentally misplaced müllerian tissue of Sampson – tend not to invade the normal organs in which they have been misplaced during organogenesis. Menstrual effusion from developmental choristomas containing endometrium is not considered invasive.

In sum, adenomyosis and endosalpingiosis are phenotypic expressions of direct or internal endometriosis. Endometriosis and peritoneal endosalpingiosis are phenotypic expressions of indirect or external endometriosis. All are invasive *acquired* müllerian diseases derived from mature müllerian tissue. In the sense that they are *invasive* as well as *acquired* müllerian diseases, adenomyosis, endosalpingiosis, and endometriosis differ from *noninvasive*, *developmental* müllerian diseases. On the other hand, both acquired müllerian diseases and developmental müllerian diseases may be considered as simply different phenotypic expressions of misplaced müllerian tissue and – in that all inclusive sense – the same disease process.

The research efforts of Cullen, Novak, Meyer, Grünwald, Goodall, and Sampson, and scores of other investigators illustrate once again the difficulty of defining pathology and pathogenesis of benign chronic disease in the interior of the human body at mid-twentieth century.

---

[108] Sampson JA. Heterotopic or misplaced endometrial tissue. Am J Obstet Gynecol 1925;10:649–664:649–650.

[109] Kelly HA. William Wood Russell, M.D. 1866–1924. Trans Am Gynecological Society 1924;49:383–384.

[110] Meyer R. *Autobiography of Dr. Robert Meyer (1864–1947): A Short Abstract of a Long Life* [New York: Henry Schuman, 1949], 33.

[111] Marshall VF. Endometrial tissue in the kidney. J Urology 1943;50:652. This was the same Victor Marshall of the Marshall, Marchetti, Krantz operation for stress urinary incontinence in women. Certainly, Marshall was familiar with female pelvic pathology.

[112] Robert Meyer, *Autobiography of Dr. Robert Meyer (1864–1947): A Short Abstract of a Long Life* [New York: Henry Schuman, 1949], 34. "In 1897 and 1898, I demonstrated some malformations and accessory adrenal tissue in the broad ligament of both fetus and adult. (The continuation of these studies is found in *Zeitschr. f. Geb. u. Gyn. 41*). Robert Meyer, *Autobiography of Dr. Robert Meyer (1864–1947): A Short Abstract of a Long Life* [New York: Henry Schuman, 1949], 86." "Cysts in the Vaginal Wall of Fetuses of 3–5 months." *Arch. f. Gyn.* 151 [1932]. "Those cysts from the Müllerian epithelium lie in the median plane as do also the cysts in the uterus."

[113] William Henry Welch, *Pathology, Preventive Medicine*, vol. 1 of *Papers and Addresses by William Henry Welch* [Baltimore, MD: Johns Hopkins Press, 1920], 432–3. Johnston, George B. Osteo-Fibromyoma of the Uterus. Am Gynaec & Obst. J., N.Y., 1901, XVIII, 307–308.

11 Scientific Objectivity

The Philosophy of Kant

> The need to unravel the skein of politics by starting from the subjects' duties rather than the citizens' rights has recently been stressed. Likewise it is diseases which have stimulated physiology; and it is not physiology but pathology and clinical practice which gave medicine its start. The reason is that as a matter of fact well-being is not felt, for it is the simple awareness of living, and only its impediment provokes the force of resistance. It is no wonder then that Brown begins by classifying diseases. Kant[1]

Scientific objectivity had to be restored to nineteenth century European medical science before diseases – such as endometriosis, adenomyosis, endosalpingiosis, and developmentally misplaced endometrium – could be identified from among the myriad of chronic diseases that ravaged the interior of the human body. Objective research in the biological sciences in many European centers had ground to a virtual standstill during the late seventeenth and early eighteenth centuries as many medical scientists succumbed to the nature philosophy of Friedrich Schelling (1775–1854).[2] Schelling's was a philosophy that deduced all of nature from pure reason.[3]

The German philosopher Immanuel Kant (1724–1804) laid the foundation for the restoration of scientific objectivity in his mature work of 1790, the *Critique of Judgment*. Johann Friedrich Blumenbach, professor of medicine at the University of Göttingen from 1778 to 1835, directly incorporated Kant's philosophy of scientific objectivity into his teaching.[4] No less an authority than Kant himself regarded Blumenbach "as

[1] Kant, *Werke,* Akdemie Ausgabe, 15(2), Anthropologie, in the ‚Handschriftlicher Nachlass', circa 1798, p. 964. Kant cited by Georges Canguilhem, *The Normal and the Pathological.* Trans. Carolyn R. Fawcett in collaboration with Robert S. Cohen [New York: Zone Books, 1991], 141.

[2] Karl Sudhoff, "Goethe and Johannes Müller," in *Essays in the History of Medicine* trans. by various hands and ed. Fielding H. Garrison [New York: Medical Life Press, 1926], 371. "As if lost in dreams, the medicine and natural history of those days rested quietly in the shadow of the system of Nature Philosophy expounded by the gifted Friedrich Wilhelm Joseph Schelling. This system evolved all natural phenomena from the idea of the absolute and endeavored to spiritualize all natural laws and turn them into laws of perception and cogitation, in consequence of which all natural phenomena seemed to disappear. Even the greatest investigators had fallen before the power of this theory and research came to a standstill, as people were chiefly concerned with bringing everything into line with this system. In this confused era, Goethe, the scientist, had kept himself free from all such philosophic fragments of imagination. Upon him fell the task of saving the great principle of observation." See also: Erna Lesky, *The Vienna Medical School of the 19th Century* [Baltimore, MD: Johns Hopkins University Press, 1976], 80.

[3] Friedrich Wilhelm Joseph Schelling, *First Outline of a System of the Philosophy of Nature.* Trans. Keith R. Peterson [Albany, NY: State University of New York Press, 2004].

[4] Timothy Lenoir, The Strategy of Life: Teleology and Mechanics in Nineteenth-Century German Biology [Chicago, IL: University of Chicago Press, 1989], 13. See: J. Bronowski and Bruce Mazlish, "Kant and Hegel: The Emergence of History." In *The Western Intellectual Tradition [*Dorset Press, 1986], 472–3. Kant founded the tradition of philosophy in Germany. "The problems of philosophy in the seventeenth and eighteenth centuries were related to the advance of science then. Much work in philosophy was an attempt to find foundations for the new science, and many philosophers were scientists. Kant was among these, and his philosophy was such an attempt to close a gap in the foundations of science which had been opened unexpectedly in his boyhood." J. Bronowski and Bruce Mazlish, 477. "Kant himself was trained as a mathematician and physicist, and for much of his life he

R.E. Batt, *A History of Endometriosis*,
DOI 10.1007/978-0-85729-585-9_11, © Springer-Verlag London Limited 2011

one of the most profound biological theorists of the modern era."[5] Blumenbach in turn taught or directly influenced Johann Wolfgang von Goethe, Alexander von Humboldt, and Johann Friedrich Meckel. Students and associates of Blumenbach in turn influenced Johannes Müller and Rokitansky. Such was the philosophical background and scientific genealogy fundamental to the emergence of objectivity in medical science, objectivity necessary for the discovery of adenomyosis and endometriosis.

For years, Rokitansky practiced macroscopic scientific objectivity during thousands of autopsies before he slowly embraced microscopy to examine more closely unusual cases that caught his attention. Such were the circumstances that lead to Rokitansky's discovery and description of three different phenotypes of endometriosis all containing benign endometrial stroma and glands. One invaded the uterine muscular wall (*cystosarcoma adenoids uterinum*) and was accompanied by myometrial hypertrophy; another invaded the endometrial cavity forming a polyp (*cystosarcoma adenoids uterinum polyposum*).[6] The third phenotype was an ovarian endometrioma (cystosarcoma adenoids ovarii uterinum.[7] Recall that at mid-nineteenth century Rokitansky, the first full-time pathologist, had defined sarcoma as benign tissue. Thus, in 1860–1861, Rokitansky identified internal endometriosis: adenomyosis, and a phenotype of external endometriosis: an ovarian endometrioma. His former assistant Chiari described endosalpingiosis in 1887, also known as salpingitis isthmica nodosa.[8]

The birth of surgical pathology at the end of the nineteenth century facilitated research into this enigmatic disease, research that required the interaction of clinic and laboratory such as that between the gynecologist Carl Ruge and the gynecologic pathologist Robert Meyer, and between the gynecologist Wilhelm Alexander Freund and the pathologist Friedrich von Recklinghausen.[9] With specimens provided by Freund, von Recklinghausen popularized Rokitansky's *cystosarcoma adenoids uterinum* and Chiari's salpingitis isthmica nodosa, which he renamed adenomyoma of the uterus and tube, respectively in 1895.[10] Cullen challenged von Recklinghausen the following year, a

earned his living as a lecturer in physics. He made an original contribution to science in 1775, when he put forward for the first time the theory that the planets have been condensed from a mass of gas, which Laplace formulated more accurately in 1796. Only at the age of 45, in 1769, did Kant begin to trouble himself with the philosophical difficulties in the foundations of science which Hume had thrown up. In that year Kant had the great revelation, that some knowledge must be a priori in order to make empirical science possible at all, which turned his career to philosophy. In the following year, in 1770, Kant was elected to the chair of logic and metaphysics in his native university of Konigsberg in East Prussia, and he outlined his approach in his inaugural lecture and published it fully in his book *The Critique of Pure Reason* in 1881." J. Bronowski and Bruce Mazlish, 479. "The question that drove Kant was, 'How does it come about that the human mind so naturally understands what goes on outside it.'" J. Bronowski and Bruce Mazlish, 477. Kant greatly influenced German scientists in the nineteenth century. See also. Ronald H. Brady, "The Idea in Nature: Rereading Goethe's Organics." In *Goethe's Way of Science: A Phenomenology of Nature,* edited by David Seamon and Arthur Zajonc, 83–111:90. [Albany, NY: State University of New York Press, 1998], 83–111:90.

[5] Timothy Lenoir, The Strategy of Life: Teleology ad Mechanics in Nineteenth-Century German Biology [Chicago, IL: University of Chicago Press, 1989], 17, 18.

[6] Carl Rokitansky, Ueber Uterusdrüsen-Neubildung in Uterus- und Ovarial-Sarcomen. Zeitschift Gesellschaft der Aerzte in Wien. 1860;16:577–581. See also: Emge LA. The elusive adenomyosis of the uterus: its historical past and its present state of recognition. Am J Obstet Gynecol 1962;83:1541–1563:1542.

[7] Carl Rokitansky, Lehrbuch der Pathologischen Anatomie III. Auflage 1855–1861. III. Band p. 488–491. Also cited by Pick L. Arch f Gynaek 1905;lxxvi:251–275, and Sampson JA. Heterotopic or misplaced endometrial tissue. Am J Obstet Gynecol 1925;10:649–664:655.

[8] Chiari H. Zur pathologischen Anatomie des Eileiter-Catarrhs. Pager Ztschr. Heilkunde 1887;8:457–473. That same year, Martin reported cases similar to Chiari. Martin. Uber Tubenkrankung. Zeitschr für Geb und Gynak 1887;13. S. 299. Martin cited by: Cuthbert Lockyer, *Fibroids and Allied Tumours (Myoma and Adenomyoma): Their Pathology, Clinical Features and Surgical Treatment* [London: Macmillan and Company, 1918], 284.

[9] Robert Meyer, *Autobiography of Dr. Robert Meyer (1864–1947): A Short Abstract of a Long Life.* With a Memoir of Dr. Meyer by Emil Novak, MD. [New York: Henry Schuman, 1949], 33. Friedrich v. Recklinghausen, *Die Adenomyome und Cystadenome der Uterus- und Tubenwandung ihre Abkunft von Resten des Wolff'schen Korpers. Im Anhang: Von W. A. Freund, Klinische Notizen zu den voluminosen Adenomyomen des Uterus* [Berlin: Verlag von August Hirschwald, 1896.]

[10] Von Recklinghausen F. Ueber die Adenomyome des Uterus und der Tuba. Wiener Klinische Wochenschrift 1895;29:530. In 1925, Oskar Frankl recommended that the designation "adenomyoma uteri" be reserved for encapsulated adenomyoma and that diffuse adenomyosis be called "adenomyosis." Frankl O. Adenomyosis uteri. Am J Obstet Gynecol 1925;10:680–684. See also: Benagiano G, Brosens I. History of adenomyosis. Best Practice Research Clinical Obstet Gynaecol 2006;20:449–463.

challenge that brought immediate recognition to the fledgling gynecologic pathologist; the scientific debate that ensued introduced the study of endometriotic disease into North America.[11]

Over a period of 25 years, Cullen studied with varying degrees of intensity all the common phenotypes of endometriosis in the pelvis and abdomen. The Englishman Cuthbert Lockyer wrote an important monograph that summarized the research in all manifestations of endometriosis recognized prior to World War I.[12] Cullen arranged for Casler to present his unique case of the menstruating ovary to the American Gynecologic Society in 1919. From this case, John Sampson drew his initial insight for the implantation theory of peritoneal endometriosis. Sampson evolved his complete three-step theory of pathogenesis of peritoneal endometriosis over a 10-year period of intense research. He implicated both uterine and fallopian tubal mucosa in the pathogenesis of peritoneal and ovarian endometriosis as well as the pathogenesis of endometriotic adhesive disease. Sampson also postulated venous and lymphatic dissemination of endometriosis. In debate with supporters of the theory of coelomic metaplasia for a quarter of a century, he strove without success to prove his theory.[13]

In 1949, just 3 years after Sampson died, Carl Javert noted "there has been a great tendency to favor only one [theory]; namely, the coelomic–metaplasia theory of Iwanoff, Meyer, and Novak."[14] Javert argued that "no single theory entirely explains the pathogenesis of endometriosis."[15] He combined several theories into a composite theory.[16] In 1949, Robert Meyer also addressed the validity of Sampson's theory. "Let us not forget the impulse that gave us Sampson's theory of endometriosis. Who is right is of no importance; what is right is what matters. This axiom I applied then, forty years ago [with reference to von Recklinghausen]. It is more important that the work of a man stimulates others to go on working than that his own conceptions become established. It is true that I have now changed my mind with respect to the question of adenomyosis. Some critics maintain that this is not right and stress the fact that the new points of view were reached indirectly, in the theory of adenomyosis as well as other problems. I have always thought that as long as a man can change his clothes standing up and can change his mind he is not yet really old."[17]

Early in his career, Sampson had noted: "cancer of the cervix…unfortunately is a disease of midlife, occurring most frequently between the ages of thirty and fifty years."[18] At about the same time, Cullen came to the conclusion that uterine fibroids and uterine adenomyoma also occurred most frequently between the ages of 30 and 50 years. The regular occurrence of uterine fibroids, cervical cancer, uterine adenomyoma, and adenomyoma of the rectovaginal septum all within the same time frame in a woman's life, led to the perception that all such were midlife diseases. Consequently, it was not until 1946 that endometriosis was diagnosed at laparotomy in adolescents,[19] and not until the 1970s and 1980s – with laparoscopy – that adolescent endometriosis was recognized more widely.

[11] Friedrich v. Recklinghausen, *Die Adenomyome und Cystadenome der Uterus- und Tubenwandung ihre Abkunft von Resten des Wolff'schen Korpers. Im Anhang: Von W. A. Freund, Klinische Notizen zu den voluminosen Adenomyomen des Uterus* [Berlin: Verlag von August Hirschwald, 1896.] Cullen, TS. Adeno-myoma uteri diffusum benignum. Bulletin Johns Hopkins Hospital 1896;6:133–157:139.

[12] Cuthbert Lockyer, *Fibroids and Allied Tumours (Myoma and Adenomyoma): Their Pathology, Clinical Features and Surgical Treatment* [London: Macmillan and Company, 1918],

[13] During Sampson's life time, Robert Meyer, Emil Novak, Peter Grünwald, GH Gardiner, Brooks Ranney, and Joe V Meigs supported the theory of coelomic metaplasia. See Robert Meyer, *Autobiography of Dr. Robert Meyer: (1864–1947): A Short Abstract of a Long Life* [New York: Henry Schuman, 1949], 78. "Peter Grünwald, the embryologist in Boston, insists that endometriosis may arise from coelomic epithelium."

[14] Javert CT. Pathogenesis of endometriosis based on endometrial homeoplasia, direct extension, exfoliation ad implantation, lymphatic, and hematogenous metastasis. (Including five case reports of endometrial tissue in pelvic lymph nodes). Cancer 1949;2:399–410:407.

[15] Javert CT. Cancer 1949;2:399–410:407.

[16] Javert CT. Cancer 1949;2:399–410. See: Benagiano G, Brosens I. History of Adenomyosis. Best Practice & Research Clinical Obstetrics and Gynaecology 2006;20:449–463:460. See also Brosens IA, Brosens JJ. Endometriosis. Eur J Obstet Gynecol Reprod Biol 2000;90:159–164. Though much of the twentieth century research has "focused on the finding evidence for Sampson's regurgitation theory…the underlying mechanism, implantation, and/or induction, remains unsolved."

[17] Robert Meyer, *Autobiography of Dr. Robert Meyer: (1864–1947): A Short Abstract of a Long Life* [New York: Henry Schuman, 1949], 33.

[18] Sampson JA. The clinical manifestations of uterine cancer. International Clinics 1908;(Series 18(2):176–201:199.

[19] Fallon J. Endometriosis in youth. JAMA 1946;131:1405.

At Sampson's death in 1946, diagnosis was based principally on an acquired awareness of endometriosis, its signs and symptoms, and by careful pelvic and rectal examination. There were no ancillary diagnostic modalities; peritoneoscopy (laparoscopy) had been abandoned due to poor equipment. Surgical treatment remained the same as Sampson practiced: conservative surgery for infertility on a selective basis, otherwise hysterectomy and removal of both tubes and ovaries when symptomatic treatment failed. In 1944, Miller advocated the use of testosterone hormone prior to operation to aid surgical treatment.[20] An attempt at medical suppression of endometriosis using diethylstilbestrol would not be introduced by Karnaky until 1948.[21] The concept of prevention developed relatively late. In 1948, Meigs, an early advocate of the prevention of endometriosis-associated infertility, recommended early marriage and pregnancy, urging parents to subsidize newlyweds instead of leaving them an inheritance. This may be considered a first attempt to prevent the disease by a cultural strategy.[22] On the other hand, great strides were made in continuing medical education for returning WWII veterans eager for specialty training in gynecology and obstetrics.[23]

Physician awareness and empathy for patient's complaints increased dramatically when gynecologists could diagnose endometriosis following the reintroduction of laparoscopy in North America in the 1960s by Melvin R Cohen,[24] and the popularization of laparoscopy in 1970s by Jordan M. Phillips.[25] Direct patient involvement began auspiciously in 1980 with the initiative of Mary Lou Ballweg, founder of the Endometriosis Association with International Headquarters in Milwaukee, Wisconsin.[26] From the beginning, this organization provided information to patients with endometriosis and within the first decade sponsored sophisticated research into the pathophysiology of endometriosis, especially as related to environmental toxicology.[27]

Maurice A. Bruhat and Michel Canis of Clermont-Ferrand, France with Veasy C. Buttram of Houston, Texas; Paul Dmowski of Chicago, Illinois; and Alain Audebert of Bordeaux, France convened the First International Symposium on Endometriosis at Clermont-Ferrand, France, November 19–21, 1986. The organizers recognized the need for more coordinated and sophisticated research, in order to achieve a "deeper understanding of this many-sided disease. By bringing together in Clermont-Ferrand the most advanced specialists in the world in this field and giving them three days to tackle all the facets of this mysterious ailment, they would be able to compare hopes and disappointments, come to a consensus on certain points, and agree on the major lines for research in the future."[28]

In the preface to the proceedings of the First International Symposium on Endometriosis, Professor Bruhat revealed the circumstances that lead to the Symposium. "Why did Endometriosis 1986, International Symposium come into being? Because the remarkable work of one of the doctors in our department meant that we read 500 articles on endometriosis. To our astonishment we found that the pathogenesis was not always clearly perceived, even if some workers have made some progress in the fields of immunology and hormonology; that the evaluation of endometriosis goes no further than a 'geographical' description, which is necessary, yes, but how limited! For how then can microscopic forms be taken into

[20] Miller JR. Preoperative use of testosterone propionate as aid to surgical treatment of endometriosis. JAMA 1944;125:207–208.

[21] Karnaky, KJ. Use of stilbestrol for endometriosis: preliminary report. South M J 1948;41:1109.

[22] Meigs JV. Endometriosis. Ann Surg 1948;127:795–809:805.

[23] Catch-up and continuing medical education for returning WWII veterans was provided by Joe Vincent Meigs and Somers H. Sturgis, editors of *Progress in Gynecology.* New York: Grune & Stratton, 1946. Also in 1946, Nicholas J. Eastman and Emil Novak founded and edited the *Obstetrical and Gynecological Survey.*

[24] Cohen MR. Culdoscopy vs. peritoneoscopy. Obstet Gynecol 1968;31:319–21.

[25] In 1971, Jordan Phillips founded the American Association for Gynecological Laparoscopy, and through the AAGL taught laparoscopic and later microsurgical skills to thousands of gynecologists. Ronald E. Batt. Jordan M Phillips, MD – Postdoctoral educator-at-large. Journal of Reproductive Medicine 1992;37:626–628. (Translated by Dr. Han Yu Chi of Tianjin Medical, College Library People's Republic of China for the Translation Journal, 1993). Ronald E. Batt. Jordan Matthew Phillips, MD: Visionary, Founder of the AAGL, Organizational Genius. Journal of Minimally Invasive Gynecology 2007; 14:536–7.

[26] Endometriosis Association. International Headquarters, 8585 N. 76th Place, Milwaukee, Wisconsin, USA 53223.

[27] Rier SE, Martin DC, Bowman RE, Dmowski WP, Becker JL. Endometriosis in rhesus monkeys (Macaca mulatta) following chronic exposure to 2,3,7,8-tetrachlorodibenzo-p-dioxin. Fundam Appl Toxicol 1993;21:433–41.

[28] Maurice A. Bruhat and Michel Canis, eds. *Endometriosis* [Basel, Switzerland: Karger, 1987], ix–x.

account? How can the evolutivity of a lesion be assessed? That treatments were judged by subjective criteria such as pain, or were often poorly assessed as in the case for sterility!"[29]

Who had performed that remarkable work? It was Michel Henri Jean Canis, now Professeur Michel Canis of the C.H.U. Clermont-Ferrand Polyclinique, Clermont-Ferrand, France. His thesis for the Doctorate in Medicine provided the stimulus for the pathbreaking International Symposium in 1986.[30] Surely, his must be the most powerful academic thesis ever written on the subject; for in the ensuing years, research in all phases of endometriosis: pathogenesis, pathology, pathophysiology, genetics, environmental influences, evolutionary developmental biology, improved diagnostic techniques, laparoscopic and robotic surgery, and new medical treatments flowed from the concerted academic coordination of clinical and laboratory research. Ten World Congresses on Endometriosis were held in countries in the four corners of the world between 1986 and 2008. Under the leadership of Professor Hans Evers, The World Endometriosis Society will sponsor the Eleventh World Congress on Endometriosis in Montpellier, France, September 4–7, 2011.[31]

[29] Maurice A. Bruhat, "Preface," in Maurice A. Bruhat and Michel Canis, eds. *Endometriosis* [Basel, Switzerland:Karger, 1987], ix–x.

[30] Michel Henri Jean Canis, Thesis pour le Doctorat en Medecine (Diplome d'Etat) par CANIS Michel, Henri, Jean. Ne le 3 Octobre 1957 a Chamalieres (PUY-DE-DOME) Presentee et soutenue publiquement le 30 octobre 1894. "TENTATIVE DE MISE AU POINT SUR L'ENDOMETRIOSE EN 1984." [Doctorat en Medicine. Universite de Clermont I Faculte de Medicine, 1984]. [An Attempt to Launch an Investigation into the State of Endometriosis].

[31] The World Endometriosis Society was founded in 1998 to promote the exchange of clinical experience, scientific thought, and investigation among gynaecologists, endocrinologists, scientists, biologists, and other qualified individuals interested in advancing the field of endometriosis.

Epilogue

12

The Foundational History of Endometriosis

This essay is offered as a foundational history for the field of endometriotic diseases. It is addressed to an international professional audience of physicians and scientists, their younger colleagues, fellows and residents, medical students and nurses, and importantly, historians of medicine and science and their graduate students. The scholarly apparatus contains informational and explanatory as well as documentary notes.

The complexity of endometriosis is easier to understand when viewed as the major expression of five closely related benign müllerian diseases: endometriosis, adenomyosis, endosalpingiosis, endocervicosis, and müllerianosis. From this perspective, this is a story of lumping and sorting, of imposing order on individual expressions of disease in order to devise a program for diagnosis and treatment. For 500 years, there was an attempt at statistical grouping of signs and symptoms on the basis of objectivity. The shift from treating symptoms to treating diseases brought order out of chaos through the application of macroscopic morbid pathology and microscopic surgical pathology. Creation of endometriotic disease as a clinical entity – which explained why patients had endometriosis-associated pain, infertility, and health problems and how physicians could relieve some of the problems – was a giant leap forward during the era from 1860 to 1946.

The future of endometriosis research is unknown. However, the past can be captured to anchor the history of the disease and highlight the intellectual quest to understand endometriotic diseases. In doing so, we are consolidating what we know and do not know. John Sampson's rich contribution to the pathology and pathogenesis of endometriosis and endosalpingiosis has been reduced to a caricature in textbooks, where his theory of retrograde menstruation and implantation is mentioned among other theories of pathogenesis. Thomas Cullen's formidable contributions to the pathology of uterine adenomyosis and extrauterine adenomyomas are seldom mentioned. European contributions that preceded those of Cullen have been largely forgotten. It took 86 years to move from the morbid pathology of Rokitansky to the pathophysiology of Cullen and Sampson, and then another 64 years of consolidation till now, we are preparing for another leap forward to personalized medicine. We are entering an era of new understanding and it is time to take stock of where we have been and to understand what we have done. Ivo Brosens insightfully noted that most of the twentieth century was spent trying to prove the implantation theory of Sampson.

In the twenty-first century as medicine moves from treatments based on statistical evidence-based medicine and returns to the Hippocratic concept of individual dyscrasias, of personal disease based on the individual's genome and environmental exposures, organized medicine must reorder ideas for the future. However, for the time under consideration – 1860 to 1946 – the pathophysiology of endometriosis only began to be understood during the era of Thomas Cullen and John Sampson, an era when surgery was the only treatment.

The story is real and I understand the reality of that time. I have treated thousands of patients with endometriosis. Field research for this history began in the early 1970s when I developed a close professional relationship with my professor of pathology, Kornel Ludwig Terplan. I learned that Dr. Terplan traced his ancestry in

R.E. Batt, *A History of Endometriosis*,
DOI 10.1007/978-0-85729-585-9_12, © Springer-Verlag London Limited 2011

academic pathology directly to Carl Rokitansky. Terplan was the premier assistant of Anton Ghon, who was the assistant of Anton Weichselbaum, who in turn was the assistant of Joseph Engel, the most brilliant assistant of Carl Rokitansky. Dr. Terplan introduced me to central European pathology. During that time, I took mini-sabbaticals to study surgery on the service of Professor Husslein at the II Frauenklinik, University of Vienna; at the University of Graz, Austria with Professor Navratil; and at the University Hospital in Strasbourg, Alsace, France. This preliminary fieldwork helped immensely. It is the author's hope that this scholarly essay will open the history of endometriosis to critical debate, refinement, and further contributions.

Appendix I: Glossary of Terms, Definitions and Theories

Adenomyoma "The term 'adenomyoma' implies a new formation composed of gland-elements, hyperplastic cellular connective tissue [stroma], and smooth muscle."[1]

Adenomyoma "An isolated area of endometrial glands and stroma in the uterine musculature that can be identified grossly."[2]

Adenomyosis "The growth of endometrial glands and stroma into the uterine myometrium to a depth of at last 2.5 mm from the basalis layer of the endometrium."[3]

Adenomyosis "Adenomyosis may be defined as the benign invasion of endometrium into the myometrium. This invasion produces a diffusely enlarged uterus which microscopically exhibits ectopic, nonneoplastic, endometrial glands and stroma surrounded by hypertrophic-hyperplastic musculature. Some of the historical synonyms for adenomyosis are: endometriosis interna, adenomyoma, adenomyomatosis, adenometritis, adenomyositis, and [briefly] von Recklinghausen's disease."[4]

Bildung "The nine-year-long *Gymnasium* with an emphasis on training in classical studies and then the university with its philosophical faculty, complemented by faculties for medicine, theology, and jurisprudence, became the places to devote oneself seriously to *Bildung*. Academic scholarship in all fields was expected to serve the higher moral aims laid out by idealism and neo-humanism. Professors therefore had to be more than simply purveyors of knowledge. They were seen as moral models and agents of creativity, restlessly aiming at expanding the limits of knowledge, disregarding any utilitarian purpose or social constraints, and guided only by their free will."[5]

Chocolate cyst "A cystic area of endometriosis in the ovary."[6]

Choristoma A choristoma is a mass of histologically normal tissue that is "not normally found in the organ or structure in which it is located." Müllerian choristomas are a subset of non-müllerian choristomas found throughout the body.

Coelomic Metaplasia "The potential ability of coelomic epithelium to develop into several different histologic cell types."[7]

Coelomic metaplasia The abnormal transformation of adult, fully differentiated tissue lining the peritoneal

[1]Cuthbert Lockyer, *Fibroids and Allied Tumours (Myoma and Adenomyoma): Their Pathology, Clinical Features and Surgical Treatment* [London: Macmillan and Company, 1918], 265.

[2]Morton A. Stenchever, William Droegemueller, Arthur L. Herbst, and Daniel R. Mishell. *Comprehensive Gynecology*. 4th edition. [St. Louis, MI: Mosby, 2001], 531.

[3]Morton A. Stenchever, William Droegemueller, Arthur L. Herbst, and Daniel R. Mishell. *Comprehensive Gynecology*. 4th edition. [St. Louis, MI: Mosby, 2001], 531.

[4]McElin TW, Bird CC. Adenomyosis of the uterus. In Ralph M. Wynn, Ed. *Obstetrics and Gynecology Annual*. Vol. 3. New York: Appleton-Century-Crofts, 1974:425–441.

[5]Andreas W. Daum, "*Wissenschaft* and knowledge," in *The Short Oxford History of Germany: Germany 1800–1870* [Oxford: Oxford University Press, 2004], 137–161:145.

[6]Morton A. Stenchever, William Droegemueller, Arthur L. Herbst, and Daniel R. Mishell. *Comprehensive Gynecology*. 4th edition. [St. Louis, MI: Mosby, 2001], 531.

[7]Morton A. Stenchever, 531.

R.E. Batt, *A History of Endometriosis*,
DOI 10.1007/978-0-85729-585-9, © Springer-Verlag London Limited 2011

cavity into a differentiated tissue of another kind, such as endometrial tissue.

Emergence "Emergence…refers to the arising of novel and coherent structures, patterns, and properties during the process of self-organization in complex systems. Emergent phenomena are conceptualized as occurring on the macro level, in contrast to the micro-level components and processes out of which they arise. In a wide variety of scientific and mathematical fields, grouped together loosely under the title 'complexity theory,' a intense search is now under way for characteristics and laws associated with emergent phenomena observed across different types of complex systems."[8]

Endometrioma "A small area of endometriosis that can be identified macroscopically."[9]

Endometriosis "The presence and growth of glands and stroma identical to the lining of the uterus in an aberrant location."[10]

Endometriosis Sampson's definition of endometriosis – 1940: "The term endometriosis was introduced to indicate the presence of ectopic tissue which possess the histologic structure and function of the uterine mucosa. It also includes the abnormal conditions which may result not only from the invasion of organs and other structures by this disease, but also from its reaction to menstruation."[11]

Germinal epithelium Germinal epithelium of the ovary consists of low flat mesothelial cells on the surface of the ovary, similar to those lining the peritoneal cavity. Mesothelial cells are derived from the mesoderm which gives rise to the gastrointestinal and reproductive organs.

Gymnasium The *Gymnasia* "were meant to create environments where students would learn, through active participation to think for themselves and develop new ideas. The focus on the individual's creative potential, and more so, on the importance of providing an educational environment aimed at stimulating this potential, is fully consistent with the humanistic conception of *Bildung*."[12]

Heteroplasia Heteroplasia, on the other hand, is the development of cytologic and histologic elements that are not normal for the organ or part in question, as the growth of bone in a site where there is normal fibrous connective tissue.[13] Heterotopia means cells or tissue displaced to an abnormal location.

Metaplasia Metaplasia is the abnormal transformation of an adult, fully differentiated tissue of one kind into a differentiated tissue of another kind; metaplasia is an acquired condition in contrast to heteroplasia.[14]

Müllerian duct Müllerian duct, also known as the paramesonephric duct, arises from the urogenital ridge in the fetus to form the fallopian tubes, uterus, cervix, and upper vagina.

Müllerian rest The paired müllerian tubes – primitive vertebrate fallopian tubes, uterus, cervix, and upper vagina – comprise two elongated masses in the early vertebrae embryo. A müllerian rest represents a group of cells or a portion of the müllerian that has become displaced and lies embedded in tissue of another character that persists as an embryonic remnant in the adult.

Müllerianosis Müllerianosis may be defined as an organoid structure of embryonic origin; a choristoma composed of müllerian rests – normal endometrium, normal endosalpinx, and normal endocervix – singly or in combination, incorporated within other normal organs during organogenesis. "A choristoma is a mass of histologically normal tissue that is not normally found in the organ or structure in which

[8]Goldstein, Jeffrey. Emergence as a construct: history and issues. Emergence 1999;1:40–72. See also: John H. Holland, *Emergence: From Chaos to Order* [New York: Basic Books, 1998].

[9]Morton A. Stenchever, 531.

[10]Morton A. Stenchever, 531.

[11]Sampson JA. The development of the implantation theory for the origin of peritoneal endometriosis. Am J Obstet Gynecol 1940;40:549–557.

[12]Arleen Marcia Tuchman, Science, Medicine, and the State of Germany: The Case of Baden, 1815–1871 [New York: Oxford University Press, 1993], 41.

[13]*Illustrated Stedman's Medical Dictionary*. 24th ed. [Baltimore, MD: Williams & Wilkins, 1982], 647.

[14]*Illustrated Stedman's Medical Dictionary*, 864.

[15]Stedman's Medical Dictionary. 28th Edition. Philadelphia: Lippicott Williams & Wilkins, 2006: 371.

[16]Batt RE, Smith RA, Buck Louis GM, Martin DC, Chapron C, Koninckx PR, Yeh J. Müllerianosis. Histol Histopathol 2007; 22:1161–1166.

[17]Knud Faber, *Nosography in Modern Internal Medicine* [New York: Paul B. Hoeber, Inc., 1923], v.

it is located."[15] Müllerian choristomas are a subset of non-müllerian choristomas found throughout the body.[16] They represent *les formes frustes* of the cervix, uterus, and fallopian tubes.

Nosography Faber defines nosography as "the description of diseases."[17]

Nosology Nosology, the classification of disease, is based on the "assumption that the way in which things [are] organized into groups [reflects] something about their actual relationships in nature."[18]

Ontological concept of disease Ontology views "disease as an entity that invaded the healthy organism and followed its own peculiar course of development." Ontological concept of disease was advocated by the Paris clinical school.[19] Ontology also stands for "fixed categories of diseases."[20]

Physiological concept of disease Physiological view of disease stresses "the uniqueness of each person's illness, defining the illness as the consequence of an alteration of the normal organic functions. Symptoms were not the signs of an alien disease entity living out its own life cycle within the sick individual, but rather the result of a disturbance of the body's normal physiological processes."[21]

Retrograde Menstruation "The flow of menstrual blood, endometrial cells, and debris via the fallopian tubes into the peritoneal cavity."[22]

Sarcoma At mid-nineteenth century, Rokitansky wrote that he had "selected the term *sarcoma* to designate the benign growths, not because of any especial analogy with muscle-flesh, but in order to fix and define a name familiarized by long usage, and also by no little abuse. The malignant we shall leave in possession of their ancient characteristic appellation *cancer, – carcinoma.*"[23]

Serosal metaplasia Serosal metaplasia is a more restricted term that refers to the abnormal transformation of adult, fully differentiated tissue covering the surface of pelvic and abdominal organs – such as the uterus – into a differentiated tissue of another kind, such as endometrial tissue.

Wissenschaft Daum equated the German term *Wissenschaft* with [self-directed] scholarship and research, which included "the sciences, social sciences, and humanities."[24]

Wissenschaft "*Wissenschaft* [is] a difficult term to define not least because its meaning underwent several changes through the years. Once identified closely with another nebulous term, *Bildung*, *Wissenschaft* originally signified the search for a holistic understanding of all knowledge aimed at cultivating the individual's personality by developing one's moral and intellectual sensitivities. In this earlier formulation, *Wissenschaft* had an inward focus, but as the century progressed, the focus turned outward and *Wissenschaft* came to refer to the production of new knowledge through in-depth scholarly work in a specialized area of research. Accompanying this transition was an increased appreciation of the importance of acquiring practical experience; by the late nineteenth century, at least in the sciences and medicine, the revered *Wissenschaftler* was one who could manipulate sophisticated instrumental apparatus and gain in this way control over laboratory conditions and, presumably, over nature."[25]

Wolffian or mesonephric rest The mesonephros – the primitive vertebrate kidney – comprises two elongated masses in the early vertebrate embryo. A Wolffian rest represents a group of cells or a portion of the

[18]Peter Dear, *The Intelligibility of Nature: How Science Makes Sense of the World* [Chicago: University of Chicago Press, 2006], 45.

[19]Tuchman, Arleen Marcia Tuchman, *Science, Medicine, and the State of Germany: The Case of Baden, 1815–1871* [New York: Oxford University Press, 1993], 60.

[20]Knud Faber, 95–96. Peter Dear, 53.

[21]Tuchman, Arleen Marcia Tuchman, *Science, Medicine, and the State of Germany: The Case of Baden, 1815–1871* [New York: Oxford University Press, 1993], 60.

[22]Morton A. Stenchever, William Droegemueller, Arthur L. Herbst, and Daniel R. Mishell. *Comprehensive Gynecology.* 4th edition. [St. Louis, MI: Mosby, 2001], 531.

[23]Carl Rokitansky, *A Manual of Pathological Anatomy*, Volume I. *General Pathological Anatomy.* trans. William Edward Swaine [Philadelphia, PA: Blanchard & Lea, 1855], Volume I. 189, 190.

[24]Andreas W. Daum, "*Wissenschaft* and knowledge," in *The Short Oxford History of Germany: Germany 1800–1870* [Oxford: Oxford University Press, 2004], 137–161:137.

[25]Arleen Marcia Tuchman, *Science, Medicine, and the State of Germany: The Case of Baden, 1815–1871* [New York: Oxford University Press, 1993], 14–15.

mesonephros (Wolffian body) that has become displaced and lies embedded in tissue of another character that persists as an embryonic remnant in the adult.

****

Between 1860 and 1946 and even to this day, ambiguity and confusion surrounded proper terminology for pelvic floor anatomy in the female.

Posterior fornix of the vagina Posterior fornix of the vagina is that space bounded anteriorly by that portion of the uterine cervix that protrudes into the vagina and posteriorly by the rectovaginal pouch of Douglas.[26]

Pseudo-retrocervical septum A pseudo-retrocervical septum may be formed – above the anatomic (true) rectovaginal septum – by dense obliterative adhesions that cement together the anterior and posterior walls of the rectovaginal pouch of Douglas as well as cement together the posterior surface of the uterus to the anterior surface of the rectum to produce a frozen pelvis.[27]

Retrocervical septum I have coined a new term "*retrocervical septum*" by combining Adamyan's anatomically correct term "retrocervix" with the time-worn but anatomically correct term "septum" that connotes a dividing wall or partition between the posterior vaginal fornix and the rectovaginal pouch of Douglas. If this new term is considered for academic use, then endometriosis of the "retrocervical septum" may replace the anatomically incorrect terminology: endometriosis of the "rectovaginal septum."[28]

Recto-genital space (Lockyer) = rectovaginal pouch of Douglas (RVPD) = culdesac.

Rectovaginal septum Rectovaginal septum is among the most misused terms found in the medical literature. With minor exceptions, the anatomically incorrect terminology endometriosis of the rectovaginal septum has been used throughout the late nineteenth and twentieth centuries, and on into the twenty-first century for endometriotic lesions of the "*retrocervical septum*" that separates the posterior vaginal fornix from the anterior rectovaginal pouch of Douglas.[29] The incorrect terminology endometriosis or adenomyoma of the *rectovaginal septum* had become so entrenched that several authorities called attention to the error beginning in the latter third of the twentieth century.[30] Thomas Cullen, borrowing from Lockyer, introduced the anatomically incorrect terminology "endometriosis of the rectovaginal septum" into the North American medical literature. Cullen observed that the earliest lesions of extrauterine adenomyomas (endometriosis) in the lower pelvis originated on the anterior portion of the rectovaginal pouch of Douglas, the "*retrocervi-*

---

[26]See *Illustrated Stedman's Medical Dictionary*. 24th ed. [Baltimore, MD: Williams & Wilkins, 1982], 555. The vaginal fornix or fornix uteri is "the recess at the vault of the vagina; it is divided into a pars anterior, pars posterior, and pars lateralis with respect to its relation to the cervix of the uterus."

[27]Footnote from Chapter 17, Adenomyoma of RV Septum. "Beneath the peritoneum and beneath the peritoneal reflection" refer *not* to the normal floor of the rectovaginal pouch of Douglas, but to the false floor of the rectovaginal pouch of Douglas created *above* the invasive disease by the fusion of the serosa of the posterior cervix to the serosa of the anterior rectum. Thus the vertical pseudo-rectovaginal septum is actually formed by fusion of diseased cervix and uterus to rectum, all located *above* the floor of the anatomical rectovaginal pouch of Douglas.

[28]The term retrocervical septum was coined on June 8, 2010 during the final editing of this manuscript for publication as a book.

[29]The author has coined the term "*retrocervical septum*" to combine the descriptive term "retrocervical" introduced by Lejla V. Adamyan with the entrenched term "septum" adopted by common usage. See Lejla V. Adamyan, "Additional international perspectives," in Gynecologic *and Obstetric Surgery,* ed. David H. Nichols [St. Louis, MO: Mosby, 1993], 1167–1182:1173, 1176.

[30]Milley PS, Nichols DH. A correlative investigation of the human rectovaginal septum. Anat Rec 1969;163–443. David H. Nichols and Paul S. Milley, "Clinical anatomy of the vulva, vagina, lower pelvis, and perineum," in *Gynecology and Obstetrics* [Hagerstown, MD: Harper & Row, 1977], 1–16. See also: Nichols DH, Milley PS, 15. Figure 1-12. "The rectovaginal septum. Sections showing the partly dissected rectovaginal septum. It extends from the pouch of Douglas to the perineal body and forms the anterior surface of the rectovaginal space. Its adherence to the posterior vaginal wall is illustrated along with its posterolateral curve. (From Nichols DH, Milley PS: Surgical significance of the rectovaginal septum. Am J Obstet Gynecol 108:215–220:215, 1970.)" Ronald E. Batt and James M. Wheeler, "Endometriosis: advanced diagnostic laparoscopy," in *Atlas of Female Infertility Surgery,* ed. Robert B. Hunt, 2nd ed. [St. Louis, MO: Mosby Year Book, 1992], 422–435:422–424, see Figure 25–2. Lejla V. Adamyan, "Additional international perspectives," in *Gynecologic and Obstetric Surgery,* ed. David H. Nichols [St. Louis, MO: Mosby, 1993], 1167–1182:1173, 1176. Ronald E. Batt, "Abdominopelvic diagnostic laparoscopy," in *Text and Atlas of Female Infertility Surgery,* ed. Robert B. Hunt, 3rd ed. [St. Louis, MO: Mosby, 1999], 372–385:372–274. Martin DC, Batt RE. Retrocervical, retrovaginal pouch, and rectovaginal septum endometriosis. Journal of American Association of Gynecologic Laparoscopists. 2001;8:12–17. Martin DC, Batt RE, Chapron C, Swoboda J. Distribution of

cal septum" that separated the rectovaginal pouch of Douglas from the posterior vaginal fornix. He erroneously termed this location the rectovaginal septum, apparently unaware of the location of the true rectovaginal septum demonstrated by Denonvilliers in 1836.[31] The true anatomic rectovaginal septum of Denonvilliers is a strong sheet of fibrous tissue that separates the vagina anteriorly from the rectum posteriorly. "It extends from [the floor of] the rectovaginal pouch of Douglas to the perineal body and forms the anterior surface of the rectovaginal space."[32] The rectovaginal space permits the rectum and vagina to distend independently. The incorrect terminology, endometriosis of the rectovaginal septum, became so embedded in the medical literature that only in the late twentieth century have some authors begun to use Adamyan's anatomically correct term "retrocervix," or the cumbersome terminology, endometriosis of the retrocervical portion of the rectovaginal pouch of Douglas.[33]

rectovaginal endometriosis 1903 – 1922. Poster presentation at the IX World Congress on Endometriosis. Maastricht, The Netherlands, 14–17 September 2005.

[31]Denonvilliers, CPD. Bull Soc Anatomy of Paris (Series 3) 1836:20:105.

[32]Nichols DH, Milley PS. "Clinical anatomy of the vulva, vagina, lower pelvis, and perineum. In *Gynecology and Obstetrics,* Vol. 1. [Hagerstown, MD: Harper & Row Publishers, Inc., 1977], 15. Figure 1–12. "The rectovaginal septum. Sections showing the partly dissected rectovaginal septum. It extends from the pouch of Douglas to the perineal body and forms the anterior surface of the rectovaginal space. Its adherence to the posterior vaginal wall is illustrated along with its posterolateral curve. (From Nichols DH, Milley PS: Surgical significance of the rectovaginal septum. Am J Obstet Gynecol 108:215, 1970.)"

[33]Lejla V. Adamyan, a Russian professor of obstetrics and gynecology, introduced the term "retrocervix" as well as a classification for retrocervical endometriosis in 1993. See Lejla V. Adamyan, "Additional international perspectives," in Gynecologic *and Obstetric Surgery,* ed. David H. Nichols [St. Louis, MO: Mosby, 1993], 1167–1182:1173, 1176.

Appendix II: English Translation of Carl Rokitansky's Ueber Uterusdrusen-Neubildung in Uterus-und Ovarial Sarcomen

Translation by
Dr. Franz Glasauer
Emeritus Professor of Neurosurgery
State University of New York at Buffalo
Buffalo, NY, USA

New Growth of Uterine Glands in Sarcomas of the Uterus and Ovaries

By

Reg.-Rath. Prof. Dr. C. Rokitansky

Among connective tissue tumors affecting the uterus are those containing glandular tubules such as uterine glands. If these tubules are a new growth, then among others they are a *Sarcoma adenoides uterinum*. As all new glandular growth first appears in the original gland or in its vicinity in the uterus, so it may also be found in the ovaries. This observation of growth was suggested in my earlier description in a tumor of the liver consisting of newly formed liver tissue (Wiener allg. Med. Ztg., April 1859, #14). The degeneration of these glandular tubules to cysts confirm the existence of a *Cystosarcoma adenoides uterinum*.

Of the existing connective tissue tumors of the uterus, the round fibroids are to be differentiated from the so-called fibrous polyps of the uterus in which glandular tubules are found. These are connective tissue tumors rooted in the basal stroma of the uterus and cannot be shelled out (Paget's continuous growth) in contrast to the well-circumscribed fibrous tumors. They commonly develop within or from the submucosal stratum and grow into the uterine cavity as so-called polyps of various shapes (cylindric-, pear-, or club-shaped) and are covered by an adherent uterine mucosa. The various changes in its texture may appear identical to the changes seen as a result of chronic inflammation. In contrast to the easily removable fibrous tumors, we commonly consider these connective tissue tumors as *sarcoma*, here specifically as *uterus sarcoma*. These tumors growing into a mucosal cavity generally retain their old name of *polyp* and *uterus polyp* and, according to the discussion above, would be distinguished from the round fibroids prolapsed into the uterine cavity. As round fibroids may develop within the inner tissue layers of the uterus, so can sarcomas on rare occasion develop from a mucosal-free outer layer.

In view of the above discussion, it is important to recognize the changes occurring in the mucosa and the submucosal stratum of the uterus as a consequence of chronic inflammation. Emphasis is on the findings of elongation of normal uterine glands versus new growth of the glands. Therefore, before presenting cases of glands – containing uterus – and ovarian sarcoma, it is advisable to consider the underlying causes of uterus sarcoma (polyp) and those of chronic inflammation. These changes are as follows:

1. A smooth mucosa or in places a predominantly bunched section with spongy stringy, areolar (decidua-type), at times also of granulated, papillary appearance is caused by the exuberant growth between the elongated and enlarged uterine glands.
2. Circumscribed hypertrophy of the mucosa and its glands.
   (a) The mucosa hypertrophies in one or more circumscribed places accompanied by elongation of glands producing the bulge (ref.: H. Mueller: Verhandl. D. phys. Med. Gesellschaft in Würzburg, 4. 1854). This bulge eventually protrudes above the neck and promptly prolapses sometimes on a stalk, into the uterine cavity. In these polypous pouches – mucous polyp of the uterus – frequently, the elongated glandular tubules partly desiccate. In these isolated sections millet- or pea-sized cysts develop, containing a single or layered colloid ball of gelatin-type mucus. This structure then consists of an aggregate of round and facetted cysts which are deposited in scaffolding areas of nuclei rich

R.E. Batt, *A History of Endometriosis*,
DOI 10.1007/978-0-85729-585-9, © Springer-Verlag London Limited 2011

connective tissue. They represent the so-called *Cell- or Vesiclepolyp.* The larger superficial cysts intermittently dehisce and are replaced by adjacent ones.

(b) On rare occasions the elongation of the uterine glands extend in both directions, toward the uterine cavity as well as into the parenchyma. In this case the incumbent bulge acts as a plug of parallel fibers driven into the uterus. Such a picture was encountered in the thick walled uterus of an older woman. Below the left tubal opening was a club-shaped, smooth polyp, about 1′ 2‴ long, with a 1 1/2″ diameter in the neck, and enlarging to 4–5‴ at the free end. A cut through the entire mass showed that the neck penetrated in a wedge-shaped fashion into the uterus to a depth of 4″. The cut surface appears as thready-fibers in its entire length and can be unraveled in that direction. This arrangement is provided by extremely long glandular tubules kept together by nuclei rich connective tissue.

3. Circumscribed hypertrophy of the submucosa of the uterus to connective tissue pouches – sarcomas – gradually give rise to the fibrous polyps. Inside, one frequently finds parts of intruding, elongated uterine glands or newly formed glandular tubules which degenerate into cysts and thus represent the structures under discussion.
4. Sometimes uterine mucosa degenerates into a notable thick, rigid, indurated connective tissue stratum containing more or less compact nuclei and fibrous strands in which the glands perished. Frequently it is interspersed by small mucous, or colloid, cysts caused by separated sections of the glands. The peripherally located cysts for the greater part have already burst.
5. In places, adhesions of the uterine walls are caused by connective tissue arising from the mucosa, rich in nuclei and striped fibers. This especially occurs in the presence of polypous mucosal pouches, vesicular polyps, and small and larger sarcomas (fibrous polyps). At times the uterine cavity is obliterated or invaded by large, already adherent sarcomas.

Following these remarks, I now turn to the description of examined cases. There are *three* extirpated uterine polyps which were sent to me from an Obstetrical Clinic. The specimens had been preserved for some time in wine-spirits. The *fourth* case is that of an ovarian cystosarcoma obtained by autopsy.

(a) *A large uterine polyp,* 3 1/2–6″ in diameter with a smooth and bulbous surface. With the exception of a notable thick neck portion, the free surface is covered with a thin, fine stringy and grainy appearing layer with adherent white drusen of fat crystals. The uterine mucosa, which is inverted into the uterine cavity, consists of a thin stroma of nuclei rich connective tissue of an areolar structure without a trace of tubular glands, except for a few areoli in the depth. Adjacent to this layer is the densely interwoven mass of the sarcoma. This consists of an inert, fibrous stroma interspersed by elongated nuclei. The stroma is arranged in bundles of various sizes which crisscross in different directions. In places, the stroma is less compact and spongy. In the lower wall there appears within the tumor mass, a dense nodule, the size of a goose-egg, but located so that it can be shelled out. For the most part, its surface adheres to the wall of a cavity by threads and is in only one place continuous with the tumor mass. In addition, especially within circumscribed areas one notes many cyst-like spaces, from poppy-seed to bean sized, without epithelium but with either smooth or delicate stringy inner linings. Some of these clefts are confluent and some are clustered into groups of 2–3 and are separated by delicate perforated membranes. A section of the tumor from the deep layers is scattered with small spaces and microscopically reveals a collection of rigid connective tissue bundles crisscrossing in different directions. These contain smaller or larger, round or oblong clefts which, except for a barely visible hyaline rim, show no other lining. However, there are spaces that are filled with atrophied cells – an epithelial layer – and on cross section appear to represent tubular structures.

(b) *A lobulated uterine polyp the size of a child's head.* The polyp is covered by uterine mucosa, with the exception of its neck, and preens areas of a discolored, friable, spongy, stringy layer. This layer extends into the depth as a spongy, succulent layer of 3–5‴ thickness and is perforated by numerous clefts of varying sizes (needle-point to millet size). Further into the depth the tissue becomes more fibrous and is scattered with millet size to larger size lumps. Everywhere there are, sometimes in nests, from small, barely visible to larger, round or irregular clefts with smooth or stringy inner walls.

The external layer appears as a horizontally removed segment, perforated by variable sized round or distorted spaces. This segment consists of nuclei rich connective tissue and in places is disintegrated into an opaque detritus.

Layers taken from the succulent, spongy stroma present as a thin or thick meshwork structure of the same nuclei rich connective tissue, containing round or oblong spaces of various sizes. In addition to these spaces, finally there are tubular structures lined with epithelial cells. Evidently, the former are cross – or oblique – sections of the latter.

In addition to the epithelial line spaces, one observes here and in the deep, porous sections of tumor clefts invaded by conical- or club-shaped excrescences, which deform them to lacunar shapes. Adjacent to the clefts and especially in the excrescencies, the tissue consists of streaky, nuclei rich connective tissue; otherwise it is a thread-like connective tissue with crisscrossing fiber bundles and notable areas which look like inserted cut fiber balls.

(c) *A third case* of a goose egg–sized uterine polyp is identical to the one described in (a).

(d) *An Ovarian – Cystosarcoma.* The autopsy performed on March 2, 1859 on a 68-years-old, malnourished female yielded the following: the body is small and thin, both lungs for the most part are adherent, in the right upper lobe there is a walnut-sized cavity with extensive, indurated desiccation of the tissue and an incorporated yellow, cheesy nodule. In the lung there are numerous thickened, airless areas infiltrated by tenacious, yellow–brownish pus. The ventricles of the heart contain loose fibrin clots. The liver is enlarged and fatty, the spleen is small, the stomach, bowels, and kidneys are pale; in the capsule of the left kidney there is a white fibroid node and the bladder is empty. A small, retroflexed uterus is situated in the left recto-vaginal space whereas its fundus is wedged between the cervix and the left ovarian tumor. The latter is degenerated to a fist-sized tumor, the right half presents as a dense, fibrous mass, whereas the left half consists of an aggregate of serous cysts. The largest of the cysts partially protruded into a cavity of the fibrous mass. The remaining small cysts were adherent to the rest of the surface. The entire tumor was twisted by its sheltered position so that the cystic portion pointed to the right. The tube was somewhat stretched over the tumor and fixed to it up to its fimbriated end. The right ovary was dense, atrophied, and contained a bean-sized cyst which protruded through the surface. Closer examination of the fibrous part of the tumor disclosed on cross section, especially around the cysts, a glandular appearance with scattered, delicate vesicles and grainy nodules. In addition, it contained individual mucous containing cysts of millet to hemp corn size. The microscopic examination revealed numerous tubular, epithelial lined structures within a thick, connective tissue layer. On cross section of these tubular structures, individual slit-like, lacunar clefts were evident into which papillary excrescences of connective tissue intruded.

The conclusions drawn from these observations are:

1. Among the fibrous uterine polyps are some that contain glandular tubules.
2. These tubules represent elongated glands of the uterine mucosa, isolated sections of them, or new growth. The latter transform the *sarcoma* to an *adenoides uterinum.*
3. Above all, as new growths are considered (1) large polyps in the depth and (2) those found in great distance from similarly lined uterine mucosa. That such a new growth actually takes place becomes less doubtful, as one may also observe tubular structures very similar to uterine glands in ovarian sarcoma.
4. In the cell-polyp of the uterus these tubules degenerate to cysts in the same manner as do isolated sections of uterine glands in the desiccated uterine mucosa – *Cystosarcoma adenoides uterinum.*
5. Sarcoma tissue in the form of papillary excrescences grow into the space of the cyst-like, degenerated tubules. The slit-like, lacunar clefts scattered within the sarcoma produce on cross section a granular appearance. The circumscribed nodes, which can be shelled out, and appear incorporated in the sarcoma mass doubtless originate from the filling of the greater cyst spaces by intruding tumor tissue – a common appearance, which is especially pronounced in cystosarcoma adenoides mammarium.
6. A sarcoma, containing uterine glandular tubules, is also found in the ovaries and some cystic structures of the ovaries, therefore become a *cystosarcoma adenoides uterinum.*
7. The ones in question and the mucosa lined uterine polyps as a whole undergo changes in their texture

which similarly occur in the uterine mucosa in the course or as the end result of chronic inflammation. In the *first* case described, the uterine mucosa is a stroma of areolar structure in which, except for a few deeper areoli, no tubular glands are present. In the *second* case, the mucosa is a large, spongy layer similar to the stratum of cell polyps. On a simple, fist-sized uterine polyp without glands (I examined the specimen fresh!), the mucosal lining presents a spongy, very fine, stringy layer, in which especially above and in proximity to the stalk numerous poppy- to millet-sized cysts are present which are frequently confluent and contain clear, tenacious mucus. On microscopic examination the mucosa appears to be a porous, nuclei rich membrane and its pores are encircled by a corresponding vascular mesh which frequently produces papillary, elevated loops. In the depth one finds numerous, epithelial lined, round vesicles – isolated sections of desiccated tubular glands. It is lined by epithelium consisting of pavement – and low cylindrical – cells.

Bibliography

Manuscript Primary Sources

- Sampson, John A. *Gynecology.* Albany Medical College Archives, Albany, New York

Printed Primary Sources

- American Journal of Clinical Pathology
- American Journal of Medical Genetics
- American Journal of Obstetrics and Diseases of Women and Children
- American Journal of Obstetrics and Gynecology
- American Medicine
- Annals of Clinical and Laboratory Medicine
- Anatomic Record
- Archives für Gynaekologie
- Archives Pathological and Laboratory Medicine
- Archives of Surgery
- Best Practice Research Clinical Obstetrics Gynecology
- Boston Medical and Surgical Journal
- British Journal History of Science
- Bulletin American College of Surgeons
- Bulletin History of Medicine
- Bulletin Johns Hopkins Hospital
- Canadian Medical Journal
- Clinical and Experimental Obstetrics and Gynecology
- Clio Medica
- Contributions to Embryology
- Current Medical Digest
- Current Problems in Obstetrics and Gynecology
- Deutsche Medicinische Wochenschrift
- Emergence
- Environmental Health Perspective
- European Journal of Obstetrics, Gynecology and Reproductive Biology
- European Urology
- Fertility and Sterility
- Fundamentals of Applied Toxicology
- Gynecologic and Obstetric Investigation
- Heart
- Histology and Histopathology
- Hong Kong Medical Journal
- Human Reproduction
- International Clinics
- International Journal of Gynecological Pathology
- Journal of American Medical Association
- Journal of Laboratory and Clinical Medicine
- Journal of Minimally Invasive Gynecology
- Journal of Obstetrics and Gynaecology British Empire
- Journal of Reproductive Medicine
- Medicinische Jahrbucher des kaiserl. konigl osterreichischen
- Memphis Lancet
- New York State Journal of Medicine
- Obstetrics and Gynecology
- Obstetrics and Gynecology Clinics of North America
- Obstetrical and Gynecological Survey
- Pager Zeitschrift fur Heilkunde
- Pathologica
- Pediatrics
- Pennsylvania Medical Journal
- Philosophical Transactions of the Royal Society of London
- Proceedings Royal Society Medicine
- Seminars in Diagnostic Pathology
- Southern Medical Journal
- Surgery Gynecology and Obstetrics
- Transactions of American Gynecological Society
- Transactions of Southern Surgical and Gynecological Association
- Virchow's Archive for Pathological Anatomy

R.E. Batt, *A History of Endometriosis*,
DOI 10.1007/978-0-85729-585-9, © Springer-Verlag London Limited 2011

- Western Journal of Surgery, Obstetrics and Gynecology
- Wiener Klinische Wochenschrift
- Zeitschift der k. k. Gesellschaft der Arzte zu Wien

Dissertations

- Canis, Michel Henri Jean. "Tentative de Mise au Point sur L'Endometriose en 1984." Doctorat en Medicine. Universite de Clermont I Faculte de Medicine, 1984. [An Attempt to Launch an Investigation into the State of Endometriosis].
- Miciotto, Robert Joseph. "Carl Rokitansky: Nineteenth-Century Pathologist and Leader of the New Vienna School." PhD Dissertation The Johns Hopkins University, 1979.
- Smith, Dale Cary. "The Emergence of Organized Clinical Instruction in the Nineteenth Century American Cities of Boston, New York and Philadelphia. PhD Dissertation. The University of Minnesota, 1979.

Bibliography Secondary Sources

- Ackerknecht, Erwin H. *Medicine at the Paris Hospital 1794–1884.* Baltimore, MD: Johns Hopkins Press, 1967.
- Ackerknecht, Erwin H. *A Short History of Medicine.* New York: Ronald Press, 1968.
- Allen RM. *The Microscope.* New York: D. Van Nostrand Company, 1940.
- Baas, Johann Hermann. *Outlines of the History of Medicine and the Medical Profession.* Translated by H. E. Henderson. Huntington, NY: Robert E. Krieger Publishing Co., 1971. [Original edition 1889, one volume; Reprint 1971, two volumes).
- Barash P., B. Cullen and R. Stoelting. eds. *Clinical Anesthesia*, 5th ed. Philadelphia: Lippincott Williams & Wilkins, 2005.
- Barry, John M. *The Great Influenza: The Epic Story of the Deadliest Plague in History*. New York: Penguin Books, 2005.
- Berglas, Alexander. *Cancer: Nature, Cause, and Cure.* Paris: Institute Pasteur, 1957.
- Black, Henry Campbell. *Black's Law Dictionary: Definitions of the Terms ad Phrases of America and English Jurisprudence, Ancient and Modern.* Sixth Edition by the Publisher's Editorial Staff. St. Paul, MN: West Publishing Co., 1990.
- Blaustein, Ancel. ed. *Pathology of the Female Genital Tract.* New York: Springer-Verlag, 1977.
- Bliss, Michael. *William Osler: A Life in Medicine.* Oxford, UK: Oxford University Press, 1999.
- Broman, Thomas H. *The Transformation of German Academic Medicine 1750–1820.* Cambridge: Cambridge University Press, 1996.
- Bronowski, J. and Bruce Mazlish. *The Western Intellectual Tradition.* Dorset Press, 1986.
- Browne, Janet. *Darwin's Origin of Species.* New York: Atlantic Monthly Press, 2007.
- Breus, Carl. *Uber Wahre Epithel Führende Cystenbildung in Uterusmyomen.* Leipzig und Wien: Franz Deuticke, 1894.
- Bruhat, Maurice A. and Michel Canis. eds. *Endometriosis.* Basel, Switzerland: Karger, 1987.
- Buchanan, Scott. *The Doctrine of Signatures: A Defense of Theory in Medicine.* 2nd ed. Urbana, IL: University of Illinois Press, 1991.
- Bynum W. F. and Roy Porter. *Companion Encyclopedia of the History of Medicine.* Vol. 1. London: Routledge, 1997.
- Canguilhem, Georges. *The Normal and the Pathological*. Translated by Carolyn R. Fawcett in collaboration with Robert S. Cohen. New York: Zone Books, 1991.
- Carroll, Sean B. *Endless Forms Most Beautiful: The New Science of Evo Devo and the Making of the Animal Kingdom.* New York: W. W. Norton & Company, 2005.
- Carter, K. Codell. *The Rise of Causal Concepts of Disease: Case Histories.* Burlington, VT: Ashgate, 2003.
- Chadha D. and V. Buttram. eds. *Current Concepts in Endometriosis. Progress in Clinical and Biological Research*, New York: Alan R. Liss, 1990.
- Clendening, Logan (ed.). *Source Book of Medical History.* New York: Dover/Henry Schuman, 1960. Reprint
- Conant, James and John Haugeland. eds. Kuhn, Thomas S. *The Road Since Structure: Philosophical Essays, 1970–1993, with an Autobiographical Interview.* Chicago, IL: University of Chicago Press, 2000.
- Coulter, Harris L. *Divided Legacy: A History of the Schism in Medical Thought. Volume II: The Origins*

of Modern Western Medicine: J. B. Van Helmont to Claude Bernard. Berkeley, CA: North Atlantic Books, 1977, 2000.

- Cruveilhier, Jean. *Anatomie Pathologique du Corps Humain.* Livraison XIII, Planche IV, Paris, 1835.
- Cullen, Thomas Stephen. *Cancer of the Uterus: Its Pathology, Symptomatology, Diagnosis, and Treatment. Also the Pathology of Diseases of the Endometrium.* New York: Appleton and Company, 1900.
- Cullen, Thomas S. *Adeno-Myome des Uterus.* Berlin: Verlag von August Hirsch, 1903.
- Cullen, Thomas Stephen. *Adenomyoma of the Uterus.* Philadelphia: WB Saunders, 1908.
- Cullen, Thomas Stephen. *Cancer of the Uterus: Its Pathology, Symptomatology, Diagnosis, and Treatment; also The Pathology of Diseases of the Endometrium.* Philadelphia: W. B. Saunders, 1909.
- Cullen, Thomas S. *Embryology, Anatomy, and Diseases of the* Umbilicus. Philadelphia: W. B. Saunders, 1916.
- Cullen, Thomas S. *Henry Mills Hurd, the First Superintendent of the Johns Hopkins Hospital.* Baltimore, MD: Johns Hopkins Press, 1920.
- Curtis, Ludwig. *Goethe, Wisdom and Experience.* Translated by Herman John Weigand. New York: Pantheon, 1949.
- Cushing, Harvey. *The Life of Sir William Osler.* Oxford, UK: Clarendon Press, 1926.
- Daston, Lorraine and Peter Galison. *Objectivity.* New York: Zone Books, 2007.
- Davis, Audrey W. *Dr. Kelly of Hopkins: Surgeon, Scientist, Christian.* Baltimore, MD: Johns Hopkins Press, 1959.
- Dean, John. W. *Warren G. Harding.* The American Presidents Series. New York: Times Books, Henry Holt and Co., 2004.
- Dear, Peter. *The Intelligibility of Nature: How Science Makes Sense of the World.* Chicago, IL: University of Chicago Press, 2006.
- Diamond, Jared. *Guns, Germs, and Steel: The Fates of Human Societies.* New York: W. W. Norton and Company, 1997.
- Donnez J, Donnez O, Squifflet J, and M. Nisolle. eds. *An Atlas of Operative Laparoscopy and Hysteroscopy,* 2nd edition. New York: Parthenon Publishing Group, 2001.
- Duffin, Jacalyn. *History of Medicine: A Scandalously Short Introduction.* Toronto: University of Toronto Press, 2000.
- Eskes, T.K.A.B. and L.D. Longo. eds. *Classics in Obstetrics and Gynecology: Innovative Papers that Have Contributed to Current Clinical Practice.* Pearl River, NY: Parthenon Publishing Group, 1994.
- Faber, Knud. *Nosography in Modern Internal Medicine.* New York: Paul B. Hoeber, Inc., 1923.
- Fagan, Brian. *The Little Ice Age: How Climate Made History 1300–1850.* New York: Basic Books, 2002.
- Fleming, Donald. *William H. Welch and the Rise of Modern Medicine.* Boston, MA: Little, Brown and Company, 1954.
- Flexner, Abraham. *Medical Education in the United States and Canada.* New York: Carnegie Foundation for the Advancement of Teaching, 1910.
- Flexner, Abraham. *Universities: American, English, German.* New York: Oxford University Press, 1930.
- Flexner, Simon and James Thomas Flexner, *William Henry Welch and the Heroic Age of American Medicine.* Baltimore, MD: Johns Hopkins University Press, 1993.
- Garrison, Fielding H. *An Introduction to the History of Medicine.* 4th edition, reprinted. Philadelphia: W. B. Saunders, 1914.
- Garrison, Fielding H. *Essays in the History of Medicine* trans. by various hands and ed. Fielding H. Garrison. New York: Medical Life Press, 1926.
- Garrison, Fielding H. *Contributions to The History of Medicine.* New York: Hafner Publishing Company, 1966.
- Gilchrist, Francis G. *A Survey of Embryology.* New York: McGraw-Hill Book Company, 1968.
- Glaser, Hermann. ed. *The German Mind in the Nineteenth Century: A Literary & Historical Anthology.* New York: Continuum, 1981.
- Godlee, Rickman John, *Lord Lister.* 3d ed., rev. Oxford: Clarendon Press, 1924.
- Goodall, James Robert. *A Study of Endometriosis, Endosalpingiosis, Endocervicosis, and Peritoneo-ovarian Sclerosis: A Clinical and Pathologic Study.* Philadelphia: JB Lippincott, 1943.
- Gross, Samuel D. *Autobiography of Samuel D. Gross: With Sketches of His Contemporaries.* Edited by His Sons in Two Volumes. New York: Arno Press & The New York Times, 1972. Reprint Series: *Medicine & Society in America.*
- Gould, Stephen Jay. *Eight Little Piggies: Reflections in Natural History.* New York: WW Norton & Company, 1993.

- Gould, Stephen Jay. *I Have Landed: The End of a Beginning in Natural History.* New York: Harmony Books, 2002.
- Gould, Stephen Jay. *The Structure of Evolutionary Theory.* Cambridge, MA: Belknap Press of Harvard University Press, 2002.
- Gray, Peter. *The Encyclopedia of the Biological Sciences.* 2nd ed. New York: Van Nostrand Reinhold Company, 1961.
- Greaves, Mel. *Cancer: The Evolutionary Legacy.* Oxford: Oxford University Press, 2000.
- Haberling, W. *German Medicine.* Clio Medica. Translated by Jules Freund. New York: Paul B. Hoeber, 1934.
- Haeckel, Ernst. *The Last Link: Our Present Knowledge of the Descent of Man. With Notes and Biographical Sketches by Hans Gadow.* London: Adam and Charles Black, 1898.
- Hannaway Caroline and Ann La Berge. *Constructing Paris Medicine.* Amsterdam, NL: Editions Rodopi B. V., 1998.
- Helferich, Gerard. *Humboldt's Cosmos: Alexander von Humboldt and the Latin American Journey That Changed the Way We See the World.* New York: Gotham Books, 2004.
- Hellemans, Alexander and Bryan Bunch. *The Timetables of Science: A Chronology of the Most Important People and Events in the History of Science.* Touchtone Edition. New York: Simon & Schuster, 1988.
- Himmelfarb, Gertrude. *The New History and the Old.* Cambridge, MA: The Belknap Press of Harvard University Press, 1987.
- Holland, John H. *Emergence: From Chaos to Order.* New York: Basic Books, 1998.
- Hollenbeck, Zeph J. R. and John I. Hollenbeck. *Profiles in Surgery, Gynecology and Obstetrics.* Flushing, NY: Medical Examination Publishing Company, 1973.
- Hudson, Robert P. *Disease and Its Control: The Shaping of Modern Thought.* Westport, CT: Greenwood Press, 1983.
- Huisman, Frank and John Harley Warner. eds. *Locating Medical History: The Stories and Their Meaning.* Baltimore: MD: Johns Hopkins University Press, 2004.
- Hull, David L. *Science as a Process: An Evolutionary Account of the Social and Conceptual Development of Science.* Chicago, IL: University of Chicago Press, 1988.
- Hunt, Lynn. *The New Cultural History.* Berkeley, CA: University of California Press, 1989.
- Hunt Robert B. ed. *Atlas of Female Infertility Surgery,* 2nd ed. St. Louis, MO: Mosby Year Book, 1992
- Hunt, Robert B. ed. *Text and Atlas of Female Infertility Surgery,* 3rd ed. St. Louis, MO: Mosby, 1999.
- Hunter, Robert S. *Federal Trial Handbook: Civil.* 4th ed. Danvers, MA: Thomson West, 2003.
- *Illustrated Stedman's Medical Dictionary.* 24th ed. Baltimore, MD: Williams & Wilkins, 1982.
- Kelly, Howard A. and Charles P. Noble, eds. *Gynecology and Abdominal Surgery.* 2 Vols. Philadelphia: WB Saunders Company, 1907.
- Kelly, Howard A. and Thomas S. Cullen. *Myomata of the Uterus.* Philadelphia: WB Saunders, 1909.
- Kenny, Anthony. ed. *The Oxford History of Western Philosophy.* Oxford: Oxford University Press, 1994.
- King, Helen. *The Disease of Virgins: Green sickness, chlorosis, and the problems of puberty.* New York: Routledge, 2004.
- King, Lester S. *The Medical World of the Eighteenth Century.* Huntington, NY: Robert E. Krieger Publishing Co., 1958, Reprint 1971.
- King, Lester S. *Medical Thinking: A Historical Preface.* Princeton, NJ: Princeton University Press, 1982.
- King, Rolf. *Goethe on Human Creativeness and other Goethe Essays.* Athens, GA: University of Georgia Press, 1950.
- Kiple, Kenneth F. *The Cambridge World History of Human Disease.* Cambridge: Cambridge University Press, 1993.
- Knapp, Vincent J. *Disease and Its Impact on Modern European History.* Lewiston, NY: Edwin Mellon Press, 1989.
- Laubichler, Manfred D. and Jane Maienschein. *From Embryology to Evo-Devo: A History of Developmental Evolution.* Cambridge, MA: MIT Press, 2007.
- Lemay A. and R Maheux, eds. *Understanding and Managing Endometriosis: Advances in Research and Practice.* New York: The Parthenon Publishing Group, 1999.
- Lenoir, Timothy. *The Strategy of Life: Teleology and Mechanics in Nineteenth-Century German Biology.* Chicago, IL: University of Chicago Press, 1989.
- Lesky, Erna. *The Vienna Medical School of the 19th Century.* Baltimore, MD: Johns Hopkins University Press, 1976.

- Lightman, Bernard. ed. *Victorian Science in Context.* Chicago: University of Chicago Press, 1997.
- Lockyer, Cuthbert. *Fibroids and Allied Tumours (Myoma and Adenomyoma): Their Pathology, Clinical Features and Surgical Treatment.* London: Macmillan and Company, 1918.
- Long, Esmond R. *A History of American Pathology.* Springfield, IL: Charles C. Thomas, 1962.
- Longnecker, D. and D. Brown, M. Newman, W. Zapol. Principles of Anesthesiology. New York: McGraw-Hill, 2008.
- Loudon, Irvine. *Western Medicine.* Oxford: Oxford University Press, 1997.
- Ludmerer, Kenneth M. *Learning to Heal: The Development of American Medical Education.* New York: Basic Books, 1985.
- Ludmerer, Kenneth M. *Time to Heal: American Medical Education from the Turn of the Century to the Era of Managed Care.* Oxford: Oxford University Press, 1999.
- MacCallum, WG. *William Stewart Halsted: Surgeon.* Baltimore, MD: Johns Hopkins Press, 1930.
- Macdougall, Doug. *Frozen Earth: The Once and Future Story of Ice Ages.* Berkeley, CA: University of California Press, 2004.
- Maulitz, Russell C. *Morbid Appearances: The Anatomy of Pathology in the Early Nineteenth Century.* New York: Cambridge University Press, 1987.
- Meigs, Joe V. and Somers H. Sturgis. *Progress in Gynecology.* New York: Grune & Stratton, 1946.
- Meyer, Robert. *Autobiography of Dr. Robert Meyer (1864–1947): A Short Abstract of a Long Life.* With a Memoir of Dr. Meyer by Emil Novak, MD. New York: Henry Schuman, 1949.
- Mills, Stacey E., ed. *Sternberg's Diagnostic Surgical Pathology,* 4th ed., vol. 2. Philadelphia: Lippincott Williams & Wilkins, 2004.
- Müller, Frank Lorenz. ed. *The Short Oxford History of Germany: Germany 1800–1870.* Oxford: Oxford University Press, 2004.
- Müller, Johannes. *Bildungsgeschichte der Genitalien aus anatomischen Untersuchungen an Embryonen des Menschen und der Thiere.* Düsseldorf: Arnz, 1830.
- Müller, Johannes. *Handbuch der Physiologie des Menschen.* 3rd ed. 2 vols. Koblenz: J. Holscher, 1838–1840.
- Needham, Joseph. *A History of Embryology.* 2nd ed. New York: Abelard-Schuman, 1959.
- Neuburger, Max. "Johann Peter Frank as Founder of the Pathology of the Spinal Cord," in *Essays in the History of Medicine.* Trans. By various hands and edited with foreward by Fielding H. Garrison. New York: Medical Life Press, 1930.
- Nichols, David H. *Gynecologic and Obstetric Surgery.* St. Louis, MO: Mosby, 1993.
- Nisolle, Michelle and Jacques Donnez. *Peritoneal, Ovarian and Recto-vaginal Endometriosis: The identification of three separate diseases.* New York: Parthenon Publishing Group, 1997.
- Novak, Emil. *Gynecological and Obstetrical Pathology, with Clinical and Endocrine Relations.* Philadelphia, PA: WB Saunders Co., 1947.
- Nuland, Sherwin B. *Doctors: The Biography of Medicine.* New York: Alfred A. Knopf, 1988.
- Numbers, Ronald L. ed. *The Education of American Physicians.* Berkeley, CA: University of California Press, 1980.
- O'Dowd, Michael J. and Elliott E. Philipp. *The History of Obstetrics and Gynaecology.* New York: Parthenon Publishing Group, 1994.
- O'Malley C. D. ed. *The History of Medical Education.* Berkeley, CA: University of California Press, 1970.
- O'Malley, John W. *Four Cultures of the West.* Cambridge, MA: Belknap Press of Harvard University Press, 2004.
- Otis, Laura. *Müller's Lab.* Oxford: Oxford University Press, 2007.
- Park, Roswell. *An Epitome of the History of Medicine.* 2nd ed. Philadelphia: F. A. Davis Company, 1908.
- Porter, Roy. ed. *The Cambridge Illustrated History of Medicine.* Cambridge: Cambridge University Press, 1996.
- Porter, Roy. *The Greatest Benefit to Mankind: A Medical History of Humanity.* New York: W. W. Norton & Company, 1998.
- Porter, Roy. *Blood and Guts: A Short History of Medicine.* New York: W. W. Norton & Company, 2002.
- Rather, LJ. *The Genesis of Cancer: A Study in the History of Ideas.* Baltimore, MD: Johns Hopkins University Press, 1978.
- Recklinghausen, Friedrich von. *Die Adenomyome und Cystadenome der Uterus- und Tubenwandung ihre Abkunft von Resten des Wolff'schen Korpers.* Im Anhang: Von W. A. Freund, Klinische Notizen

zu den voluminosen Adenomyomen des Uterus. Berlin: Verlag von August Hirschwald, 1896.

- Ritter, Harry. *Dictionary of Concepts in History.* New York: Greenwood Press 1986.
- Robertson, John George. *The Life and Work of Goethe: 1749–1832.* New York: Haskell House Publishers, 1973.
- Robinson, Judith. *Tom Cullen of Baltimore*. London, Toronto, New York: Oxford University Press, 1949.
- Roger, Jacques. *The Life Sciences in Eighteenth-Century French Thought*. Edited by Keith R. Benson and translated by Robert Ellrich. Stanford, CA: Stanford University Press, 1997.
- Rokitansky, Carl. *Handbuch der allgemeinen Pathologischen Anatomie.* Wien: Braumüller & Seidel, 1846.
- Rokitansky, Carl. *A Manual of Pathological Anatomy.* Volume I. *General Pathological Anatomy.* Trans. William Edward Swaine. Philadelphia, PA: Blanchard & Lea, 1855.
- Rokitansky, Carl. *A Manual of Pathological Anatomy.* Volume II. *The Abdominal Viscera.* Trans. Edward Sieveking. Philadelphia, PA: Blanchard & Lea, 1855.
- Rokitansky, Carl. *Lehrbuch der pathologischen Anatomie.* Wien: Braumüller, 1861.
- Rosai, Juan, ed. *Ackerman's Surgical Pathology,* 8th ed., vol. 1. St. Louis: Mosby, 1996.
- Rosai, Juan. ed. *Guiding the Surgeon's Hand: The History of American Surgical Pathology*. Washington, DC: Armed Forces Institute of Pathology, 1997.
- Rosenberg, Charles E. and Janet Golden. eds. *Framing Disease: Studies in Cultural History.* New Brunswick, NJ: Rutgers University Press, 1991.
- Rosenmüller, JC. *Quaedam de Ovariis Embryonum et Foetuum Humanorum.* Leipzig: C. Tauchnitz, 1802.
- Rothstein, Edward. *Emblems of Mind: The Inner Life of Music and Mathematics.* Chicago, IL: University of Chicago Press, 2006.
- Sachs, Aaron. *The Humboldt Current: Nineteenth-Century Exploration and the Roots of American Environmentalism.* New York: Viking, 2006.
- Schelling, Friedrich Wilhelm Joseph. *First Outline of a System of the Philosophy of Nature.* Translated by Keith R. Peterson. Albany, NY: State University of New York Press, 2004.
- Schlesinger, Jr., Arthur M. *The Cycles of American History.* Boston, MA: Houghton Mifflin Company, 1986.
- Schwarz, Vanessa R. *Spectacular Realities: Early Mass Culture in Fin-de-Siecle Paris.* Berkeley, CA: University of California Press, 1999.
- Scott, Joan Wallach. "Gender: A useful category of historical analysis." In *Feminism and History*, edited by Joan Wallach Scott, 152–180. Oxford: Oxford University Press, 1996.
- Seamon, David and Arthur Zajonc eds. *Goethe's Way of Science: A Phenomenology of Nature*. Albany, NY: State University of New York Press, 1998.
- Sedivy, Roland. *Carl Freiherr von Rokitansky: Wegbereiter der Pathologischen Anatomie.* Vienna: Verlag Wilhelm Maudrich, 2002.
- Sigerist, Henry E. *Man and Medicine: An Introduction to Medical Knowledge.* Translated by Margaret Galt Boise. New York: W. W. Norton & Company, 1932.
- Sigerist, Henry E. *The Great Doctors: A Biographical History of Medicine.* Translated by Eden and Cedar Paul. New York: W. W. Norton & Company, 1933.
- Smith, John Maynard. *Genes, Embryos and Evolution.* New Haven, CT: Yale University Press, 1999.
- Speert, Harold. *Obstetric & Gynecologic Milestones: Illustrated.* New York: Parthenon Publishing Group, 1996.
- *Stedman's Medical Dictionary*. 28th Edition. Philadelphia: Lippicott Williams & Wilkins, 2006.
- Stenchever, Morton A. and William Droegemueller, Arthur L. Herbst, Daniel R. Mishell. *Comprehensive Gynecology.* 4th edition. St. Louis, MO: Mosby, 2001.
- Strathern, Paul. *A Brief History of Medicine from Hippocrates to Gene Therapy. New York: Carroll & Graf, 2005.*
- Sudhoff, Karl. *Essays in the History of Medicine*. Translated by various hands and edited with foreward and biographical sketch, by Fielding H. Garrison. New York: Medical Life Press, 1926.
- Talbott, John H. *A Biographical History of Medicine: Excepts and Essays on the Men and Their Work.* New York: Grune & Stratton, 1970.
- Taylor, E. Stewart. *Essentials of Gynecology.* Philadelphia: Lea & Febiger, 1958.
- Temkin, Owsei. *The Double Face of Janus and Other Essays in the History of Medicine*. Baltimore, MD: Johns Hopkins University Press, 1977.
- Tuchman, Arleen Marcia. *Science, Medicine, and the State of Germany: The Case of Baden, 1815–1871.* New York: Oxford University Press, 1993.

- Tudge, Colin and Josh Young. *The Link: Uncovering Our Earliest Ancestors.* New York: Little, Brown and Company, 2009.
- Turner, Frederick Jackson. ed. *The Early Writings of Frederick Jackson Turner.* Madison WI: 1938.
- U. S. Department of Health and Human Services Centers for Disease Control and Prevention: National Center for Health Statistics, National Vital Statistics System. United States Life Tables, 2004. National Vital Statistics Reports: Volume 56, Number 8, December 28, 2007.
- Virchow, Rudolf. *Die Cellularpathologie in ihrer Begründung auf physiologische und pathologische Gewebelehre.* Berlin: Hirschwald, 1858.
- Wadepuhl, Walter. *Goethe's Interest in the New World.* New York: Haskell House Publishers, 1973.
- Wangensteen, Owen H. and Sarah D. Wangensteen. *The Rise of Surgery: From Empiric Craft to Scientific Discipline.* Minneapolis, MN: University of Minnesota Press, 1978.
- *Webster's New Biographical Dictionary.* Springfield, MA: Merriam-Webster Inc., 1988.
- Welch, William Henry. *Pathology, Preventive Medicine, Vol. 1 of Papers and Addresses by William Henry Welch.* Baltimore, MD: Johns Hopkins Press, 1920.
- Worboys, Michael. *Spreading Germs: Disease Theories ad Medical Practice in Britain, 1865–1900.* Cambridge, UK: Cambridge University Press, 2000.
- Wynn, Ralph M. ed. *Obstetrics and Gynecology Annual.* Vol. 3. New York: Appleton-Century-Crofts, 1974.
- Yourgrau, Palle. *A World Without Time: The Forgotten Legacy of **Gödel** and Einstein.* New York: Basic Books, 2005. **Edit**
- Ziporyn, Terra. *Nameless Diseases.* New Brunswick, NJ: Rutgers University Press, 1992.

Key Primary and Secondary Sources

- Mayer, Ueber Verdoppelungen des Uterus und ihre Arten, nebst Bemerkungen uber Hasenscharte und Wolfsrachen. Journal der Chirurgie und Augen Heilkunde 1829;13:525–564.
- Von Prof. Dr. Rokitansky, Über die sogenannten Verdoppelungen des Uterus. Medicinische Jahrbucher des kaiserl. konigl osterreichischen Staates 1838;26:S39-77.
- Rokitansky, Carl. Ueber Uterusdrüsen-Neubildung in Uterus- und Ovarial-Sarcomen. Zeitschift Gesellschaft der Aerzte in Wien. 1860;16:577–581.
- Chiari H. Zur pathologischen Anatomie des Eileiterkatarrhs. Pager Ztschr. Heilk 1887;8:457.
- Recklinghausen, Friedrich von. *Die Adenomyome und Cystadenome der Uterus- und Tubenwandung ihre Abkunft von Resten des Wolff'schen Korpers.* Im Anhang: Von W. A. Freund, Klinische Notizen zu den voluminosen Adenomyomen des Uterus. Berlin: Verlag von August Hirschwald, 1896.
- Cullen, TS. Adeno-myoma uteri diffusum benignum. Bulletin Johns Hopkins Hospital 1896;6:133–157.
- Iwanoff NS. Adeno-myome de l'uterus. Inaug.-Diss. Petersburg. (Russisch.) Vergl. auch Frommel's Jahresberichte für 1897. S. 103 u.
- IwanoffNS.DrusigescystenhaltigesUterusfibromyom compliciert durch Sarcom und Carcinom. Monatsschr. Geburtsh u. Gynak. 1898;7:295.
- Russell, William Wood. Aberrant portions of the müllerian duct found in an ovary. Johns Hopkins Hospital Bulletin 1899; 10:8–10.
- Pick L. Arch f Gynaek 1905;lxxvi:251–275.
- Cuthbert Lockyer. *Fibroids and Allied Tumours (Myoma and Adenomyoma): Their Pathology, Clinical Features and Surgical Treatment.* London: Macmillan and Company, 1918.
- Cullen TS. The distribution of adenomyomas containing uterine mucosa. Archives of Surgery 1920;1:215–283.
- Sampson JA. Perforating hemorrhagic (chocolate) cysts of the ovary: their importance and especially their relation to pelvic adenomas of endometrial type ("Adenomyoma" of the uterus, rectovaginal septum, sigmoid, etc.) Archives of Surgery 1921;3:245–323.
- Sampson JA. Ovarian hematomas of endometrial type (perforating hemorrhagic cysts of the ovary) and implantation adenomas of endometrial type. Boston Medical and Surgical Journal 1922;186:445–56.
- Sampson JA. Heterotopic or misplaced endometrial tissue. Am J Obstet Gynecol 1925;10:649–664.
- Sampson JA. Peritoneal endometriosis due to the menstrual dissemination of endometrial tissue into the peritoneal cavity. Am J Obstet Gynecol 1927;l4:422–469.
- Sampson JA. The development of the implantation theory for the origin of peritoneal endometriosis. Am J Obstet Gynecol 1940:40:549–557.
- James Robert Goodall. *A Study of Endometriosis, Endosalpingiosis, Endocervicosis, and Peritoneo-ovarian Sclerosis: A Clinical and Pathologic Study.* Philadelphia: JB Lippincott, 1943.

Index

R.E. Batt, *A History of Endometriosis*,
DOI 10.1007/978-0-85729-585-9, © Springer-Verlag London Limited 2011

S

T

U

V